Health Impact Assessment

OXFORD

UNIVERSITY PRESS

Great Clarendon Street, Oxford, ox2 6DP,
United Kingdom

Oxford University Press is a department of the University of Oxford.
It furthers the University's objective of excellence in research, scholarship,
and education by publishing worldwide. Oxford is a registered trade mark of
Oxford University Press in the UK and in certain other countries

© Oxford University Press 2013
Chapter 31© World Health Organization 2013

The moral rights of the authors have been asserted

First Edition published in 2013

Impression: 1

British Library Cataloguing in Publication Data
Data available

Library of Congress Cataloging in Publication Data
Library of Congress Control Number: 2012944657

ISBN 978–0–19–965601–1

Printed and bound by
Ashford Colour Press Ltd., Gosport, Hants.

Health Impact Assessment

Past Achievement, Current Understanding, and Future Progress

Edited by

John Kemm

Director, JK Public Health Consulting,
Stoke Prior, Bromsgrove, England

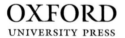

OXFORD
UNIVERSITY PRESS

Dedication

This book is dedicated to the memory of Emma,
my darling daughter.

Preface

The idea of health impact assessment (HIA) really took root in the 1990s. The idea that one should try to predict the health consequences of a proposal before implementing it was obviously reasonable and if environmental impact assessment had protected the environment could not HIA do the same for health? This book describes how that simple idea has been developed.

The Gothenburg consensus statement published in 1999 summarized ideas about HIA at that time. Five years later *Health Impact Assessment: Concepts, theories, techniques and application* (Oxford University Press 2004) attempted to map progress up to that time and showed that thinking about HIA had developed and that HIA was being applied in many different situations. Ideas and understanding have now moved on further, and much more experience has been gained. Some former problems have been solved and new problems have become apparent.

This book is not a manual on how to do an HIA and if it were it would be misguided because one thing that has become very clear is that each HIA has to be designed to match the questions it is seeking to answer and the circumstances in which it takes place. Instead the book attempts to describe a wide range of methods that have been used in various HIAs so that the reader can choose the mix of methods which best suits their situation. The book is not the definitive description of HIA but a description of current knowledge. Ideas about HIA continually evolve and improve as more people undertake them.

One area of progress is the realization that HIA is a decision support tool not a decision-making tool. It exists to help decision makers, not to replace them. One theme running through the book is therefore how those doing HIAs should relate to the decision makers and how one should attempt to ensure that decision makers find the HIA relevant and useful. Another theme is whether HIA can be impartial rather than an advocacy tool. Such issues raise questions of ethics and power.

HIA claims to be able to predict the future. This has been challenged by some and assessors are becoming more aware of the audacity of their claim to be able to predict. Certainly it is wise for assessors to think it possible that they may be wrong. The book considers on what basis predictions can be made and how one can reduce the likelihood of error with both quantitative and qualitative methods.

This book is arranged in two parts. The first part is written by the editor and gives his opinions based on his experience on the various issues in HIA. There are of course many areas of controversy and where this is so the book attempts to describe the alternative opinions. However, the first part of the book is one person's opinion.

The second part of the book covers experience of HIA in many different parts of the world from many different authors, but although it has contributions from 20 different countries there are many more countries where HIA is carried out that are not mentioned (New Zealand, other Scandinavian countries, many African countries, many South American countries, and many South East Asian countries to name a few). This second part of the book illustrates how HIA has been adapted to fit different contexts and cultures. It also makes clear that different authors have different opinions, which in many cases are different to those of the editor. This should help the reader appreciate the issues of disagreement in HIA and therefore the areas where there is likely to be progress in the future.

Like its predecessor this book attempts to map out the current state of knowledge about HIA. It is to be hoped that it will help to clarify the issues for those working in the field and for those coming to it anew and will serve as a stepping stone for those who in the future will make further advances in HIA.

Contents

Contributors

Elena Aldosoro
Department of Health and
Consumer Affairs. Basque
Government, Vitoria-Gasteiz, Spain

Carlos Artundo
Andalusian School of Public Health,
Granada, Spain

Kwaku Poko Asante
Kintampo Health Research Centre,
Kintampo, Ghana

Fabrizio Bianchi
National Research Council,
Institute of Clinical Physiology,
Unit of Epidemiology, Pisa, Italy

Marie Louise Bistrup
Institut for Folkesundhedsvidenskab,
Copenhagen, Denmark

Henrik Brønnum-Hansen
Institut for Folkesundhedsvidenskab,
Copenhagen, Denmark

Nicola Cantoreggi
University of Geneva, Geneva,
Switzerland

Chloe Chadderton
Cardiff Institute of Society and
Health (CISHE), Cardiff,
Wales, UK

Siriwan Chandanachulaka
HIA Division, Ministry of Public
Health, Nonthaburi, Thailand

Harrison Ng Chok
Centre for Primary Health Care and
Equity, University of New South
Wales, New South Wales, Australia

Liliana Cori
National Research Council,
Institute of Clinical Physiology,
Unit of Epidemiology, Pisa, Italy

Andrew Dannenberg
Consultant, Healthy Community
Design Initiative, National Center
for Environmental Health, Centers
for Disease Control and Prevention,
Georgia, USA

Lea den Broeder
RIVM, Bilthoven, the Netherlands

Mark Divall
SHAPE Consulting Ltd, Pretoria,
South Africa

Carlos Dora
Public Health and the Environment
Department, World Health
Organization, Geneva, Switzerland

Margaret Douglas
Consultant in Public Health,
NHS Lothian, Edinburgh,
Scotland, UK

Eva Elliott
Cardiff Institute of Society and
Health (CISHE), Cardiff, Wales, UK

Rainer Fehr
Landesinstitut fur Arbeitsgestaltung
des Landes Nordrhein-Westfalen,
Dusseldorf, Germany

Yoshihisa Fujino
University of Occupational and
Environmental Health, Fukuoka,
Japan

Liz Green
Public Health Wales, Croesnewydd
Hall, Wrexham, Wales, UK

Gabriel Gulis
Unit for Health Promotion Research,
University of Southern Denmark,
Esbjerg, Denmark

Fiona Haigh
Centre for Primary Health Care and
Equity, University of New South
Wales, New South Wales, Australia

Elizabeth Harris
Centre for Primary Health Care and
Equity, University of New South
Wales, New South Wales, Australia

Patrick Harris
Centre for Primary Health Care and
Equity, University of New South
Wales, New South Wales, Australia

Ben Harris-Roxas
Centre for Primary Health Care and
Equity, University of New South
Wales, New South Wales, Australia

Claire Higgins
Institute of Public Health in Ireland,
Forestview, Belfast, Northern Ireland

Martin Higgins
NHS Lothian, Waverley Gate,
Edinburgh, Scotland, UK

Eunjeong Kang
Department of Health
Administration and Management,
Soon Chun Hyang University,
Choong Nam, Korea

John Kemm
JK Public Health Consulting,
Bromsgrove, England

Gary Krieger
NewFields LLC,
Colorado, USA

Teresa Lavin
Institute of Public Health in Ireland,
Redmond's Hill, Dublin, Ireland, UK

Odile Mekel
Landesinstitut fur Arbeitsgestaltung
des Landes Nordrhein-Westfalen,
Dusseldorf, Germany

Anika Mendell
National Collaborating Centre for
Healthy Public Policy, Quebec,
Canada

Owen Metcalfe
Institute of Public Health in Ireland,
Redmond's Hill, Dublin, Ireland, UK

Seth Owusu-Agyei
Kintampo Health Research Centre,
Kintampo, Ghana

Nicolas Prisse
Ministry of Health, Paris, France

Ana Rivadeneyra
Andalusian School of Public Health,
Granada , Spain

Jean Simos
University of Geneva, Geneva and
WHO Healthy Cities collaborating
centre, Rennes, France

Burton Singer
Emerging Pathogens Institute,
University of Florida, Florida, USA

Louise St-Pierre
National Collaborating Centre for
Healthy Public Policy, Quebec,
Canada

Brigit Staatsen
RIVM, Bilthoven, the Netherlands

Marcel Tanner
Department of Epidemiology and
Public Health, Swiss Tropical and
Public Health Institute, Basel,
Switzerland

Jüerg Utzinger
Department of Epidemiology and
Public Health, Swiss Tropical and
Public Health Institute, Basel,
Switzerland

Aaron Wernham
Director, Health Impact Project,
The Pew Charitable Trusts,
Pennsylvania, USA

Gareth Williams
Cardiff Institute of Society and
Health (CISHE), Cardiff,
Wales, UK

Mirko Winkler
Department of Epidemiology and
Public Health, Swiss Tropical and
Public Health Institute, Basel,
Switzerland

Marilyn Wise
Centre for Primary Health Care and
Equity, University of New South
Wales, Australia

Abbreviations

AC	autonomous communities	FOPH	Federal Office of Public Health
CDC	US Centers for Disease Control and Prevention	GDP	gross domestic product
CDS	Conference of Sanitary Directors	GSG	General Secretariat of the Government
China Exim Bank	Export-Import Bank of China	HIA	health impact assessment
		HTA	health technology assessment
CMNS	Consorzio Mario Negri Sud	IFC	International Finance Corporation
CSDH	Commission on Social Determinants of Health	IFC-CNR	Institute of Clinical Physiology of the National Research Council
DALY	disability adjusted life year		
DHSSPS	Department of Health and Social Services and Public Safety	IIA	integrated impact assessment
		IPCC	International Panel on Climate Change
DSS	demographic surveillance system	IPH	Institute of Public Health in Ireland
EES	European employment strategy	IPPC	integrated pollution prevention and control
EFHIA	equity-focused health impact assessment	KIHASA	Korea Institute for Health and Social Affairs
EHIA	environmental health impact assessment	LHB	local health board
EIA	environmental impact assessment	LIHEAP	Massachusetts Low Income Home Energy Assistance Program
EIS	environmental impact statement		
EMRO	Eastern Mediterranean Regional Office	MHSPE	Ministry of Health, Social Policy, and Equity
		MONRE	Ministry of Natural Resources and Environment
EPFI	Equator Principles Financial Institutions		
EPHIA	European policy HIA	MSSS	Ministry of Health and Social Services
EQIA	equality impact assessments	NEPA	National Environmental Policy Act 1970
ESHIA	environmental, social, and health impact assessment	NOx	nitrogen oxides
ETS	environmental tobacco smoke	NPHS	National Public Health Service for Wales

NRC	National Research Council		RCT	randomized controlled trial
NSW	New South Wales		RFNP	Ruhr Regional Land Utilisation Plan
ONEP	Office of Natural Resources and Environmental Policy and Planning		RHA	regional health agency
			RIVM	National Institute for Public Health and the Environment
PATH	people assessing their health		SEA	strategic environmental assessment
PAHO	Pan American Health Organisation		SHIAN	Scottish Health Impact Assessment Network
PEEM	Panel of Experts on Environmental Management		SIA	social impact assessment
			SOPHIA	Society of Practitioners of Health Impact Assessment
PERS	pre-environmental review system			
PHAC	Public Health Agency of Canada		UBA	German Federal Environment Agency
PHARE	Programme of Community Aid to Countries of Central and Eastern Europe		UCLA	University of California, Los Angeles
			UNECE	United Nations Economic Commission for Europe
Piedmont ARPA	Regional Environment Protection Agency		VOC	volatile organic compounds
PNG LNG	Papua New Guinea liquid natural gas		WCfH	Wales Centre for Health
QALY	quality adjusted life year		WHIASU	Wales Health Impact Assessment Support Unit
QRA	quantitative risk assessment		WLGA	Welsh Local Government Association
RCHA	regional conferences for health and autonomy			

Part 1

Introducing HIA

Chapter 1

Origins and outline of health impact assessment

John Kemm

Health impact assessment (HIA) is intended to contribute to public health by allowing those who make decisions on behalf of the public to anticipate how those decisions will affect people's health. The decision makers are then able to take health into consideration along with the other objectives that they are aiming to achieve for the public good. HIA is a decision support tool not a decision making tool.

An idea whose time has come

HIA was first discussed in the context of development projects in the early 1990s.[1] The role of WHO in these early developments is described in Chapter 31, Page 285.

In 1996 Alex Scott-Samuel[2] popularized HIA in England with a paper entitled 'Health Impact Assessment: An idea whose time has come'. Future developments showed that his title was very apposite. In 1996 very few HIAs had been undertaken and interest in HIA was limited to only a few countries. Since then the number of HIAs undertaken has grown hugely and interest in HIA has spread to many different countries. Centres of HIA expertise have grown up in many places and the community of people interested in HIA has steadily increased. The first HIA was held in Liverpool in 1998 and this has now evolved into a regular international conference the 12th and most recent being held in Quebec in 2012. HIA is truly an idea whose time has come.

What is HIA?

HIA has two essential features:

+ It seeks to predict the future consequences for health of possible decisions.
+ It seeks to inform decision making.[3]

A more complex definition was produced by the Gothenburg consensus conference in 1999,[4] which stated that HIA is 'a combination of procedures, methods and tools by which a policy, program or project may be judged as to its potential effects on the health of a population and the distribution of effects within the population'.

The two bullet points above and the term 'potential' in the Gothenburg definition make it clear that HIA is about prediction. The Gothenburg definition further makes clear that HIA is not a single method but a combination of procedures, methods, and tools. In this book we will describe many of these procedures, methods, and tools. The Gothenburg definition also talks about the distribution of effects within populations, thereby raising the issue of equity, which is discussed in Chapter 6. The International Association for Impact Assessment[5] extended the Gothenburg definition by adding the sentence 'HIA identifies appropriate action to manage those effects' (i.e. the effects on health and distribution of health).

Some would further argue that participation is an essential feature of HIA but this is contentious and is discussed in Chapter 4. The definition of HIA produced by Williams and Elliot (see Chapter 12, page 122), while retaining the idea of prediction, additionally talks of different kinds of evidence and dialogue between relevant stakeholders. These ideas are developed and discussed in Chapter 4.

If one accepts these definitions then it is clear that there are many activities that call themselves HIAs but are not HIAs. Equally, many activities that do not call themselves HIAs are in fact HIAs. However, for public health the important issue is that the health consequences of decisions are considered, not the name that is given to that process or the precise means by which it is done.

One confusing aspect of some of the early literature on HIA is the use of the terms 'prospective', 'concurrent' and 'retrospective'. If HIA is concerned with prediction then clearly it is prospective and the term 'prospective HIA' is tautologous, while the terms 'concurrent HIA' and 'retrospective HIA' make no sense. Those activities that were called retrospective HIAs should more accurately be called evaluation and those that were described as concurrent HIA should more accurately be described as monitoring.

An HIA considers health in a broad sense, being informed by the WHO definition:[6] 'Health is a state of complete physical, mental and social well-being and not merely the absence of disease or infirmity'. The notion of 'complete health' has been criticized as being unrealistic, unattainable, and impossible to measure.[7] Using a broad definition of health has the advantage that it steers HIA away from a narrow focus on disease. However, it could also be interpreted as meaning that almost anything people do not like has a negative impact on their health. This may make it difficult to limit the scope of an HIA. In HIA health is usually viewed as being synonymous with 'well-being'.

HIA and decision making

HIA exists to support and assist decision making and where there is no decision to be made there is no HIA. HIA always compares two or more possible decisions. At the very least one compares the do something and the do nothing/business as usual options, and usually there are many more possible options. The HIA must consider the health impacts under each option. Often under the business as usual option the future health state may be expected to change so that the HIA has to predict changes under this option as well as under the do something option. It is not helpful to explore one option in depth if the consequences of choosing the other options are ignored.

HIA cannot usefully begin until the general outline of the options has been clarified. As first conceived HIA was applied to a near-finalized proposal to assess whether it was better than the do nothing option but HIA can be usefully applied at a much earlier stage, helping to refine and improve the options and rule out those which are clearly not optimal. HIA in parallel with decision making is further discussed in Chapter 5, page 60.

Evaluation, monitoring, and community development

There are several public health activities which have something in common with HIA. These activities are all important and worthwhile but they are not HIAs.

Evaluation consists of looking at the effect of some service or intervention in order to see if it has affected (improved) health. It looks not only at outcomes but also at processes in order to understand if the service or intervention has been successful why it has been successful, and if it has not been successful why not. The key difference between evaluation and HIA is that evaluation is about what has happened (the past) while HIA is about what will happen (the future). Of course good evaluation is planned before the service or intervention is begun but observation and data collection can only occur after the intervention has taken place. The logic processes for evaluation and HIA are different. Evaluation is an inductive process in which one makes observations and then moves to general theory (the intervention did or did not work). HIA is a deductive process[8] in which one starts with general principles (a view of how the world works and how the proposal would be expected to change the world) and moves to particular conclusions (how health will be impacted).

Monitoring (or surveillance) is the process of observing the health of a population after a particular change has been implemented. It thus allows any deviations from the expected outcome to be detected so that remedial action can be taken. It differs from HIA in that it is an inductive process based on observation of the present not prediction of the future. An HIA often makes recommendations about how the outcome of a decision should be monitored.

Community development is another important public health activity and certain types of community development may be confused with HIA. Community development workers may work with communities to study and understand how their health is influenced by their surroundings and conditions of living. They then identify how things could be changed to improve the health of the community.[9] As in HIA, causal chains are constructed to assess how environmental factors influence health. The difference from HIA is that in this situation there is no proposal whose health impacts are being assessed. Rather proposals are being developed de novo in order to improve community health.

The benefits of HIA

HIA is intended to inform decisions and assist decision makers, therefore its main benefit must be decisions that are better for health and equity, and reduced risk of decisions having unexpected negative health impacts. Clarifying the health impacts of different options should enable decision makers to make the trade-offs necessary when choosing between options and allow them to optimize their decision.

HIA can not only improve the final decision but also improve the decision process. Where there is participation of those who will be affected by the decision, HIA makes the decision process more open and allows those affected to understand how the decision was made even if they do not like it.

A further benefit of HIA is that it builds understanding between different authorities and decision makers. There are numerous examples of local authorities and primary care trusts (health authorities) working together on HIAs. Where this has happened invariably the health authority officers arrive at a better understanding of the workings of the local authority and vice versa.

Equally, where organizations and staff unfamiliar with public health become involved with an HIA they develop a better understanding of health issues. Even if the HIA does not affect the decision immediately under consideration it is likely that the increased understanding of health issues will linger and affect future decisions, leading to better health.[10,11]

The origins of HIA

The term 'HIA' suggests that HIA may have much in common with environmental impact assessment (EIA). Just as increased awareness of environmental damage resulting from unwise decisions led to the introduction of EIA, could increased awareness of the possibility of health damage resulting from unwise decisions have led to HIA? While this idea is plausible there are many differences between the methods used and the practice of EIA and HIA. There is undoubtedly considerable overlap between EIA and HIA, and the scope for integrating these assessments is discussed in Chapter 9, but most EIA practitioners in UK would consider health as outside the scope of their assessment,[12,13] Part 2 of this book contains many examples of countries where EIA has been much more ready to consider health issues.

The roots of HIA can be better found in policy science and the healthy public policy literature. Milio[14] and others pointed out how economic, educational, housing, trade, and many other conditions were determinants of health and argued that health should be considered when making policy decisions in these domains. The approach used in HIA has more in common with the policy appraisal process[15] than with EIA. Those who make decisions on behalf of the public have always tried to review the options open to them, to assess the consequences of choosing each of those options, and then to choose the option that is best for the communities that they serve. HIA builds on this process by allowing more thorough and systematic review of the health consequences.

Application to policy, project, and programme

A policy is an expression of intent, desired outcomes, and general direction, with some indication of how these are to be achieved. Sometimes policy is formally stated in legislation, at other times it may be no more than a guiding philosophy and tendency to act (or not to act) in a general direction. A project is a defined set of actions, such as building a motorway, constructing a new supermarket, or refurbishing a housing estate. A programme is a collection of projects. The term 'proposal' is used in this book to describe a policy, programme, or project. While HIA claims to be applicable to a policy, programme, or project, nearly all the first HIAs were related to projects and it is only recently that policy makers have explored its use. In consequence much of the literature on how to carry out HIAs describes the HIAs of projects. Application of HIA to policy is discussed in Chapter 8.

Some easily available collections of HIA reports are listed in Box 1.1.

Inside and outside the fence

In large construction and industrial projects developers will make detailed plans for construction and operation. These will include measures to prevent accidents and catastrophic events such as fire, explosion, and release of toxic materials. They will also include occupational health plans to care for the health of the

---

Box 1.1 Some easily available collections of HIA reports

HIA Gateway	http://www.hiagateway.org.uk
IMPACT	http://www.liv.ac.uk/ihia/IMPACT_HIA_Reports.htm
Wales HIA Support Unit	http://www.wales.nhs.uk/sites3/page.cfm?orgid=522&pid=10108
HIA Connect	http://www.hiaconnect.edu.au/completed_hia.htm
New Zealand HIA	http://www.health.govt.nz/our-work/health-impact-assessment/completed-nz-health-impact-assessments
San Francisco bay area HIA collaborative	http://www.hiacollaborative.org/case-studies
The Health Impact Project	http://www.healthimpactproject.org/
EIS platform	http://www.impactsante.ch (French and German)
Centro de Recursos en Evaluación del Impacto en Salud, CREIS	http://www.creis.es/experiencias-eis (Spanish)

All links accessed 26 March 2012.

---

workforce. Such plans are often referred to as 'inside the fence' while consideration of the consequences for surrounding communities is referred to as 'outside the fence'. Although many of the issues considered in 'inside the fence' plans might be regarded as issues that could be considered in an HIA, there is no sense in covering them in an HIA if they are already being considered elsewhere.

Steps in HIA

There is no shortage of guides on how to carry out an HIA (for example the Mersey guidelines[16] or the West Midlands guide[17]), most of which are guides to HIAs of projects. One could argue that there are far too many 'how to do it' guides for HIA. This book is a further addition to the 'how to do an HIA' literature, but it places more emphasis on the underlying theory and is more critical than is usually the case.

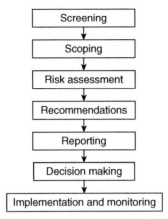

Fig. 1.1 Stages of HIA.

There are seven steps in a typical HIA and these are illustrated in Figure 1.1. The screening step seeks to answer the question 'Does this proposal warrant an HIA?'. In the scoping step the underlying problems are outlined, the baselines are described, the people involved are identified, and a plan for assessing the impacts is made. The assessment step is the main stage where the various possible health impacts are identified and their magnitude is assessed. In the next step recommendations are made to remove or minimize negative impacts and maximize positive impacts. The findings of the assessment and the recommendations are then reported to the decision maker. The penultimate step is making the decision and implementing it. Finally comes monitoring, in which the effects of the decision are monitored to see if predicted impacts materialize and to allow early corrective action if required.

These steps are described in much more detail in Chapters 2–5.

Types of HIA

HIAs come in a spectrum of intensities ranging from rapid (mini) through standard to comprehensive (maxi).

A rapid HIA may simply consist of thinking through in a systematic way what will change as a result of the proposal and how these changes could affect health. There is no participation or consultation with the people affected. The assessors rely on their knowledge and understanding of public health and there is no literature search. Readily available routine statistics may be consulted but there is no gathering of new data. Such an HIA might involve two or three people and be completed in an afternoon.

At the other end of the spectrum is a comprehensive HIA, which might involve collection of new data and extensive literature searches in four or five different topic areas. It could also involve interviews with dozens of key informants and efforts to obtain the views of people affected with interviews, focus groups, and surveys. Models might also be built to estimate the health effects of various aspects of the proposal. The whole study might take two or three years and involve many people from several different organizations. An HIA of a controversial major infrastructure project such as a new airport might need to be comprehensive.

Most HIAs come in the middle of this spectrum. They involve some literature searching, some participation of the people who will be affected by the proposal, and perhaps some reanalysis of existing routine data. They might involve five or six people for two or three months.

The choice of what level of HIA is required will be made at the scoping stage. It will depend on the size and complexity of the proposal and whether or not it is controversial. It may also depend on the resources available. Certainly, a rapid HIA should not be scorned and in many situations it is adequate for what is required.[18] The return on investment in HIA follows a law of diminishing returns. An HIA which costs £100,000 will probably give more information than one which costs only £10,000 but it is most unlikely to give ten times more information.

Stakeholders

The term 'stakeholder' is widely used in HIA. Stakeholders are all those who will be affected by or have an interest in the decision. Thus the proposers and the decision makers are stakeholders. Equally, all the people who live close to a proposed development or who will gain or lose employment or who will gain or lose income as a result of the proposal or who will be in any other way affected by it are stakeholders. The politicians and others who claim to represent these people are also stakeholders. Campaigning groups with special interests such as environmental groups (for example Friends of the Earth, Greenpeace and the Royal Society for the Protection of Birds), groups concerned with culture and heritage buildings, and groups concerned with amenity are all stakeholders. HIAs seek to take account of the wishes and fears of all these people, which are an important part of the evidence used in an HIA. The involvement of stakeholders is discussed further in Chapter 4.

Roles in HIA

There are three roles involved in an HIA:

+ proposer
+ assessor
+ decision maker.

The analogous roles are clear for EIAs in the context of UK planning applications. The proposer is the developer who wishes to build something and has applied for planning permission. The decision maker is the planning committee who will allow or refuse the application and may ask for an EIA to help them before they make the decision. The assessor is the person who undertakes the EIA (usually a commercial firm paid for their work by the developer).

In HIAs the situation is more complex and less well defined. It is common for the same organization to play two of the roles or even all three. For example, a local authority may propose a scheme to upgrade a housing estate, perform its own HIA and decide to proceed. However, if the local authority asks someone else to perform the HIA for them or if a health authority decides to undertake an HIA on a proposal put forward by another organization then it is important to realize that the assessment and the decision will be made by different people. In this situation the relationships between proposer, assessor and decision maker are crucial and these three people have to work together. The ethical issues raised by the separate roles and the possible conflicts of interest are discussed in Chapter 6.

The legal framework for HIAs

In UK there is often no legal framework for HIAs, unlike EIAs, and the circumstances in which there is a legal framework for HIAs are very limited. Where an HIA is part of a planning application planning committees have to abide by strict rules and if they depart from them there is likely to be a legal challenge. Planning committees are not required to ask for an HIA although health is a legitimate consideration for them and a proposer may include an HIA in the evidence they submit.[19] Proposals for large infrastructure projects frequently result in planning enquiries and an HIA may be presented as evidence to these, in which case they are subject to the laws governing enquiries.

A similar situation occurs in integrated pollution prevention and control (IPPC), where a proposer applies to the Environment Agency or the local authority for an operating licence for an industrial process or facility.[20] Health is an important consideration in these applications and an HIA may be part of the evidence. Legislation covers how applications under IPPC are to be considered and again any deviation from the law is likely to result in challenge. Applications involving HIAs have on occasion been subject to judicial review (a process in which a judge reviews the legality of the process followed in reaching a decision).

There is also legislation covering how the impact of UK national policies is to be assessed (impact assessment) and this is described in Chapter 8. Strategic environmental assessment, which incorporates consideration of health, is also governed by a legal framework. This is discussed in Chapter 9.

Apart from these limited examples, most HIAs in the UK take place outside any legal framework. Often an HIA is undertaken jointly between a health authority (primary care trusts) and a local authority. Local authority planners are becoming increasingly aware of the health implications of spatial planning and are often ready to consider health impacts as part of the planning application. Where new health infrastructure, such as a hospital, is proposed it is common for the health authorities to include an HIA in their business case. Sometimes HIAs are commissioned by people who wish to oppose a proposal; at other times they are commissioned by people who wish to support one.

Where there is no legal framework it is entirely up to the decision maker whether they consider the HIA or not. It is therefore essential that those carrying out the HIA liaise closely with those whom they wish to advise. They have to be aware of and address the decision makers' concerns (although they may of course raise other issues) and they must conform to the timetable constraints of the decision makers. (It is no use presenting an HIA report a week after the crucial committee meeting at which it might have been considered). Working with the decision makers is further discussed in Chapter 5.

This section has described the legal framework in England. In the other countries described in Chapters 12–31 the legal systems and frameworks are often different.

Plan of the book

This book is organized in two parts. The first part (Chapters 1–11) describes the various methods that could be used when undertaking an HIA. It then considers the ethics of HIAs and how they should be evaluated before discussing the application of HIA to policy, integration with other impact assessments, and application to projects in different areas. Finally it considers the conditions that are needed to make HIAs more widely used.

The second part of the book (Chapters 12–31) draws on experience from across the world and describes how HIAs are applied in different countries. These chapters show how HIA faces different problems in different settings and is developing new solutions for new problems. The authors contributing to this section have been encouraged to express their own views and these do not always agree with the views expressed in the first part of the book. Such debate is a sign that HIA is a healthy and growing field.

References

1. Birley M. History of HIA, Chapter 3 in Birley M, Health Impact Assessment: Principles and Practice, Abingdon: Earthscan, 2011.

2. Scott-Samuel A. Health Impact Assessment: An idea whose time has come. British Medical Journal 1996; 313: 183–84.

3. Kemm JR. Perspectives on Health Impact Assessment. WHO Bulletin 2003; 81: 367.

4. WHO European Centre for Health Policy. Health Impact Assessment: main concepts and suggested approach—Gothenburg consensus paper. Brussels: WHO European Centre for Health Policy, 1999.

5. Quigley R, den Broeder L, Furu P, Bond A, Cave B, Bos R. Health Impact Assessment Best Practice Principles Special Publication Series No 5. Fargo: International Association for Impact Assessment, 2006.

6. World Health Organization Constitution. Geneva: WHO, 1946.

7. Sarracci R World Health Organization needs to reconsider its definition of health. British Medical Journal 1997; 314: 1409.

8. Veerman JL, Mackenbach JP, Barendregt JJ. Validity of predictions in health impact assessment. Journal of Epidemiology and Community Health 2007; 61: 362–66.

9. Mittelmark MB. Promoting social responsibility for health: health impact assessment and healthy public policy at the community level. Health Promotion International 2001; 16: 269–74.

10. Davenport C, Mathers J, Parry J. Use of health impact assessment in incorporating health considerations in decision making. Journal of Epidemiology and Community Health 2006; 60: 196–201.

11. Wismar H, Blau J, Ernst K. Is HIA effective? A synthesis of concepts, methodologies and results, in Wismar M, Blau J, Ernst K, Figueras J. (eds), The effectiveness of health impact assessment: Scope and limitations of supporting decision making in Europe. Brussels: European Observatory on Health Systems and Policies, 2007, pp 15–36.

12. Burns J, Bond A. The consideration of health in land use planning; barriers and opportunities. Environmental Impact Assessment Review 2008; 28: 128–37.

13. Harris PJ, Harris E, Thompson S, Harris-Roxas B, Kemp L. Human health and well being in environmental impact assessment in New South Wales Australia: Auditing health impacts with environmental assessment of major projects. Environmental Impact Assessment Review 2008; 29: 310–18.

14. Milio N. Promoting health through public policy. Ottawa: Canadian Public Health Association, 1986.

15. Bullock H, Mountford J, Stanley R. Better policy making. London: Centre for management and Policy Studies, 2001.

16. Scott-Samuel, A, Birley, M, Ardern, K. (2001) The Merseyside Guidelines for Health Impact Assessment. Liverpool: International Health Impact Assessment Consortium, 2001. Available at http://www.liv.ac.uk/ihia/IMPACT%20Reports/2001_merseyside_guidelines_31.pdf.

17. Kemm J. More than a statement of the crushingly obvious: A critical guide to HIA. Birmingham: West Midlands Public Health Observatory, 2007. Available at http://www.apho.org.uk/resource/item.aspx?RID=44422.

18. Parry JM, Stevens A. Prospective Health impact assessment: Problems, pitfalls and possible ways forward. British Medical Journal 2001; 323: 1177–82.

19. Higgins M, Douglas M, Muir J. Can health feasibly be considered as part of the planning process in Scotland? Environmental Impact Assessment Review 2005; 25: 723–36.

20. Ahmed B, Pless-Mulloli T, Vizard C. HIA and pollution control: What they can learn from each other? Environmental Impact Assessment Review 2005; 25: 307–18.

Chapter 2

Screening and scoping
John Kemm

Screening

The first step in HIA is screening, that is, deciding whether or not a proposal needs an HIA. This involves deciding if the proposal is likely to affect health directly or indirectly by affecting determinants of health such as environment, employment, income, social cohesion, and so on. If the answer to this questions is yes and if there is some prospect of influencing the decision maker then an HIA is probably indicated.

Several screening tools consisting of a series of questions that could be used to examine proposals have been suggested. A large number can be found on the HIA Gateway website.[1] The checklist for policies produced by the English Department of Health[2] has much to recommend it and has the added merit of being short (a fuller version of this list is given in Box 8.1 on page 86):

- Will the proposal have a direct impact on health, mental health, or well-being?

- Will the proposal have an impact on social, economic, and environmental living conditions that would indirectly affect health?

- Will the proposal affect an individual's ability to improve their own health and well-being?

- Will there be a change in demand for or access to health and social care services?

(*Note*: The printed version of the second question refers to policy rather than proposal.)

It is sometimes said that every proposal involving a public body should be screened to see if an HIA is required but this is clearly impractical. For a time the Netherlands had an Intersectoral Policy Office, which attempted to screen for HIA all documents produced by the Netherlands government. The volume of documents was vast and they introduced automated word-searching software to help in this task. It is not clear how successful this venture was and the unit has now been discontinued (see Chapter 15).

In reality screening does not take long and is not arduous. There can be very few proposals that could not be said to affect health or the determinants of health in some way. HIAs are usually undertaken because someone wants one to be done. This may be the decision maker or the proposer or someone who is strongly opposed to the proposal. Capacity to undertake HIAs is limited and if no-one is asking for an HIA of a proposal one has to consider carefully whether it would be worth doing it. If someone wants an HIA one then has to decide if there are likely to be impacts that are not immediately obvious, and whether the decision maker is likely to be influenced or could be persuaded to be influenced by an HIA. If the answer to these questions is yes then one has to consider if the required resources are available.

Some real-life screening questions are:

- Could the proposal possibly affect health?
- Are any of these possible impacts not immediately obvious?
- Is there anyone who wants an HIA?
- Will the decision makers be influenced by the HIA?
- Can resources be found to do the HIA?

Scoping

Having decided that an HIA should be done the next step is scoping, that is, planning how the HIA should be done. First one needs to know the answers to these questions:

- What is the proposal?
- What are the options (do it, don't do it, do it differently)?
- Who is the decision maker?
- When will the decision be made?
- What is the decision process?

Timing

Having identified the decision process and when the decision is to be made it is possible to begin to plan the HIA. The HIA report must be presented to the decision makers before they make their decision. Knowing when the report has to be submitted, one can work back from that date to plan the dates by which the various preceding steps have to be completed. An HIA that reports after the decision has been made is totally useless and a waste of everyone's time.

Stakeholders

The definition of stakeholders was discussed in Chapter 1 (page 10) and early in the process it has to be decided who these are. Once all the stakeholders have been identified one has to find a way of communicating with them. Even with a fairly small project the number of stakeholders may be several thousand (for example for a proposed road to bypass a town the stakeholders will include residents of the town being bypassed, residents of the area through which the bypass will go, and all those who will use the bypass). Ways of involving stakeholders are discussed in Chapter 4, and it is also desirable to have some representative stakeholders involved in the scoping.

Steering groups

Communication is the key to a satisfactory HIA. Early in the scoping stage it is advisable to set up a steering group who can advise on the various decisions and be used to test the emerging shape of the HIA. The steering group needs to be large enough to contain necessary skills and interests, and small enough to be workable. It should include the person who is going to lead or do most of the work for the HIA, probably a representative of the organization the HIA is intended to advise, probably a representative of the proposer, a selection of stakeholders (residents and special interest groups), and representatives of organizations such as health and local authorities. It should not be dominated by either proponents or opponents of the project. The composition of the groups may need to be negotiated since opponents may be reluctant to sit in a group with the proposer.

The steering group will first oversee the scoping stage and then keep an eye on the assessment. It may receive and comment on draft reports. It will probably meet three or four times during the course of the HIA, although this depends on the duration of the HIA and how it is progressing. The steering group can be very helpful in giving access to expertise and other information. As the HIA proceeds the steering group may want to recruit additional members if it becomes clear that it is missing some relevant expertise or influence. The steering group does not do the HIA but it can be a very useful sounding board and can at times ease the way for the HIA.

Geographic scope

Often people think of a proposal as something that just affects their locality but the impacts can be extensive. A new road will not only impact on those who live near it but also on all those who will travel on it or whose business will be made more or less viable by the road. Increased production in one place may impact on the financial viability of businesses elsewhere (including in other countries) who previously supplied the product. Emissions to the upper atmosphere from a factory with a tall stack may affect countries far away (e.g. acid rain). Proposals which increase or decrease carbon emissions (which includes almost anything that uses energy) will contribute to or reduce climate change and therefore sea level, a matter that seriously affects the millions of people throughout the world who live close to the coast. It is very easy to argue that an HIA should consider the health impact on the whole world, but this is not practical. The problem is made worse because often the impact on different areas varies. Often the immediate neighbourhood suffers negative impacts while more distant areas benefit, for example a waste disposal facility may inconvenience those living near it but be of great benefit to the much wider area whose waste is disposed of.

One therefore has to decide the area and population for which impacts will be considered and the areas and populations which will be out of scope. Often the overall balance of benefit and harm will change as the geographical scope is increased. A compromise has to be drawn between considering only the immediate locality of the proposal (Not In My Back Yard) and the ever widening circles of impact. There is no easy answer to the question of geographic scope but one has to be ready to give reasons for whatever scope is decided on.

Temporal scope

HIA is concerned with the future, but how far into the future? Some impacts will occur immediately or soon after the implementation of the proposal, others will occur decades or centuries later. Some toxic chemicals and radioactive isotopes persist for many years. There is also the possibility of depleting non-renewable resources. Sustainability argues that we have to be concerned with the health of not only the current generation but also of future generations. Again the balance of positive and negative impacts may differ depending on the time period considered. Often the current generation will reap benefits but future generations may be harmed.

It is therefore necessary to agree the temporal scope of an HIA. To what extent is it limited to impacts on those who are currently alive and what weight should be given to the impact on future generations? Again there is no easy answer to the question of temporal scope but one has to be ready to give reasons for whatever scope is decided on. Most HIAs limit themselves to consideration of the current generation.

Construction, operation and commissioning phase

In any project that involves construction three phases must be considered: construction, operation, and decommissioning. The construction phase may be associated with considerable negative impacts, such as the movement of heavy vehicles, noise, and dust, as well as the positive impact of the creation of a number of jobs. This phase is relatively short (a few months or years) and at its end many of the negative environmental impacts may be rehabilitated.

After the construction phase whatever was constructed (housing, industrial plant, retail development, transport infrastructure etc.) will operate for a number of years. Operation will be associated with a completely different set of impacts and will probably involve a different and much smaller workforce. The operational phase may continue for many years.

Finally, many projects will have a decommissioning phase when operational use has ended because raw materials are exhausted or the plant has exceeded its useful life or has been superseded by some newer technology. This decommissioning phase may be associated with further negative impacts. It is obvious that there are negative impacts associated with decommissioning of nuclear power plants or plants which used toxic materials (this includes most industrial plants). When planning the HIA both the construction and operational phases must be considered and, if relevant, the decommissioning phase.

Limits of enquiry (in scope and out of scope)

In addition to deciding geographical and temporal scope it is likely that there will need to be agreement on various issues that are in or out of scope for the assessment. Projects are conceived in a context of national policy that limits or constrains options. Frequently proponents or opponents of a project wish to revisit the national policy affecting the project. At the scoping stage one needs to agree what constraints will be taken as given and which will be the subject of further enquiry.

It may also be agreed that some causal pathways are too unlikely or will have such small impacts that they do not deserve further investigation. Clear decisions as to what is in and out of scope will allow the HIA to concentrate on what is important and susceptible to change.

Policy analysis

An important part of the scoping process is analysing current policies and plans relevant to the proposal. Are there existing national or local strategies which constrain the proposal? Construction of transport infrastructure will have to conform to national transport policy. Construction of energy plant will have to be compatible with national energy policy. Regional spatial plans broadly specify the types of development that can take place. National and regional policies give broad objectives (such as increasing physical activity, reducing obesity, and reducing smoking). The HIA and any recommendations need to be mindful of and conform to these national and local policy frameworks.

Causal diagram

The HIA will need to consider the various ways in which the proposal could impact on health. The proposal will change various things (intermediate factors) and these will in turn directly or indirectly impact on health (Figure 2.1). An example of a causal diagram is given in Figure 2.2. Each causal path can be looked at to decide if it is important or is likely to be trivial and can be neglected in the HIA. The causal diagram will also help make clear what topics require literature searches or further investigation. It will also suggest what expert help might be required. For example, if it looks as if some impacts are due to traffic one might wish to ensure that advice from traffic engineers is available. If emissions look as if they could be an important cause of impacts then one might wish to ensure that advice could be obtained on the process producing pollutants and the dispersion of emissions. If income and employment appear in the causal diagram then one might wish to have the advice of economists.

The causal diagram constructed at the scoping stage is only a first attempt and it is likely that after further investigation it will be revised. Nonetheless a causal diagram is a very helpful way of organizing and exchanging ideas with others about how they think the proposal could impact on health. Causal diagrams are discussed further in Chapter 3 (page 25).

Types of evidence

Having outlined possible causal paths one can sort them into those that are already fully understood and those for which further evidence is required.

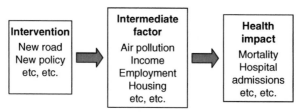

Fig. 2.1 Causal paths.

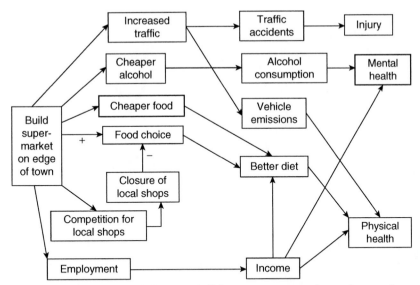

Fig. 2.2 Example of a causal diagram—building a new supermarket. +, increase in choice; –, decrease in choice.

At the scoping stage one key issue is to decide how much to seek socially constructed truth by relying on participatory methods exploring how people think, feel, fear, and hope the proposal will impact and how much to seek 'scientific' (note the quotes) truth, which it is assumed can be found by consulting experts, searching the literature, and other methods. Neither of these approaches is right or wrong. Each is better suited to investigating some causal paths and less suited to investigating other paths. The different types of evidence are discussed further in Chapters 3 and 4. At the scoping stage the important issue is to reach agreement as to which approaches should be applied to which paths. The steering group will probably have opinions as to which types of evidence convince them and will give them greater confidence in the findings of the HIA.

Assessing resources

The next step is to consider what resources are available for the HIA. There is no point in planning an immensely complex HIA unless you have the resources to carry it out. Commercial firms are very practiced at working out what it will cost to perform each step and quoting an appropriate price. Those working in public service tend to be less business-like, borrowing resources from all sorts of pockets. This is all very well as long as it works but all too often this approach results in an abandoned or incomplete HIA. Even if the resources are not formally costed it is essential to plan ahead.

If the first rough causal path has identified particular expert knowledge as necessary, are people with this knowledge willing to help or will experts have to be hired in? How many person hours are going to be needed to search the evidence, analyse it, and write the report? If there is to be community participation are the people and facilities (travel costs, crèche, refreshments, room hire) available? Can the cost of office functions and facilities be covered? Are there paid staff available and willing to undertake these functions and is it possible to cover other expenses from existing budgets?

Having assessed available and needed resources one is in a position to approach potential funders of an HIA for the funds or other resources identified as being necessary. It is very likely that the final HIA plan will be a compromise between what you would like to do given unlimited resources and what you can do with the resources you have. The question of how HIAs are paid for is discussed further in Chapter 11.

There is surprisingly little information on the cost of doing an HIA. One study[3] suggested that costs for six HIAs were between £3,000 and £60,000 but these figures must be regarded as unreliable.

Using different skills

The causal path diagram will have identified pathways that are not covered by public health training. Forecasting traffic flows, impacts on economy and employment, furnace emissions, plume distribution, and many other topics require specialist expert knowledge. If the assumptions made about these early stages are wrong then the predictions of health impacts based on them will also be wrong. It is essential that health impact assessors recognize the limits of their competence and do not guess at things they do not understand.

When working with local authorities or other public bodies very often these specialist skills are available within the organization and can be given to the HIA. Often the proposer will have expert knowledge. Those proposing to build an industrial plant will know a great deal about how it works, likely emissions, and possible hazards but they may also have an interest in a particular outcome of the impact assessment. When the conclusions of an HIA are based on matters outside the competence of the assessor it is essential that the assessor makes clear who was responsible for this part of the assessment and point out that the accuracy of the HIA prediction is dependent on the prediction of change in these intermediate factors.

Planning the report

The report should be considered at an early stage. How are the findings to be communicated to the decision makers? Will there be supplementary reports for different groups such as residents and informants? The various options for reporting are discussed further in Chapter 5.

On to the assessment

If the scoping has been thoroughly done the assessment can be carried out in a business-like fashion. One has to be prepared to revisit some of the decisions made at the scoping stage in the light of issues that become apparent as the assessment proceeds but it is best to start off with a plan even if it needs to be refined later.

Describing the baseline

A first step in understanding how a proposal will impact on health is knowing the initial state (the baseline). One needs to know the current state of health and the determinants of health in the population affected by the proposal. State of health may be indicated by measures such as death rate, hospital admission rate, and prevalence of disease, and the state of the determinants of health by measures such as prevalence of smoking and heavy drinking, unemployment, housing, and quality of environment. It is likely that a start will be made on compiling the baseline report during the scoping stage and that it will be further refined during the assessment stage.

Routine statistics may provide a lot of information on the health of administrative regions. For example, in England death rates, hospital admission rates, employment rates, and crime rates can be obtained for local authority areas (see, for example, the health profiles that are published each year for local authorities,[4] the health data for smaller areas (Middle Super Output Areas),[5] and neighbourhood statistics[6]). Similar datasets can be found for most high-income countries. For many lower- and middle-income countries some data are usually available at the national level[7] but may be unavailable below this level. For HIAs of local-level projects it will usually be necessary to conduct baseline surveys at individual, household, and community level. Strategies and methods for doing this in complex settings have been described.[8,9]

Often the available information may refer to populations far larger than the population that will be affected by the proposal. Equally, given that one is concerned with unequal impacts on different sections of the affected population there should be separate baselines for the groups which will experience different impacts. There is likely to be considerable variation in health between the different sections of larger populations and average health figures are often unreliable indicators of the health of smaller groups within these populations. Health impact assessors can do no more than make the best estimates that they can for small population groups. Public health departments and local statisticians may be able to help with gathering baseline information.

When compiling the baseline report it is essential to remember that its purpose is to identify the key problems that might be addressed by the proposal and the indicators that might change if the proposal is implemented and they should therefore be monitored. Too often the baseline section of an HIA report is no more than a collection of all the statistics that can be found vaguely relevant to the population and no reference is made to them in the rest of the report.

References

1. Tools for HIA. http://www.apho.org.uk/resource/view.aspx?RID=44541.
2. Herriot N. Williams C. A guide to carrying out a health impacts assessment of new policy as part of an Impact Assessment. London: Department of Health, 2010. www.apho.org.uk/resource/view.aspx?RID=96531.
3. York Health Economics Consortium. Cost benefit Analysis of Health Impact Assessment: Final Report. London: Department of Health, 2006. Available at http://www.apho.org.uk/resource/item.aspx?RID=44796.
4. Association of Public Health Observatories. Health Profiles for Local Authorities. Available at http://www.apho.org.uk/default.aspx?RID=49802.
5. APHO. Small area statistics for Joint Strategic Need Assessment. Available at http://www.apho.org.uk/RESOURCE/VIEW.ASPX?RID=87735.
6. Office of National Statistics. Neighbourhood Statistics. Available at http://www.neighbourhood.statistics.gov.uk/dissemination/.
7. World Health Organization. Global Health Observatory Country Health Statistics. Available at http://www.who.int/gho/countries/en/index.html.
8. Winkler MS, Divall MJ, Krieger GR, Schmidlin S, Magassouba ML, Knoblauch AM, Singer BH, Utzinger J. Assessing health impacts in complex eco-epidemiological settings in humid tropics: Modular baseline health surveys. Environmental Impact Assessment Review 2012; 33: 15–22.
9. United Nations. Designing household survey samples: Practical guidelines. New York: Department of Economic and Social Affairs, 2008. Available at http://unstats.un.org/unsd/demographic/sources/surveys/Handbook23June05.pdf.

Chapter 3

Quantitative assessment

John Kemm

HIA claims to predict the likely consequences for health (health impacts) of implementing different options. A full description of impacts would cover:

+ the nature of the impacts (death, illness, discomfort, anxiety)

+ the direction of change (increased or decreased)

+ the magnitude of change (how many, how severely)

+ distribution—which groups will experience impacts?

Magnitude may be described in words such as big and small or major and minor (see Chapter 4, page 49) but it is better to describe it in quantitative (number) terms wherever possible. Trade-offs between options are easier when magnitude is precisely described and decision makers are more likely to be influenced when the impacts are quantified.[1]

Box 3.1 gives a simple example of an attempt to quantify the additional road injuries associated with the opening of a new attraction.

Causal diagrams

Causal diagrams provide a basis for predicting impacts and attempt to show everything that could be changed if the proposal were implemented. The diagram then shows what would happen as a result of each of the changes until a change in health is reached. For example, building a new road may change traffic flow, increasing it in some places and reducing it in others, and the changed traffic flow could increase or decrease vehicle emissions, which could change the concentration of nitrogen oxides in the air, which could change the prevalence of respiratory disease. For each step in the causal chain the direction and magnitude of the change should be determined. Often even the direction of change is uncertain, for example would loss of employment increase smoking because people are bored and anxious or decrease smoking because people cannot afford it? An example of a causal diagram to examine the effect of minimum wage legislation is shown in Figure 3.1. Other causal diagrams are shown in Figure 2.2 (page 21) and Figure 10.1 (page 99).

Box 3.1 Estimation of the additional travel casualties caused by the opening of the National Botanical Garden of Wales

The National Botanical Garden of Wales in Carmarthenshire was intended to be tourist attraction. This shows an attempt to estimate how many additional road casualties would be caused as a result of the garden opening.

Estimated number of visitors per year	250,000
Estimated number of visitors arriving by car (85%)	212,500
Estimated vehicle journeys (2.5 visitors per car)	85,000
Estimated vehicle kilometres (mean journey length 150 km)	12,750,000

Injury rates per 100 million kilometres

	Deaths per 100 million vehicle kilometres	Seriously injured per 100 million vehicle kilometres	Deaths per year travelling to garden	Seriously injured per year travelling to garden
Car occupants	0.5	5.8	0.063	0.74
Pedestrians	0.2	2.3	0.025	0.29

Conclusion: One might expect one additional serious injury of car occupant or pedestrian every year and one additional death every ten years as a result of journeys to visit the garden. Note that not all of these will be additional deaths since some of the vehicles would have made other trips if they did not come to the garden. Also note the other assumptions on which this calculation is based.

DETR Road accidents in Great Britain 1997; The Casualty Report HMSO (1997 data was used because it was the latest available at the time of the HIA).

Source: Data from Kemm J. National Botanic Garden of Wales—Health Impact Assessment report. 2001 National Botanic Garden of Wales, Carmarthenshire.

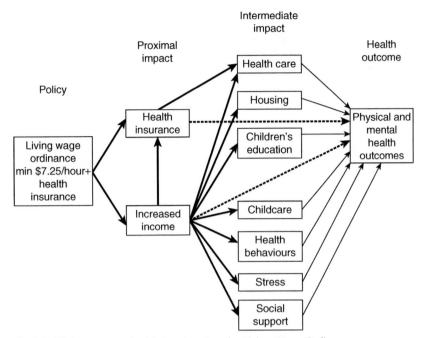

Fig. 3.1 Minimum wage legislation. Los Angeles Living Wage Ordinance Causal Paths.

Reproduced from Journal of Epidemiology & Community Health, Brian L Cole *et al.*, Projected health impact of the Los Angeles City living wage ordinance, Volume 59, Issue 1, pp. 645–650. ©2005 with permission from BMJ Publishing Group Ltd.

The DPSEEA (drivers, pressures, state, exposure, effect, actions) model developed by WHO[2] as a framework for environmental health indicators is a special case of a causal diagram.[3]

Epidemiology

Epidemiology is one of the basic disciplines contributing to HIA. Epidemiology describes the relationship between the socioeconomic and physical environment and health (or ill-health) of populations. These relationships are investigated by observing the associations between variations in the environment and health. General laws are then derived from these observations. For example, in Victorian times John Snow observed that cholera deaths were far more frequent in houses supplied by the Lambeth water company than in houses supplied by the Southwark water company. From this he concluded that something in the water of the Lambeth water company caused cholera deaths.[4,5] (Later scientific studies showed that the something in the water was cholera vibrios coming from polluted Thames water.) Similarly, it was shown that times of extreme air pollution in London were associated with increases in deaths from heart disease and respiratory disease, from which it was concluded that air pollution causes deaths from these diseases.[6,7] These are extreme examples but they illustrate the general approach.

Dose–response curves

The relationship between the environment and ill-health is usually described by a dose–response curve (Figure 3.2). The horizontal axis of a dose–response curve represents exposure, i.e. the level of environmental factor to which the individual is exposed. The vertical axis indicates the risk of ill-health. Note that these diagrams do not show what will be the outcome for any particular individual but only their probability of experiencing a health event and the overall risk for the population.

Information from the dose–response curve can be put together with the expected change in exposure level and the current prevalence of disease in the population to predict the impact of the change[8] (Figure 3.3). Thus if we correctly predict the change in exposure and the dose–response curve is correct we can predict the impact.

Evidence

In order to construct and interpret a causal diagram one needs evidence to know the nature, direction, and magnitude of the causal links. In this section

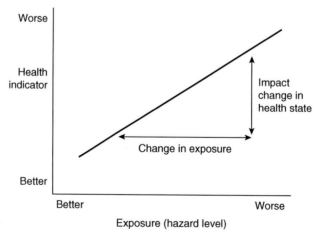

Fig. 3.2 Dose–response curve and impact.

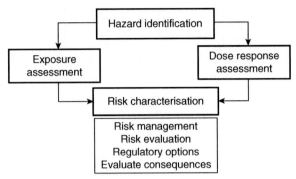

Fig. 3.3 US NRC model.

we consider evidence from the bio-medical literature and evidence from technical experts. There are other types of evidence and these are discussed in Chapter 4.

The biomedical literature is full of reports of associations between environment, lifestyle and health state. Living in damp or cold housing, living close to industrial sites, smoking, heavy drinking, and numerous other factors have been claimed or shown to be associated with poor health. However, before accepting that there is really an association rather than a chance coincidence one needs to apply the tests of association that epidemiology and statistics have developed. Having established that there really is an association one has to establish that the one factor causes the other rather than the association being caused by some other factor. People who live in bad housing or uncongenial surroundings are usually disadvantaged in many other ways, such as low income or uncongenial work. There are tests which aim to assess whether or not an association is causal (see Box 3.2).

This scepticism about the existence of associations is often a cause of dispute. If two mothers living near a waste tip have children with congenital deformities is it not obvious that the tip caused the deformities? Worried residents are likely to disbelieve any statistician who tells them that these two cases could well have arisen by chance or that there is no reason to believe that the proximity of the tip caused the deformities. It may be that the standards of proof customarily used in biomedical work are too high. They are particularly designed to prevent false-positive conclusions (type 2 errors, i.e. finding an association where in truth none exists) rather than false-negative conclusions (type 1 errors, i.e. failing to find an association where in truth one exists). There is no shortage of examples where biomedical experts have proved to be wrong. Despite these reservations biomedical evidence is an important guide to recognizing real causal links and avoiding non-existent links.

Box 3.2 Testing whether or not an association is causal (Bradford-Hill Criteria)

1. Consistency: Has the same association been reported by several different authors in several different places?

2. Specificity: Is the association with one specific disease or is it a general association with poor health?

3. Strength: Is there a strong correlation between the supposed cause and consequence?

4. Time relationship: Does the supposed consequence occur after the supposed cause?

5. Dose response: Is there a dose response between supposed cause and consequence, i.e. more disease in those exposed to higher dose?

6. Plausibility: Does the supposed causal relationship fit with our general understanding of what benefits or harms health?

None of these tests is entirely reliable, but taken together they are a good guide.

Data from Weed D.L. On the use of causal criteria. International Journal of Epidemiology 1997; 26: 1137–1141.

With interventions intended to improve health and well-being there is often uncertainty as to whether they have the desired effect. For example, will introducing alcohol education to schools decrease, have no effect on, or even increase the probability of children drinking to excess? Answering this type of question is called evaluation. The usual way to evaluate a medical treatment (decide whether it helps to cure or prevent a disease) is to conduct a randomized controlled trial (RCT) but it is often not possible to use this or similar methods to find out whether the sorts of intervention that may be the subject of HIA work[9] and one has to rely on descriptions of what happened when the intervention was tried elsewhere. There are still many gaps in the evidence and the quality of the evidence base currently available for HIA limits the soundness and completeness of its conclusions.[10]

In searching for evidence on links between environment or lifestyle and health or the likely effect of an intervention it is wise to search for articles in the biomedical literature. Using Pubmed[11] is a quick way of doing this but a trained librarian will be able to advise you how to do a much more thorough job. A good librarian can also help you to search the 'grey literature' in which many reports of interventions will be found. The internet is also a very useful source of evidence, but evidence found on the internet has to be used with care because it can produce not only a great deal of very good work but also a great deal of nonsense. Talking to knowledgeable people (key informants) is also an important way of obtaining evidence but again be careful because not every key informant is well informed or correct.

In many cases you need information from other disciplines, for example what pollutant and how much of them will come out of an incinerator or factory chimney, how will traffic flows be changed by construction of a bypass, how many jobs will be created by a development, and how will the development affect the local economy. For these and similar questions you will need to consult key informants with expertise in the relevant discipline and get them to search the relevant literature on your behalf.

Environmental health

The epidemiological dose response approach to assessing impacts is most easily applied to physicochemical agents. The relationship between air pollutants such as small particles ($PM_{2.5}$),[12] nitrous oxides,[13,14] sulphur dioxide, ozone, benzene, and various health events has been extensively studied.[15] Similar studies have shown the relationship between levels of various water and soil pollutants and health. The effects of ionizing radiation and noise on health have also been subject to extensive enquiry.

However, the epidemiological approach can also be applied to factors in the socioeconomic environment. There is a strong relationship between employment, unemployment, and loss of employment and health.[16,17] Income, both absolute and related to the income of others, is associated with major differences in health. The various aspects of social capital, such as trust of others and quality of social networks, can also be shown to be associated with health.[18,19] In theory therefore the impacts due to changes in these factors could be estimated using the epidemiological approach.

Limitations of dose–response curves

While theoretically exposure and dose response offer a robust way of estimating impacts, the reality is more problematic. First it is often difficult to estimate the future exposure and more fundamentally there is uncertainty as to what is the relevant measure of exposure. Exposure might be described in terms of peak exposure, some form of average exposure, or cumulative exposure: which of these is most relevant to health?

In many cases the dose–response curve is not fully understood. For many substances it is clear that high exposures are very harmful to health, but are small exposures slightly harmful? Is there a threshold below which there is no increase in risk? Does the risk increase linearly with exposure or exponentially? Frequently the data needed to answer these questions are not available. For many substances the evidence comes from occupational exposures, which are far higher than those likely to be encountered by general populations, and estimates of the effect of low exposures can only be made by extrapolation from the effects seen at high doses.

A further problem is that except in the laboratory it is unusual for every other factor to remain constant while one factor changes. In situations where there is exposure to one pollutant there is nearly always exposure to other pollutants and this may give rise to uncertainty as to how much of any associated health change is due to any one pollutant. This problem is known as confounding. There are statistical techniques for estimating the contributions of each factor but confounding remains a major difficulty and it is easy to conclude a relationship is causal when in fact it is due to the unrecognized influence of some other factor. Another facet of the same problem is the cocktail effect: two pollutants may individually have a fairly small effect on health but the effect when both are present is far greater than the sum of the two individual effects (that is to say the effect is synergistic). For example, the risk of cancer in those who are exposed to asbestos and smoking is very much greater that the separate effects of exposure to smoking and to asbestos.[20] Concern about possible cocktail effects is often prominent in popular worries about impacts of pollution.

If the uncertainties which attach to dose–response relationships for physicochemical agents are considerable, those which attach to dose–response relationships for socioeconomic factors are much greater but there is no fundamental reason why the same reasoning of exposure (the socioeconomic state that people experience) and dose–response curves relating these to health state should not later be extended to factors other than physicochemical ones.

Expressing uncertainty

Uncertainty always attaches to prediction and this is especially true for predictions of magnitude. Where an estimate of magnitude is given it is usually possible to set some limits around the uncertainty by stating that your best estimate is that X people will be affected but it is very unlikely to be less than Y or greater than Z. This is often done by presenting confidence limits (typically 95% confidence limits) with the central estimate. Uncertainty may arise from uncertainty about the level of exposure or uncertainty about the dose–response relationship or uncertainty about both, and there are methods of calculating confidence limits taking all these into account. Where the uncertainty arises from doubt about whether a causal relationship really exists all one can do is describe in words how great the uncertainty is.

Models

There have been attempts to estimate the magnitude of impacts by modelling the systems. If the initial states, the changes in key variables, and the relationship between these variables and health are known then it should be possible to describe the system with equations and construct a model to simulate its behaviour. For some problems modelling is the only possible solution. If one needs to investigate catastrophic events such as whether the structures would prevent disaster if a nuclear power station caught fire or a refinery exploded or an aeroplane crashed into building, it is obviously not possible to answer such questions by experiment; simulating them in a model is the only possibility. Models are also used to study the likely distribution in air of pollutants from stacks (plume distribution), the spread of pollutants through other paths, traffic flows, the effects of tax and price changes, and much else.

Numerous models have been used.[21] Early examples are PREVENT,[22] which was used to study the effect of various lifestyle changes on mortality and morbidity, and POHEM,[23] which was used for similar purposes. More recently the global burden of disease model has studied the effect of various health determinants. ARMADA[24] is a model constructed to show how the operation of incineration plants would impact on mortality. Other models and their uses are discussed in Chapters 17 (page 163) and 18 (page 171). Several models have been reviewed by Lhachimi and colleagues.[25]

Simsmoke is a model that predicts the effect of implementing different policy interventions (raising the price of cigarettes, media campaigns, clean-air laws restricting places where smoking is allowed, advertising restrictions, health warnings, and smoking cessation services) on smoking behaviour and smoking-related deaths.[26] It has been tested on data from several states in America, and various Asian and East European countries. Smoking is one of the simplest outcomes to model and Simsmoke is one of very few examples where a models is immediately applicable to policy making.

There is much to be said for models. They are extremely data hungry and force those using them to collect a great deal of data. They require the modeller to be absolutely explicit about the assumptions that underlie the model and do not allow vague thinking. They can accommodate more complex relationships such as non-linear change, delayed effects, interactions, and feedback loops. However, one has to be careful in using models. It is all too easy to concentrate on the answer produced and ignore all the underlying assumptions and complexities in the model. Often the models are difficult to understand and maybe only the modeller understands the full properties of the model. The numerical presentation of the results can give a misleading impression of accuracy. Models should not be looked on as producing precise answers but they can often produce results in 'the right ballpark'.[27] Applied with care models can be useful in indicating the likely magnitude of impacts.

Chaos

There is a further limitation on the epidemiological and modelling approach to HIA. In complex systems the relationships between the various elements is such that it is never possible to specify the initial starting conditions with sufficient precision to allow the final state of the system to be predicted. The usual illustration of this phenomenon is the suggestion that the flapping of a butterfly's wings in Brazil might cause a tornado in Texas.[28] The health of populations is a complex system and precisely predicting its final state is likely to be as difficult as predicting the ultimate consequence of the fabled butterfly's wings. However, that does not mean that one can say nothing about likely consequences for health, only that one cannot give a complete description.

Single metrics and multiple domains

One of the strengths of HIA is that it describes a range of impacts, such as deaths, illness, discomfort, and anxiety as well as positive impacts, but does not attempt to combine all these different impacts into a single metric, leaving it to others to decide whether an additional death is more or less bad than a thousand people suffering severe discomfort or whether it is compensated for by five thousand people gaining employment.

Other forms of assessment attempt to combine all the different impacts into a single metric. In cost–benefit analysis the metric is money, in comparative risk analysis the impacts are combined into disability adjusted life years (DALYs) and other approaches use quality adjusted life years (QALYs). The first problem with this approach is it can only handle impacts that can be described in numeric terms. It is therefore forced to ignore the wide range of impacts that cannot be so described, although often these turn out to be the most important impacts. Often the construction of these single metrics is presented as a technical exercise. However, despite the considerable sophistication used to develop the weightings given to different kinds of impacts, the weighting is ultimately a value judgement. While one person may consider a year of life confined to a wheelchair as of equivalent value to eight months of life with full mobility, another person may take a very different view.

Single metrics and decision making

Combining different impacts into a single metric has a further disadvantage. It turns the assessment from a decision support tool to a decision making tool. Whether the metric is the cost–benefit ratio or additional DALYs or QALYs one simply has to compare the impacts of different options expressed in a single metric and chose the one that produces the largest good metric or the smallest bad metric. The role of the decision maker is thus reduced to simply comparing numbers. Fortunately the decision maker usually realizes that there is a lot more to be considered than the single metric and takes many other factors into account. A different opinion on single metrics is expressed in Chapter 15 (page 146).

Progress with quantitative assessment

While there are many reasons to wish that impacts could be quantified it has to be recognized that this is rarely done. A survey of HIAs in 2005 found that of 98 published HIAs only 17 reported any numeric estimates of change in exposure and only 16 reported numeric estimates of change in health outcome.[29] A similar survey of HIAs done in the USA in 2011 found only 14 examples of HIAs including numeric estimates.[30] The reasons for this are that quantification is often hard or impossible. Frequently one or more of the initial conditions, the effect of the proposal, and the theoretical framework linking conditions to health outcome are not adequately known to allow use of quantitative methods. This is a challenge for HIA and a reason to try and fill the gaps in our knowledge.

References

1. Mindell J, Hansell A, Morrison D, Douglas M, Joffe M. What do we need for robust, quantitative health impact assessment? Journal of Public Health Medicine 2001; 23: 173–78.
2. WHO. Environmental health indicators for Europe: a pilot indicator based report. Copenhagen: Regional Office for Europe WHO, 2004. Available at http://www.euro. who.int/__data/assets/pdf_file/0003/140925/E82938.pdf.
3. Morris GP, Beck SA, Hanlon P, Robertson R. Getting strategic about the environment and health. Public Health 2006; 120: 889–907.
4. Snow J. On the mode of communication of cholera. 1854. Available at http://www. deltaomega.org/documents/snowfin.pdf.
5. Hempel S. The medical detective: John Snow and the mystery of cholera. London: Granta Books, 2006.
6. Ministry of Health. Mortality and Morbidity during the London Fog of December 1952. Reports on Public Health and Medical Subjects No. 95. London: Ministry of Health, 1954.

7. Bell ML, Davis DL, Fletcher T. A retrospective assessment of mortality from the London smog episode of 1952: The role of influenza and pollution. Environmental Health Perspectives 2004; 112: 6–8.

8. O'Connell E, Hurley F. A review of the strengths and weaknesses of quantitative methods used in health impact assessment. Public Health 2009; 123: 306–10.

9. Bonel C, Hargreaves J, Cousins S, Ross D, Hayes R, Petticrew M, Kirkwood BR, Alternatives to randomisation in the evaluation of public health interventions: design challenges and solutions. Journal of Epidemiology and Community Health 2011; 65: 582–87.

10. Joffe M, Mindell J. A framework for the evidence base to support Health Impact Assessment. Journal of Epidemiology and Community Health 2002; 56: 132–38.

11. Pubmed. http://www.ncbi.nlm.nih.gov/pubmed/.

12. Industrial Economics Incorporated. Expanded expert judgement assessment of the concentration-response relationship between PM2.5 exposure and mortality. Cambridge MA: US Envornmental Protection Agency, 2006. Available at http://www. epa.gov/ttn/ecas/regdata/Uncertainty/pm_ee_report.pdf.

13. Samoli E, Touloumi G, Zanobetti A, LeTertre A, Schindler C, Atkinson R, Vonk J, Rosse G, Saez M, Rabczenko D, Schwartz J, Katsouyanni K. Investigating the dose response relationship between air pollution and total mortality in the APHEA2 multicity project. Occupational and Environmental Medicine 2003; 60: 997–82.

14. Samoli E, Aga E, Touloumi G, Nisiotis K, Forsberg B, Lefranc A, Pekkanen J, Wojtynial B, Schindler C, Niciau E, Brunstein R, Dodik Fikfak M, Schwartz J, Katsouyannis K. Short term effects of nitrogen dioxide on mortality: an analysis with the APHEA project. European Respiratory Journal 2006; 27: 1129–38.

15. Committee on the Medical Effects of Air Pollution. Long term exposure to air pollution: effect on mortality. London: The Stationery Office, 2009. Available at http://www.dh.gov.uk/prod_consum_dh/groups/dh_digitalassets/@dh/@ab/documents/digitalasset/dh_108152.pdf.

16. Moser KH, Fox AJ, Jones DR. Unemployment and mortality in the OPCS longitudinal study. Lancet 1984; ii: 1324–28.

17. Lundin A, Lindberg I, Hallsten L, Ottosson J, Hemmingsson T. Unemployment and mortality: a longitudinal prospective study on selection and causation in 49,231 Swedish middle aged men. Journal of Epidemiology and Community Health 2010; 64: 22–28.

18. Berkman LF, Syme SL. Social networks, host resistance and mortality: a nine year follow-up study of Almeda County residents. American Journal of Epidemiology 1979; 109: 186–204.

19. Berkman LF, Glass T. Social integration, social networks, social support and health, in Berkman LF, Kawachi I (eds), Social epidemiology. Oxford: Oxford University Press, 2000.

20. Berry G, Liddell FDK. The interaction of asbestos and smoking in lung cancer: A modified measure of effect. Annals of Occupational Hygiene 2004; 48: 459–62.

21. Bronnum-Hansen H. Quantitative health impact assessment modelling. Scandinavian Journal of Public Health 2009; 37: 447–49.

22. Bronnum-Hansen H. How good is the PREVENT model for estimating the health benefits of prevention? Journal of Epidemiology and Community Health 1999; 53: 300–305.

23. Will BP, Bertholt JM, Nobrega KM, Flanagan W, Evans WK. Canadian population health model POHEM: a tool for performing economic evaluation of cancer control interventions. European Journal of Cancer 2001; 37: 1797–804.

24. McCarthy M, Biddulph JP, Uttley M, Ferguson J, Gallivan S. A health impact assessment model for environmental changes attributable to development projects. Journal of Epidemiology and Community Health 2002; 56: 611–16.

25. Lhachimi SK, Nusselder WJ, Boshuizen HC, Mackenbach JP. Standard tool for quantification in health impact assessment: A review. American Journal of Preventive Medicine 2010; 38: 78–84.

26. Levy DT, Bauer JE, Lee H. Simulation modelling and tobacco control: creating more robust public health policies. American Journal of Public Health 2006; 96: 494–98.

27. McMichael AJ. Integrated assessment of potential health impact of global environmental change: Prospects and limitations. Environmental Modelling and Assessment 1997; 2: 129–37.

28. Lorenz EN. Predictability: Does the flap of a butterfly's wings in Brazil set off a tornado in Texas? Paper to 139th meeting of American Association for the Advancement of Science 1972.

29. Veerman JL, Barendregt JJ, Mackenbach JP. Quantitative health impact assessment: current practice and future directions. Journal of Epidemiology and Community Health 2005; 59: 361–70.

30. Bhatia R, Seto E. Quantitative estimation in health impact assessment: Opportunities and challenges. Environmental Impact Assessment Review 2011; 31: 301–309.

Chapter 4

Qualitative assessment: lay and civic knowledge

John Kemm

The previous chapter described the epidemiological approach to predicting impacts in HIA. It is important to realizes, however, that there are other equally logical ways of thinking and different types of evidence. HIA has traditionally put great emphasis on participation, which is implied by democracy, one of four core values mentioned in the original Gothenburg consensus document. This chapter considers how participation can contribute to prediction of impacts.

Throughout this chapter we use the terms 'scientific' and 'expert' in inverted commas. By 'scientific' we mean generally based on the reasoning and methods of biomedical science. By 'expert' we mean someone who claims or is claimed to have greater knowledge of a particular subject. These terms are intended to be neutral descriptors and do not imply any approval or disapproval.

Participation

Arnstein[1] proposed a ladder of citizen participation with a range of ways in which a government could interact with its citizens. Similar ranges can be recognized for the interaction of doctors with their patients or other professionals with their clients. At one end of the spectrum is manipulation, in which government merely seeks compliant citizens. At the other end is citizen control, where citizens have complete control over decision making. There are varying degrees of informing and consultation between these extremes (Figure 4.1). Participation in HIA tries to operate closer to the citizen control end of the spectrum.

Mahoney and colleagues[2] have pointed out that the term 'participation' has been used very imprecisely and widely differing degrees of public involvement in HIA have been described as participation. They suggest that public involvement in HIA could usefully be categorized into four types:

- non-participatory HIA
- consultative HIA
- participatory HIA
- community HIA.

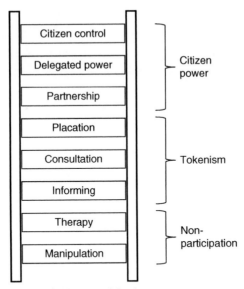

Fig. 4.1 Arnstein's ladder of citizen participation.

Reproduced with permission from Sherry R, Arnstein A, Ladder Of Citizen Participation, Journal of the American Institute of Planners, Volume 35, Issue 4, 1969, pp. 216–44 © Taylor and Francis Group.

Community HIA equates to Arnstein's highest level of citizen participation, in which the relevant community has complete ownership of the HIA process and control of the questions researched, the methods used, and the interpretation of the data. The assessor's only role is to support and facilitate the community. In participatory HIA the community are involved with all stages of the HIA, contribute to workshops, and sit on advisory and steering committees but the process is steered by the assessors. In consultative HIA the community is informed and asked to give its views on specific questions but the process and outcome is controlled by the assessors.

Reasons for participation in HIA

Participation brings five advantages to HIA:

- source of information: the people who know most about living in an area are the people who live there
- people have a right to be informed about how decisions that affect them are being made
- 'little democracy': people have a right not only to be informed but to participate in decisions that affect them

◆ conflict resolution: people are more likely to accept a decision even if they do not like it if they understand why and how it was made

◆ social learning: when people participate in an HIA they gain a greater understanding of the factors that affect their health and are better able to take control of these factors.

The Gothenburg consensus paper saw 'the right of people to participate in a transparent process for the formulation, implementation and evaluation of [decisions] that affect their life, both directly and through the elected decision makers' as a key element of democracy. (The original document refers to 'policies' rather than decisions.) There is some disagreement about the place of participation in HIA. Some regard it as the main purpose of HIA while others regard it as a tool to be used only when it adds to the power of the HIA to predict impacts and support decision making.

Fallibility of 'expert' knowledge

Communities and people have their own ideas about what affects or will affect their health and often these do not agree with the 'scientific' views based on the rules and evidence of scientific disciplines. Often these 'scientific' views are regarded as the 'expert' view and aligned with the views of authority. Sometimes an 'expert's' view is no more than the opinion of a particular person or group and is not supported by sound reasoning or evidence. The denial of illness due to water contamination in Woburn, Massachusetts,[3] illness due to soil contamination in the Love Canal area,[4] and more recently the denial that bovine spongiform encephalopathy (mad cow disease or new variant Creutzfeld–Jakob disease in humans) could cross the species barrier into humans are all cases where the 'expert' view was shown to be in error. These examples remind one that the evidence on which 'expert' views are based should always be scrutinised but do not demonstrate that the 'expert' view is always or even often wrong.

Lay knowledge

Lay knowledge can greatly enrich expert knowledge. It adds fine-grain detail to the picture, revealing the lived experience of residents and what particular issues affect their quality of life.[5] In a housing estate damp, mould, difficulty of cleaning, thin walls, vermin, noise, graffiti, litter, antisocial behaviour, excessive traffic, lack of play space for children, and insecurity of tenure may all be present but which of these are the things that really make residents' life difficult and which come lower on their priority list? What are the aspects of the place they live in that they value: living near to relatives, tight knit communities, living where they grew up, or other aspects of the place? Unless these things are understood the assessment of the situation and future may be very wrong. In many cases the community may find its own 'experts' who will advance views different to those of authorities' 'experts' and often lay claim to greater 'scientific' insight. They should not be regarded as any more reliable than 'experts' produced by the authorities or project's supporters. The importance of lay knowledge in HIA is further argued in Chapter 12.

Reaction to the proposal

Another aspect that only those affected know is how they will react if the proposal is implemented. This may be an important element in the causal chain. For example, residents may say that if an incinerator is built near them they will not allow their children to play outside. This is likely to impact on the health of the children and has to be added into the causal pathway irrespective of whether keeping the children in would be a wise decision. Equally, if people say that if a housing estate is built near them they will dislike and distrust the new residents then it is possible that there will be negative impacts on social cohesion and the health of the community. It may be that if the proposal is implemented people will not react as they have said they would but what they have said must be considered when assessing the impact. Listening to the community's views is the only way to assess how they might react to the proposal.

When lay and 'expert' knowledge differ

Sometimes the community and 'expert' opinion reach very different conclusions. In the UK many communities feel that telecommunication masts for mobile phones are dangerous and object strongly to having a mast near their homes. Generally 'expert' opinion is that the balance of evidence indicates that there is no general risk to the health of people living near these masts on the basis that exposures are expected to be small fractions of guidelines.[6] Similar disagreements often arise in relation to incinerators or any plant that produces emissions of any type. Often the community will have 'scientific' theories to explain its fears and the discussion may be framed as a 'scientific' disagreement, for example how much of each pollutant will be emitted and what the level of exposure to these pollutants will be.

As implied by Williams and Elliot's definition of HIA (page 122), the aim is to 'bring into dialogue evidence, interests, values and meanings of different stakeholders in order to imaginatively understand'. Debate as to who is 'right' is usually a dead end. Perception is more important than any 'expert' assessment of risk. If the community believes that something is a problem, then no matter how much 'experts' may demonstrate that there is no danger, it remains a problem because someone thinks it is a problem. Discussions of rival 'scientific' theories are usually not helpful since the community is frequently not convinced by the arguments that the 'experts' advance. It is better to start by accepting the fact that the community do not like the proposal and then set about understanding why they do not like it.

Empowering communities

Participation should involve much more than giving those affected by a proposal the chance to express their views. It should give them real opportunity to influence a decision that is going to affect them. This means that they should have input to all stages of the HIA, being members of the steering committee contributing to the scoping stage (Chapter 2), helping to draw up the causal diagram, and deciding what are the main issues to be addressed, the types of evidence to be used, the ways in which the impacts will be assessed, the recommendations that will be made, and how these will be reported to the decision makers (Chapter 5). The degree to which they wish to be involved will vary but if participation is to be a meaningful part of the HIA then one must make every effort to give stakeholders an opportunity to be part of all steps.

One problem is consultation fatigue and disillusionment.[7] All too often deprived communities are repeatedly asked to complete surveys and give their opinions on various subjects at the end of which nothing happens. They may have lost all trust in authorities who repeatedly seek their views although nothing changes.[8] Under these circumstances invitations to participate in an HIA may be regarded as no more likely to produce a result than the last ten consultations. Communities may need to be convinced that this time their views will really be listened to, but at the same time those invited to join in an HIA must be given a realistic view of what that HIA can achieve. Although views will be listened to there is no guarantee that the decision makers will do as the community wants or even that the HIA report will support all their views.

Conflict resolution

HIAs are often called for in situations where there is conflict. Sections of the community may be strongly opposed to a proposal and see the HIA as part of the strategy for opposing it. Sometimes opposition may be driven by NIMBYism (not in my back yard). A person may be generally in favour of a process such as wind generation or waste recycling so long as the plant is not near their home. It may be that a completed HIA will produce a report that can be used powerfully in advocacy against the proposal. However, all concerned need to understand that an HIA seeks to find evidence of good and bad impacts for the proposal and for the alternative options, not to argue the case for any particular option (see Chapter 6).

Running an HIA in such circumstances needs skill and tact. First the assessor has to make clear that they are not advocates for any party and that they are eager and willing to hear the views of all interested in the proposal. They must show respect for all parties, any suggestion that anyone's views are not being taken seriously will rapidly destroy trust. They must try and allow time for stakeholders to respond. While commercial firms and public organizations are used to reading and responding very rapidly to even complex documents, community groups may well wish to have discussions among themselves to ensure they have fully understood the issues and made precisely the response they want, and this takes time. Often the timetable is outside the control of the health impact assessor but they should make every effort to ensure that community groups have the time they need to react to developments.

Representativeness

So far we have talked about the community view, implying that everyone in the community has the same view. This is plainly nonsense and one should be talking of community views, recognizing that there are likely to be different views within the community, some of which may be directly opposed to each other. Not only are there differences between individuals but there are also differences over time as people's views evolve. To recognize this is in no way to demean community views; frequently one finds similar divergence and changes of view among 'scientific' experts.

These changes and differences in views do, however, complicate the issue of how community views are to be represented and fed into the HIA. The community may have leaders who are either self-appointed or in some way chosen by the community. Various people may put themselves forward to represent the community. Those working with the community, such as family doctors, community nurses, social workers, or voluntary sector workers, may claim to be mandated to speak for that community. Trades union representatives and faith leaders may speak on behalf of their members. Democratically elected councillors probably have a better claim than most to represent their constituents even if only a very small proportion of the electorate voted for them. Deciding which of these various people is best suited to represent the community's views in an HIA is difficult. The author does not have an answer to this question but it is important that those doing an HIA realize that there is a problem and think about how to resolve it in each situation.

One way to hear as many voices as possible is to make clear that the assessment team is eager to hear from anyone who wants to speak to them. This may well result in voices being heard that are not represented elsewhere. Another approach is to take steps to ensure that the assessors hear the 'voice of the voiceless', seeking out views that do not seem to be represented by others. While this has much to recommend it, one must recognize that it is dangerously close to paternalism since the assessor has decided that certain voices will be heard. Some have argued that representativeness may be unobtainable and the important thing is to value the insights obtained from individual cases rather than to worry about their generalizability.[9]

Tokenism

The rhetoric of HIA is strong on participation but examination of HIA reports suggests that the practice is often far less impressive.[10] All too often participation seems to consist of one or two people who are said to represent the community and were invited to express opinions on one or two occasions. This bears no resemblance to good participation where members of the HIA team use sociological skills to set about thoroughly understanding the community with which the HIA is concerned, invest time in ensuring that the community understands what the HIA is trying to do, establish relationships with members of the community who are keen to help, use rigorous methods in interviews and focus groups to explore the participants' views (usually recording responses verbatim), and then carefully analyse the data collected.

It has been argued that participation is better not done at all than done badly in a tokenistic way.[11]

Logistics of participation

The practical aspects of arranging participation are not straightforward and one has to have a process for involving those who wish to be closely involved with the HIA and for gathering information from other members of the community. Among the methods that can be used are:

- questionnaires
- interviews
- focus groups
- formal public meetings
- steering/working group meetings

- protest group meetings
- informal public meetings
- photo surveys.

Questionnaires

Questionnaires are the only way of getting information from very large numbers of people. Questionnaires may be very widely distributed by post to named addressees or by encouraging people to pick up questionnaires from public places such as libraries, bus and train stations, and so on. Widespread access to the internet means that responses can often be collected through this medium. In this way one can collect very large numbers of responses, although this is usually a very small fraction of those who could have responded and one is never sure about the characteristics of those who have responded. This makes questionnaire data difficult to interpret.

Questionnaires may include closed questions such as:

What do you think of this proposal?   Strongly support/Support/No opinion/Oppose/Strongly oppose

How often do you fly from xx airport?   1–3 times per year, 4–6 times per year, 1–2 times per month, more frequently

What gender are you?   Male/Female

or open questions such as:

How will this proposal affect you?

Closed questions are more likely to be completed but they give far less information than a fully completed open question. It is generally wise to use a mixture of open and closed questions. The questions should seek information on what the respondent thinks about the proposal and also a little about themselves so this can be related to their views on the proposal. Questionnaires are probably never suitable to be used as the only or main method of participation but they can be a very useful supplement to other methods.

Interviews

Interviews are a method of hearing the views of one or two people. For most purposes a semi-structured interview is best. This is an interview that feels like a normal conversation but the interviewer has a list of topics on which they wish to hear the interviewee's opinion and gently steers the conversation towards them in an order that fits naturally into the conversation. The interviewer needs to be careful to remain neutral, not favouring any particular view but using neutral prompts (tell me more, why do you say that, etc.) encouraging the interviewee to give their views. It is difficult both to interview and take notes at the same time so it is probably best, provided the interviewee gives their permission, to record the interview for later analysis. Through the local paper or other media one can invite people who wish to give their view to be interviewed. The interview is a very good way of getting a detailed insight into people's views but it can be labour intensive. For most key informants interview is the preferred method.

Focus groups

In a focus group a group of people are invited to discuss a proposal. The groups are chosen so that the views of different segments can be heard (young people, women, employees etc.). Again the aim is to have a natural sounding conversation that the facilitator guides to address the particular points of interest and allow all to express their points of view. Skilled facilitation of a focus group is more difficult than interviewing. As with interviews it is difficult both to facilitate and record so it is advisable either to have someone else act as recorder or to use a tape recorder. Often it is a good idea to persuade a preformed group (such as a sports group, hobby group or residents) to be a focus group since they will already have agreed to meet together. In choosing members to form a focus group there has to be a compromise between willingness to attend, interest in the topic, and the characteristics of the members. Sometimes it is necessary to specially convene groups with particular characteristics (for example young people, mothers with children, particular ethnic group). A focus group allows one to hear the views of several people in one session and also to see how they react to each other's views.

Formal public meetings

Public meetings allow a lot of views to be heard and often the community will want to use this form of input, but it has several drawbacks. Public meetings can easily be dominated by those with loud voices and public debating skills. They can readily become arenas for advocacy, with one viewpoint bringing all their supporters and seeking to overwhelm alternative views. If they are to be used they need to be chaired by a skilled person with a strong personality. It is difficult for those who are diffident or lacking in confidence to put their views in this setting. Sometimes people will demand public meetings and if they are held then the health impact assessors should attend and listen. Usually the meeting's main function is to demonstrate the strength of feeling of certain groups. Less formal styles of public meeting described later in this chapter may work better.

Steering groups and working groups

Participation of stakeholders in the HIA should not be limited to the evidence-gathering phase and ideally members of the community would be involved in all phases of the HIA. Certainly it is helpful to have them on the steering group and if one is fortunate they may also be willing to be part of the working group that is carrying out the HIA. If this is to be so then the group meetings must be arranged with this in mind. Usually group meetings are arranged in working hours, which suits professionals very well but may be impossible for community members with work or childcare commitments. The meetings need to be in places that are convenient for the group members from the community. The professional members will expect to do the work as part of their paid employment and perhaps community members of the group should be paid as well. Certainly they should be able to claim their expenses (possibly including childcare). Most of the group members will be used to committee work and probably working with each other but group members from the community may be less comfortable with this style of working and need support. These issues will all need to be recognized and solutions found if participation is to work well.

Protest group meetings

With a contentious issue, local groups of people concerned about the proposal may form protest groups. The assessment team should get to know these groups and involve them in the HIA. If possible the assessors should try to be invited to meetings of the group. They will only hear one side of the story but it is an excellent opportunity to understand people's worries and often protest groups are very knowledgeable—they tend to be familiar with articles on the internet that support their case.

Informal public meetings

Informal public meetings in which people hold discussions in small groups, rather than make speeches and statements, can work a lot better than formal public meetings. It is easy for people to drop in and out of such meetings to suit their schedule. Information is available to them about what an HIA is and what seem to be the main issues of the proposal. They can put their views forward in the form with which they are most comfortable, talking to a member of the assessment team or discussing matters among themselves. An issues wall can be used on which people can stick post-it notes with questions, issues, and comments or a graffiti wall (white board or paper and lots of marker pens) can be used for the same purpose. Those of an artistic bent can even convey their comments through drawings. Planning for real is a similar approach in which people are invited to look at a model of a proposed development and then move parts of the model around to show how they would like things to be. These sorts of events need to be in a convenient place at a convenient time, with facilities such as crèches and refreshments. They take a great deal of preparation but if they work well then people should go away having had an enjoyable and interesting time, and the assessment team should have learnt a great deal. After such an event it is a good idea to prepare some sort of summary report and feed it back to the community members.

Photo surveys

The advent of cheap disposable cameras offers another good way of gathering information. Members of the community are given a disposable camera and asked to take photos of things they like and things they dislike about their area. Most people will come back with a set of really interesting photos and they can then be asked to describe what each is and why they took it. Some people will find it much easier to communicate in this way, and the photos and descriptions will give all sorts of insights into how people feel, what bothers them, and what they value.

Meanings stories and values

The whole of this chapter has been about getting another type of knowledge that is essential to a rounded understanding of how people could be affected by a proposal. The previous chapter was about the 'scientific' way of thinking based on the biomedical disciplines and using the language of those disciplines. This is a very logical and useful way of thinking but it is not the only useful and logical way of thinking.

Many community members will want to think and talk about things in a different way. Their discourse is full of stories and the stories convey meaning and values. Effective participation requires the assessor to understand this discourse and see the underlying meanings.

Magnitude of impact and participation

One major weakness of most participatory approaches is the question of magnitude of impact. Too often this is framed as a qualitative/quantitative debate. Those who use qualitative methods declare themselves not to be interested in numbers but the question is not whether they use numbers but how they describe magnitude of impact. Any meaningful discussion of impact has to consider magnitude. Some impacts are unimportant while others are crucially

Major	Strongly positive	+++
Minor	Weakly positive	+
Negligible	No effect	O
	Weakly negative	-
	Strongly negative	- - -

Fig. 4.2 Ordinal scales to describe magnitude.

important and HIA has to be able to distinguish between them. Those who talk of prioritizing impacts are making precisely this point.

Numbers are one way of describing magnitude, but magnitude of impact can also be described in words and symbols, as shown in Figure 4.2. All these are ordinal scales—that is to say they place impacts in order—and unless we can begin to have criteria for using those scale points they have no meaning. One must be able to explain why one impact has been classified as major and another as minor. Some possible criteria for ordering magnitude of impact are discussed under prioritizing impacts in Chapter 5 (page 51). Presumably in participatory work this distinction is based on the degree to which stakeholders are disturbed by the prospect of different impacts but a better understanding of this issue is needed.

References

1. Arnstein SR. A ladder of citizen participation. Journal of American Planning Association 1969; 35: 216–24.
2. Mahoney ME, Potter J-L, Marsh RS. Community participation in HIA: Discords in teleology and terminology. Critical Public Health 2007; 17: 229–41.
3. Harr J. A civil action. New York: Random House:Vintage, 1996.
4. Brown M. Laying waste: The poisoning of America by toxic chemicals. New York: Pantheon Books, 1980.
5. Williams G, Elliott E, Rolfe B. The role of lay knowledge in HIA, in Kemm J, Parry J, Palmer S. (eds), Health impact assessment: Concepts, theories, techniques and applications. Oxford: Oxford University Press, 2004, pp 81–90.
6. Independent expert group on mobile phones. Report of the group: Mobile phones and health (The Stewart report). Oxford: National Radiological Protection Board, 2001. Available at http://www.iegmp.org.uk/report/text.htm.
7. Morrison DS, Petticrew M, Thomson H. Health impact assessment—and beyond. Journal of Epidemiology and Community Health 2001; 53: 219–20.

8. Kearney M. Walking the walk? Community participation in HIA: A qualitative interview study. Environmental Impact Assessment Review 2004; 24: 217–29.

9. Clyde MJ. Case and situation analysis. Sociological Reviews 1983; 31: 187–211.

10. Wright J, Parry J, Mathers J. Participation in health impact assessment: Objectives, methods and core values. Bulletin of World Health Organization 2005; 83: 58–63.

11. Parry J, Wright J. Community participation in health impact assessment: Intuitively appealing but practically difficult. Bulletin of World Health Organization 2003; 81: 388.

Chapter 5

Recommendations and reports
John Kemm

Bottom line or no bottom line

Having completed his or her assessment of likely impacts the assessor will probably have an opinion as to which option is best. Some decision makers will want to know which option the assessor thinks they should adopt, in which case the report should give this information. Other decision makers may feel that any suggestion of which option to choose infringes their role and want the assessor to limit themselves to stating the likely positive and negative impacts under each option, leaving the decision maker to draw their own conclusions. The health impact assessor needs to understand what the decision maker expects of them and shape the report to fit this expectation.

In reality the distinction between clearly stating a preferred option and only describing the impacts under each option is not marked. In situations where the options are evenly balanced the assessor would probably only wish to describe the strengths and weaknesses of each option. In situations where one option is clearly preferable this will be obvious from the description of positive and negative impacts whether or not the assessor finishes with a plain statement of their preferred option.

Prioritizing impacts

Where there are many impacts it may be helpful to sort (prioritize) them into those that are more important and those that are less important. Ultimately it is up to the decision maker to decide which impacts they feel are most important but it may be helpful to them to know how the assessor prioritized them.

In deciding how important or unimportant an impact is there are a number of considerations:

- How many people or what proportion of the population will be affected?
- How nasty (or nice) will the impacts be?
- How certain is it that the impacts will occur?
- Who will experience the impacts?

An impact that affects a large number of people is more important than the same impact affecting a small number of people. The proportion affected is also relevant. One additional event such as a death is probably less unacceptable if it is one in a population of one million rather than in a population of five hundred.

The nature of the impact also has to be considered. Most people would consider a death a more severe impact than loss of hearing, although all such judgements are debatable. Also relevant is the duration and reversibility of the impact—a temporary illness lasting a month being less unacceptable than one lasting a lifetime and a curable problem being less unacceptable than an incurable one. The timing of the impact also affects its acceptability—a negative impact occurring next week is less acceptable than the same impact occurring in ten years' time.

The certainty of the impact also affects its importance. A negative impact that is certain to happen is less acceptable than one that might possibly happen.

Including the criterion of who is affected is contentious. One usually takes the view that all lives are equally valuable and therefore who is affected by an impact is irrelevant. However, one may wish to modify this by saying that impacts on children, old people, or people less able to look after themselves are less acceptable than impacts on fully fit adults. If one takes the idea of equity seriously then impacts falling on the disadvantaged are less acceptable than those falling on privileged people.

Having decided all these points then one needs some calculus to combine all the different criteria to arrive at a single assessment of the impact.

Categorizing an impact as important or unimportant or in some similar way involves a large number of value judgements and different assessors will make different judgements. However, these matters have to be considered and unless the criteria are explicitly stated, ordinal scales have little meaning. An example of the criteria used by Winkler and colleagues is shown in Box 5.1.

Use of mitigation recommendations

Having identified the impacts likely to occur under the different options the next step is to try and suggest ways of modifying the options so that negative impacts can be avoided or reduced (mitigated) and any positive impacts increased (enhanced). How recommendations for mitigation are framed depends on the primary audience for the report.

In some construction and development projects funding will depend on whether the funder (for example International Finance Corporation) is satisfied that the mitigation recommendations are adequate. The mitigation

Box 5.1 Criteria for rating the impact of projects as low, medium, high, or very high

This system was developed for use with large projects in extractive industries and natural resource sectors in the humid tropics.

Step 1 Each consequence is rated for its extent, intensity, duration, and health effect.

	Consequences			
	A **Extent**	**B** **In tensity**	**C** **Duration**	**D** **Health effect**
Low (0)	Rare individual cases	Individuals hardly notice impacts	<1 month	Health effect is not perceptible
Medium (1)	Local, small, and limited A small number of households are affected	Those impacted will be able to adapt to the health impact with ease and maintain their pre-impact level of health	Short-term (1–12 months)	Health effect resulting in annoyance, minor injuries, or illness that does not require hospitalization
High (2)	Project area but not extending beyond village level	Those impacted will be able to adapt to the health impact with some difficulty and will maintain pre-impact levels of health with support	Medium term (1–4 years)	Health effect resulting in moderate injury or illness that may require hospitalization
Very high (3)	Extends beyond the project area	Those impacted will not be able to adapt to the health impact or to maintain their pre-impact level of health	Long-term/ irreversible (> 4 years)	Health effect resulting in loss of life, severe injuries, or chronic illness that may require hospitalization

The overall impact severity is calculated by summing the score for all four consequences.

Box 5.1 Criteria for rating the impact of projects as low, medium, high, or very high (continued)

Step 2 Relates impact severity to likelihood of impact

Impact severity A + B + C + D	Likelihood			
	Improbable (<40%)	Possible (40–70%)	Probable (70–90%)	Definite (90–100%)
Low (0–3)	Low	Low	Low	Medium
Medium (4–6)	Low	Medium	Medium	High
High (7–9)	Medium	High	High	Very high
Very high (10–12)	Medium	Very high	Very high	Very high

Adapted from Environmental Impact Assessment Review, Volume 30, Issue 1, Mirko S. Winkler *et al.*, Assessing health impacts in complex eco-epidemiological settings in the humid tropics: Advancing tools and methods, pp. 52–61 © 2010, with permission from Elsevier.

recommendations may well form the basis for conditions attached by the decision makers to permission to proceed with the project. In many cases the project will be required to have a health action plan, which states the measures that will be taken as part of the project and the mitigation suggestions will inform this plan. In other contexts, especially where the HIA comes fairly late in the development process, the recommendations for mitigation are no more than suggestions and will not be contractually required.

Mitigation

Adverse impacts can be mitigated in three main ways:

- ◆ Prevent and avoid the adverse impact by a change in design or modifying other details of the proposal.
- ◆ Minimize the impact by modifying details of the proposal.
- ◆ Compensate for adverse impacts by providing other benefits in place of those lost as a result of the proposal.

The recommendations for mitigation would ideally modify the proposal to change the impact without compromising the aims of the proposal. However, sometimes mitigating adverse impacts may reduce some of the benefits associated with the proposal so that the preferred option after mitigation measures have been included may be different from the preferred option before mitigation was considered.

The causal diagram is again useful since it identifies the paths by which each negative or positive impact arises and so suggests the points at which changes might modify impacts in the desirable direction. The recommendations should clearly flow from the analysis of impacts. This is not the place for the assessor to put forward their pet schemes that are unrelated to the impacts.

Mitigation may involve changes to the technical details of the proposal and for these it is likely that knowledge of many disciplines other than public health will be needed. If the impacts are produced by emissions then people with knowledge of the processes which produce the emissions (combustion experts, chemical engineers) or ways of limiting emissions (cleaning flue gases, dust suppression, filtering emissions to water, and so on) will be required. If noise is the problem then people with expertise in limiting noise (by altering noise production or fitting noise insulation at source) are needed. If the impacts are produced by traffic then impacts might be reduced by redesigning the road and its surroundings.

Mitigation may also affect the way in which the proposal is operated, for example limiting night flights and regulating aircraft flight paths at airports, modifying road access routes to avoid villages, or regulating opening hours and attaching conditions to the operation of entertainment venues. Negative impacts as a result of construction activity may be mitigated by limiting working hours, controlling dust, and other methods. Where there will be a large construction workforce, which is often an issue with major infrastructure projects in developing countries, any negative impacts resulting from their presence may be mitigated by providing proper living arrangements and leisure facilities.

Where a negative impact is unavoidable it may be mitigated by providing some compensatory benefit. For example, if open space or sports facilities have to be lost in a proposal then alternative open space and sports facilities might be provided. Where there are negative impacts due to noise, affected homes may be double or triple glazed and sound proofed in other ways. Sometimes communities may be compensated by provision of health or other public services, or public assets such as community meeting rooms.

Where a proposal is controversial the HIA might recommend reducing resentment by better engagement with the stakeholders, such as establishing liaison groups and regular provision of information in the future. The HIA of Donnington Airport[1] recommended that an independent Airport Health

Impact Group should be established to monitor impacts while the airport was operational and this became a condition attached to approval of the airport.

Enhancement

Examination of the causal chains will not only reveal steps where measures are needed to mitigate negative proposals but will also highlight opportunities to enhance the benefits of the proposal. For example, an HIA of a proposal to develop a leisure facility might include recommendations on including healthy options in the range of foods offered or local sourcing of products. An HIA of a housing development might recommend a layout that encouraged active travel (cycling and walking) rather than car use. There will be occasions when the proposer is already intending to undertake these enhancements but finds it helpful to be recommended to do so by an independent outsider.

Reporting impacts with and without mitigation

In some proposals mitigations and enhancements are a part of the proposal and the proposer is committed to implementing them. In other cases the HIA report is the first time that a mitigation or enhancement has been mentioned and there can be no certainty that they will be implemented. In describing impacts it is important to be clear which mitigations and enhancements are a committed part of the proposal and which are not. If the proposal definitely includes mitigation measures then it is reasonable to describe the impacts of the proposal with those mitigation measures in place. However, if there is no commitment to the mitigation then the impacts of the proposal without mitigation should be reported. In many HIAs in the developing world impacts both with and without mitigation are reported.

Monitoring

The HIA will have described the impacts that are considered likely to happen but in all prediction there is uncertainty. It is therefore prudent to monitor what happens after the decision has been implemented and the HIA should suggest what should be monitored and how. The HIA will have identified the anticipated changes in hazards and health, and it may suggest indicators that should be monitored to check that its assumptions were correct. For example, it may be worth setting up a surveillance system to show if a particular condition such as asthma or exposure levels to certain pollutants such as PM_{10} are as expected. One cannot monitor every indicator and monitoring is often expensive, therefore there has to be a compromise between monitoring everything that might change and monitoring nothing. As far as possible monitoring should be based on data that are already being collected and should concentrate on the indicators that are the most sensitive (i.e. will be the first to change if impacts deviate from those predicted). The purpose of monitoring is to enable any problems to be spotted early so that corrective action can be taken before there are adverse consequences.

The precautionary principle

Decision makers often invoke the precautionary principle when choosing between options but the HIA report may usefully offer some guidance as to how the precautionary principle could apply to the different options. The 1998 Wingspread Statement on the precautionary principle[2] summarizes the principle this way: 'When an activity raises threats of harm to human health or the environment, precautionary measures should be taken even if some cause and effect relationships are not fully established scientifically.' This principle states that uncertainty is not a reason for not taking precautions and further implies that the burden of proof where a proposal is suspected to be likely to cause harm lies with the proposer to show that it does not cause harm rather than with others to show it does cause harm.

However, the precautionary principle should not be taken to mean a presumption in favour of the status quo. Unthinking use of the precautionary principle can result in bad decisions. For example, knowledge of the environmental hazard of DDT led to a decision not to use DDT-impregnated sleeping nets in East Africa, a decision which led to many deaths from malaria.[3] Equally, a decision to use single-use (disposable) instruments for tonsillectomy because of the risk of transmitting prions that cause Creutzfeld–Jakob disease on non-disposable instruments had to be reversed after finding that serious complications were more common when single-use instruments were used. Considering the risks of only one option can lead to the wrong decision. The precautionary principle supports the view that when choosing between options (adopt proposal vs do not adopt proposal) one should, other things being equal, choose the option with the lowest risk. The HIA report therefore needs to make clear the uncertainties and risks of the negative impacts associated with all options so that the decision maker can then properly apply the precautionary principle.

The report

HIA reports vary from a single side of A4 to multi-volume documents. While it is difficult to see how very short reports can adequately cover the complexities, most committee members will not read very long documents. A possible content list for an HIA report is shown in Box 5.2.

Box 5.2 Contents of an HIA report

- Executive summary
- What is an HIA?
- The options for the proposal examined by the HIA
- The policy context for the decision
- The scope of the HIA: limits to the enquiry
- The types of evidence and the methods used to assess risk
- Groups given special consideration
- The local situation and the baseline conditions
- The logic diagram and the causal paths
- The intermediate variables and how they will change
- Health impacts resulting from changes in each important intermediate variable
- How special groups are affected
- Implication of impacts for equity
- Summary of positive and negative impacts through different paths
- Recommendations for mitigation, enhancement, and monitoring
- Reflections on the process of the HIA
- Resources used in performing the HIA
- Names of people who contributed to the HIA

The 1-3-25 rule has been offered as a guide for the length of HIA reports: 1 page of key bullet points, 3 pages of executive summary and 25 pages for the full report.[4] Many organizations now ask for reports to be presented in this form. While there is much to recommend the 1-3-25 rule it is no substitute for understanding what length of report the decision makers want and meeting their requirements. It is understandable that assessors want to demonstrate how many scientific papers they have read and the hours of searching interviews they have performed but if this hides the key findings of the HIA it is not helpful. There is no reason why such information should not be put into appendices which could be offered along with a 1-3-25 report (provided that the report can be understood without reference to the appendices). Those who have been paid to perform an HIA may feel that they have to produce a fat report to justify their fees but in most contexts this will not be appreciated, particularly if they are padded out with lengthy descriptions of irrelevant matter.

Where stakeholder interviews have been part of the HIA direct quotations from the stakeholders can add greatly to the report and help people understand the issues. The following quotes from the HIA report on a proposed extension to an opencast mine give a far more vivid description of residents' experiences than a descriptive passage could:[5]

> 'We could sit out and eat al fresco—can't do it now unless you want to eat coal dust sandwiches.'

> 'I am not going to be able to cope with it—I am not going to be able to keep my home clean.'

> 'There was a time when you could blow your nose and it would be a nice creamy grey colour – sometimes you blow your nose and it is actually black. Now that is not what you get in a normal healthy environment.'

Pictures and diagrams can often make a point better than words and make the report easier to read.

In addition to reporting to the decision maker it is usually desirable to produce reports for different purposes. Where residents and others have helped you with information they will want to know what has happened and it may be a good idea to produce a short (1 to 2 pages) report especially for them. Of course it should be made clear that they are also welcome to the longer report if they would like it but most will not want this. If many of the residents are not comfortable reading English it may be necessary to produce a report written in their own language. It may be that residents prefer an oral report, in which case this should be provided. There are some examples of very innovative reports for residents, such as a report in video (see page 274) or cartoon strip form.

Health impact assessors from academic institutions may feel that they need to publish a report of their HIA in a peer-reviewed journal and this is to be encouraged. However, publication in a peer-reviewed journal is generally no use for communicating with the decision makers so such publications must be additional to the main report and not a substitute for it. The sort of report that is likely to be accepted by a peer-reviewed journal is short and will probably not allow the space to describe the details that other impact assessors would like to know.

Communication with decision makers

Bearing in mind that the purpose of an HIA is to assist decision makers it is vital that the findings of the HIA are communicated to them. Ideally they will have been involved with and committed to the HIA from the start and will already have agreed how they will receive the findings of the HIA. Where the HIA is part of the evidence to be submitted for a planning application there will be clear instructions as to how and when the HIA findings are to be submitted.

Where the decision makers have not been involved with the HIA because for some reason or another they did not wish the proposals to be scrutinized in this way, communication is more difficult. First the HIA report should be sent to the decision makers in case they have changed their minds and wish to take notice of it. Second the report should be sent to all stakeholders and particularly those who are in dialogue with the decision makers. Thirdly it may be helpful to feed the findings to the media. Simply handing the report to the media is unlikely to be effective as they probably will not have the time to read it, but a well-crafted press report containing the key points could attract their interest. Once the findings are in the newspapers and on radio and television the decision makers may decide that they cannot be ignored. It is likely that the media will push the assessors to move from impartial assessment to express support for one or other option (i.e. become an advocate, see Chapter 6, page 65). For this reason it is better if the producers of the HIA allow others to communicate with the media.

HIA in parallel with decision making

When HIA is near the final step in decision making there is a danger that it is difficult or expensive to rectify negative impacts. It is better if the assessors work in parallel with the decision makers to consider health impacts as the options are being formulated and refined (Figure 5.1). This way of working ensures close cooperation between decision makers and health impact assessors, and allows mitigation and enhancement to be built into the final

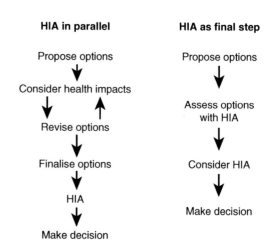

Fig. 5.1 HIA in parallel and HIA as the final step.

decision. When HIA is carried out in parallel the final report will identify few negative impacts and contain few recommendations since these will all have been dealt with earlier. Readers of the final report may therefore incorrectly conclude that the HIA has not made any difference but integrating the HIA with the decision development is an excellent idea.

References

1. Abdel Aziz MI, Radford J, McCabe J. The Finningley Airport HIA: A case study, in Kemm JR, Parry J, Palmer S. (eds), Health Impact Assessment: Concepts, theories and applications. Oxford: Oxford University Press, 2004, pp 285–298.
2. Science and Environmental Health Network. The precautionary principle: a common sense way to protect public health and the environment. Available at http://www.mindfully.org/Precaution/Precautionary-Principle-Common-Sense.htm. Accessed 21 March 2012.
3. Editorial. Caution required with the precautionary principle. Lancet 2000; 356: 265.
4. Canadian Health Service Research Foundation Communication Notes—Reader friendly writing. Undated. Available at http://www.chsrf.ca/Migrated/PDF/CommunicationNotes/cn-1325_e.pdf. Accessed 21 March 2012.
5. Golby A, Lester C. Health impact assessment to the proposed extension to Margam opencast mine Cardiff Welsh Health Impact Support Unit 2005. Available at http://www.wales.nhs.uk/sites3/Documents/522/Kenfig%20Hill%20Final%20-%20Dec%2005.pdf. Accessed 21 March 2012.

Chapter 6

Values and ethics of health impact assessment

John Kemm

The ethics of HIA are derived from the strong values held in public health. These deserve careful scrutiny. The Gothenburg consensus paper[1] identified four values and the explanation it gave for these terms is shown in Box 6.1:

+ democracy

+ equity

+ sustainability

+ ethical use of evidence.

Assessor and decision maker

In discussing the ethics of HIA we have to draw a sharp distinction between the ethical duties of the assessor and the ethical duties of the decision maker. The decision maker (person or committee) is bound by the same ethical rules as any other citizen and in this context by the ethics of public health. Thus it is to be hoped that in making their decision and deciding which impacts are acceptable and on whom these impacts will fall they will follow the principles of beneficience (doing good), non-malefience (doing no harm), promoting equity (reducing unfair inequalities), and sustainability. Utilitarianism and value for money are discussed later in this chapter.

The ethical duty of the assessor is rather different—it is to provide the decision maker with the information needed in order to make ethical decisions. This means describing existing inequalities, identifying the positive and negative impacts under each option, and describing on whom these impacts will fall. The assessor should not attempt to usurp the decision maker's role overtly or covertly. Except in conditions of anarchy, the decision maker is subject to some form of governance (democratic or otherwise) and can claim to have a mandate to take decisions on behalf of the population. The assessor has no such mandate and could be accused of paternalism if they attempt to make

Box 6.1 The Gothenburg values for HIA

Democracy, emphasizing the right of people to participate in a transparent process for the formulation, implementation, and evaluation of policies that affect their life both directly and through the elected decision makers.

Equity, emphasizing that HIA is not only interested in the aggregate impact of the assessed policy on the health of a population but also on the distribution of the impact within the population, in terms of gender, age, ethnic background, and socioeconomic status.

Sustainable development, emphasizing that both short-term and long-term as well as more and less direct impacts are taken into consideration.

Ethical use of evidence, emphasizing that the use of quantitative and qualitative evidence has to be rigorous and based on different scientific disciplines and methodologies to get as comprehensive assessment as possible of the expected impacts.

Reproduced with permission from WHO European Centre for Health Policy Health Impact Assessment, Main concepts and suggested approach, Brussels European Centre for Health Policy 1999. Available at http://www.apho.org.uk/resource/item.aspx?RID=44163. Accessed 22 March 2012.

the decisions. Of course in situations where the same individual is both assessor and decision maker things are less clear-cut but the individual should try and make it clear when they are acting as assessor and when as decision maker.

Democracy and participation

The value of democracy emphasizes that those affected by a decision have a right to be involved in the making of that decision. In HIA this has been interpreted as a requirement for participation (see Chapter 4, page 38). The difficulty in implementing this is that it is very difficult to give all stakeholders equal opportunity to participate and to avoid privileging some voices over others. Within HIA democracy has usually been understood as participative democracy and there are ethical arguments as to what extent a participative democracy arranged for the HIA should displace the representative democracy that most European countries enjoy,[2,3] The Aarhus convention ratified by all countries of the European Union and many others recognizes the right of the public to have information on and participate in the decisions of public authorities that affect the environment.[4]

Equity

Equity and inequity must be distinguished from equality and inequality.[5] Inequality means that different people have different characteristics, such as degree of wealth and state of health. Inequity means that those differences are unfair. Almost everything is unequally distributed in society, including wealth, education, capabilities, and health. Numerous studies[6-8] have demonstrated striking inequalities in health in England as measured by life expectancy, infant mortality, death rates from different disease, prevalence of different diseases, measures of subjective health, and many other indicators. The differences within other countries and between countries are as wide or wider. Some inequalities, for example the increased death rates in those who participate in high-risk sports compared to those who do not, are equitable since the risks were knowingly and willingly incurred. However, most health inequalities, such as those between different socioeconomic groups, are not equitable since they are not willingly chosen and not unavoidable. Respect for equity leads to the conclusion that negative impacts, if unavoidable, should mostly fall on those most able to bear them (i.e. the privileged and least deprived) while positive impacts should fall mostly on the under-privileged and deprived. While all would agree that the distribution of impacts should be fair, deciding what fair means and so on which groups positive and negative impacts should fall can be highly contentious.

The job of the assessor is to describe the inequalities that currently exist and describe how the negative and positive impacts under each option will be distributed between the different groups in the population. It is not their job to judge whether the current equalities and the distribution of impacts are equitable. That is the job of the decision maker.[9] Of course the assessor will probably have opinions about equity—often to describe inequalities is sufficient to demonstrate their inequity. The health impact assessor may propose mitigation measures that in their view decrease inequity.

Sustainability

Sustainable development may be defined as development that 'meets the needs of the present without compromising the ability of future generations to meet their own needs'.[10] Sustainability requires consideration of how a proposal will affect the use of non-renewable natural resources, the availability of water and fertile land, the conservation of animal and plant species, the preservation of forest and other habitats, and the pollution of air, water, and land. More recently climate change has become a major sustainability issue. Attention to sustainability means that HIA must take a long-term view considering not only impacts in the near future but also impacts that will affect future generations. Often this poses difficult questions because a proposal that brings immediate benefits may deplete the resources available to future generations. Sometimes benefit for future generations is at the cost of risks for the current generation (for example disturbing contaminated land in order to remove pollutants may benefit future generations but expose the current workforce and those near the land to those pollutants.) Prediction of future impacts is further complicated by the possibility that future technologies may offer opportunities for succeeding generations to avoid negative impacts. It is the job of an HIA to describe the positive and negative impacts for both the current generation and future generations. It is then the job of the decision makers to decide what balance of impacts on the different generations is acceptable.

Ethical use of evidence

Ethical use of evidence means that one reports and interprets all available evidence honestly and to the best of one's ability, considering not only the evidence from the scientific literature and from 'expert' opinion, but also the evidence from the views of stakeholders. Where the evidence is conflicting this must be acknowledged. Under no circumstances should items of evidence that do not support the assessor's conclusion be suppressed. Where there is uncertainty about the direction or magnitude of the impact this should be made clear.

In addition to the four values listed in the Gothenburg consensus there are other values which deserve consideration:

+ impartiality
+ openness
+ broad view of health
+ utilitarianism
+ value for money.

Impartiality or advocacy

Some authors have clearly urged that HIA should be an advocacy tool: 'HIA goes beyond just providing information—the aim of HIA is to achieve changes in policies and proposals so that they support better health and reduce health inequalities ... Many HIAs therefore overtly aim to influence the decision-making process.'[11] O'Keefe and Scott-Samuel[12] even state 'HIA can and should aim to provide tools that can capture the most deep seated systematic and global economic and environmental crimes in which humankind is complicit.'

The problem with using HIA as an advocacy tool is that it risks violating the principle of ethical use of evidence. An advocate has decided which option they prefer and will present the evidence in such a way as to support that case, possibly downplaying evidence that does not support it. Furthermore, while a good HIA makes clear the uncertainty attached to its prediction of impacts, an advocate will not emphasize the uncertainties attached to their argument.

The view that HIA should strive to be impartial is stated in other guides to HIA. 'Health impact assessment should not be used as a form of advocacy, either for or against the proposal. The HIA should be done impartially and the recommendations should be based on the evidence of health impacts rather than on a pre-existing stance.'[13] Of course interpretation of data can never be purely objective[14–16] and humans can never be perfectly impartial. We all bring values and preconceptions that colour our thinking, but an assessor should always be looking for the weaknesses in their argument and finding out what alternative interpretations are possible.

People trained in public health find it difficult to be impartial since their natural inclination is to be advocates for better health, health equity, and improving the lot of the under-privileged and deprived.

There are five main reasons why people want an HIA:

1. To demonstrate that the decision they have already taken is correct.

2. To make the case against doing something.

3. To make the case for doing something.

4. To inform a decision.

5. To obtain recommendations for mitigating or avoiding negative impacts and for enhancing positive impacts.

It should be noted that only in the last two cases (which are the least common) are the people wanting the HIA indifferent to its conclusions. In the first three cases they are looking for support in favour of or against the proposal and may be disappointed by an impartial report.

The discourse about a proposal that is subject to an HIA is a political discourse. Lasswell[17] defined politics as a debate about 'Who gets what, when and how', and deciding what will be the positive and negative impacts of a proposal is precisely about these questions. Assessors will often find themselves under considerable pressure to support one option but they should try and stand aside from the political debate.[18] Advocacy is a very right and proper function of public health but it cannot be mixed with impartiality. An HIA report may well become an important advocacy tool but it is best if the advocacy can be done by someone other than the assessor. If this is not possible then at least there should be a pause before the assessor transforms themselves into an advocate.

Openness

The value of openness derives from democracy. If people are to play a part in informing the HIA they must know what is happening, what evidence the HIA is considering, and what is being discussed. It follows that as far as possible meetings and working papers should be open to all. This doctrine of perfection needs some modification in practice. Meetings don't work if there are too many people participating and so the working group may want to do much of its work without an audience. If some informants are willing to supply information only if it is not made public ('commercial in confidence') the assessor has to decide whether they are willing to accept information under that condition. If the assessor refuses to accept information on a 'commercial in confidence' basis then there is a risk that the situation may be misunderstood and an incorrect assessment of the impacts produced. If the assessor does agree to accept information on a confidential basis then that confidence must be honoured but the other stakeholders should be informed that the assessor has some information which cannot be shared with them. Special considerations apply when discussing openness in the context of policy and these are discussed in Chapter 8 (page 83).

Broad view of health

A feature of most HIAs is that they take a broad view of health (see Chapter 1, page 4). This means that not only is the absence of disease considered but also the whole range of well-being, not simply physicochemical agents such as pollutants and noise but all the socioeconomic and environmental factors that could influence health and well-being. While this approach is widespread it has been criticized on the grounds that where developers are private companies it requires them to take account of things that they have no possibility of influencing (see Chapter 29). Developers are very good at finding design and engineering solutions but changing the balance of power within societies is generally the business of governments.[19]

Utilitarianism

Utilitarianism is often regarded as one of the key values of public health. It will be a value of the decision maker rather than the assessor but assessors need to understand it so that they can supply the decision makers with the information they need to apply utilitarian principles. Utilitarianism usually associated with

Jeremy Bentham may be succinctly stated as 'the greatest good for the greatest number'. So stated it is difficult to disagree with, but it carries the awkward corollary that some harm to a few is acceptable provided that it is counterbalanced by good for a greater number. Again this seems reasonable unless one happens to be among the few who suffer harm. While utilitarianism is widely accepted, Rawls[20] has stringently criticized the whole principle and argued that it is unethical because harm to the few cannot be justified by benefit for others.

It is very common to find in HIA that there are gainers and losers or at least some who gain more and some who gain less. It is not the place of HIA to judge whether the gains justify the losses but it must supply the decision makers with the information they need to make this decision. Furthermore, the HIA may make recommendations as to how any negative impacts suffered by the losers could be mitigated.

Value for money

The decisions that an HIA is intended to inform frequently involve the use of public money or public resources in some way (for example construction of a new highway or facility, provision of a service, or use of open space and natural resources). Those making these decisions have an ethical duty to ensure that they are obtaining the best value for that money or resource since they are disposing of public resources rather than their own. The question of value for money primarily concerns the decision maker rather than the assessor, and opportunity cost and value for money are usually outside the scope of HIA. Economics offers cost–benefit analysis and a range of other tools to assist comparisons of value in order to help decision makers in considering value for money.

Human rights

Human rights impact assessment involves comparing any benefits of a proposal with the burden (i.e. the degree to which it infringes) on any human rights[21] and a guide to human rights impact assessment has been produced.[22] The United Nations have declared that 'health is a fundamental human right indispensable for the exercise of other human rights. Every human being is entitled to the enjoyment of the highest attainable standard of health conducive to living a life in dignity' (article 12 ICESCR),[23] but this leaves open the question as to what is the highest attainable standard of health and what duties this imposes on the state and others. Certainly HIA can inform a human rights impact assessment[24] but detailed interpretation of human rights and deciding whether or not a particular impact infringes on them lies beyond the competence and probably the mandate of most health impact assessors.

Performance standards

The International Finance Corporation (IFC), part of the World Bank Group, prescribes performance standards for the development projects that it finances. These standards are another way of declaring values and enforcing them, since projects that are not deemed to meet these standards will not be funded by the IFC. The purpose of the performance standards is to ensure that projects in which the IFC invests 'do no harm' to people or the environment and that if negative impacts are unavoidable they are reduced, mitigated, or compensated for appropriately. In particular, the IFC is committed to ensuring that the costs of economic development do not fall disproportionately on those who are poor or vulnerable, that the environment is not degraded in the process, and that natural resources are managed efficiently and sustainably.[25] The problems of applying standards are further discussed in Chapter 29.

Compensation

Many proposals undoubtedly have negative impacts for those most directly affected that are not fully balanced by positive impacts such as employment, increased income, or improved living conditions. At the same time the developer may make substantial profits from the project. This is frequently the case with large infrastructure projects (mines, dams, and so on) in developing countries. Some of the developer's profits may go to the national government in taxation and other revenue. Ideally this increased revenue would benefit those who have suffered negative impacts or the general population of the country but sometimes they are siphoned off by powerful elites. In some situations the negative impacts can be mitigated while in other cases it would be more appropriate to talk of compensation with some other benefit such as improved health or education facilities or improved infrastructure (water supply, bridges, roads) being provided for the community. These compensatory benefits are often called 'social investment' and in considering the impact of the proposal the assessor is invited to consider not just the development but the development and social investment, which is part of the package. These issues are further discussed in Chapters 29 and 31.

References

1. WHO. European Centre for Health Policy Health Impact Assessment: Main concepts and suggested approach. Brussels: European Centre for Health Policy, 1999. Available at http://www.apho.org.uk/resource/item.aspx?RID=44163. Accessed 22 March 2012.
2. Cooke S, Vyas D. Votes and voices: the complimentary nature of representative and participative democracy. London: LGA Publishers, 2008.

3. Pilet J-B, Steyvers K, Delwit P, Regmaert H. Participation and direct democracy at the local level—DIY politics as a cure for all democratic problems, in Delwit P, Pilet J-B, Regmaert H, Steyvers K. (eds), Towards DIY Politics. Brugge: Vanden Broele, 2007, pp 347–360.

4. UNECE. Convention on access to information, public participation in decision-making and access to justice in environmental matters, 1998. Available at http://live.unece.org/fileadmin/DAM/env/pp/documents/cep43e.pdf. Accessed 22 March 2012.

5. Whitehead M. The concepts and principles of equity in health. International Journal of Health Services 1992; 22: 429–45.

6. Townsend P, Davidson N. Inequalities in Health—The Black Report. Harmondsworth: Pelican Books, 1982.

7. Committee chaired by Acheson. Report of independent enquiry into inequalities in health. London: Department of Health, 1998. Available at http://www.archive.official- documents.co.uk/document/doh/ih/preface.htm. Accessed 22 March 2012.

8. WHO Commission on the Social Determinants of Health CSDH. Closing the gap in a generation: health equity through action on the social determinants of health. Final Report. Geneva: World Health Organization, 2008.

9. Joffre M. How do we make health impact assessment fit for purpose? Public Health 2003; 117: 301–304.

10. United Nations. Report of the World Commission on environment and development. General Assembly Resolution 42/187, 11 December, 1987. Available at http://www.un.org/documents/ga/res/42/ares42-187.htm. Accessed 22 March 2012.

11. Taylor L, Gowman N, Quigley R (Health Development Agency), Influencing the decision-making process through health impact assessment, 2003. Available at http://www.nice.org.uk/niceMedia/documents/decision_making_hia.pdf. Accessed 22 March 2012.

12. O'Keefe E, Scott-Samuel A. Human rights and wrongs: Could health impact assessment help? Journal of Law, Medicine & Ethics 2002; 30: 734–38.

13. Health Scotland. Scottish HIA network—How to HIA guides. Available at http://www.healthscotland.com/resources/networks/HIAguides.aspx. Accessed 22 March 2012.

14. Berger JO, Berry DA. Statistical analysis and the illusion of objectivity. American Scientist 1988; 76: 159–65.

15. Vandenbroucke JP. Subjectivity in data analysis. Lancet 1991; 337: 401–402.

16. Greenland S. Accounting for uncertainty about investigator bias: disclosure is informative. Journal of Eoidemiology and Community Health 2009; 63: 593–98.

17. Lasswell HD. Politics: Who gets what, when and how. New York: Whittlesey House, 1936.

18. Veerman JL, Bekker MPM, Mackenbach JP. Health impact assessment and advocacy: a challenging combination. Society for Preventive Medicine 2006; 51: 151–52.

19. Krieger G, Utzinger J, Winkler M, Divall MJ, Phillips SD, Balge MZ, Singer BH. Barbarians at the gate: Storming the Gothenburg consensus. Lancet 2010; 375: 2129–31.

20. Rawls J. A theory of justice (revised edition). Oxford: Oxford University Press, 1990.

21. Gostin M, Mann JM Towards the development of human rights impact assessment for the formulation and evaluation of public health policy. Health and Human Rights 1994; 1: 59–80.

22. Guide to Human Rights Impact Assessment. Available at http://www.guidetohriam. org/welcome. Accessed 22 March 2012.

23. United Nations General Comment 14. The right to the highest attainable standard of health, 2000. Available at http://www.unhchr.ch/tbs/doc.nsf/(Symbol)/40d009901358b 0e2c1256915005090be?Opendocument#1. Accessed 23 March 2012.

24. Scott-Samuel A, O'Keefe E. Health impact assessment, human rights and global public policy: a critical appraisal. Bulletin of World Health Organization 2007; 85: 212–17.

25. International Finance Corporation. Policy and Performance Standards on Social and Environmental Sustainability, 2012. Available at http://www1.ifc.org/wps/wcm/ connect/topics_ext_content/ifc_external_corporate_site/ifc+sustainability/ publications/publications_handbook_pps. Accessed 22 March 2012.

Chapter 7

Evaluation and quality assurance of health impact assessment

John Kemm

This chapter addresses two questions:

How can one demonstrate that HIA fulfils its claims of being useful to decision makers?

How can one assess whether or not an individual HIA has been competently performed?

Evaluation of the HIA and the evaluation of decisions

It is essential to distinguish the evaluation of the decision from the evaluation of the HIA that informed it (Figure 7.1). Evaluation of a decision asks how implementation of that decision or the intervention that it produced have affected the health of the population. Numerous books have been written on the evaluation of public health interventions and this book will not address this issue further. Evaluation of the HIA must look at whether the HIA informed the decision, whether the prediction of impacts was correct and whether the process of decision making, in particular the involvement of stakeholders, was improved.

Effectiveness

The immediate test of effectiveness of an HIA is whether it has influenced the decision or not. However, an HIA can also be effective even when it has not affected the decision. In reviewing the effectiveness of an HIA one must ask if it was considered by the decision makers and whether it changed the decision. Wismar[1] suggested a two-way table to analyse effectiveness and this is produced in a modified form in Table 7.1. (In Wismar's version 'Indirectly effective' is called 'Generally effective' and 'Happy accident' is called 'Opportunistically effective'.)

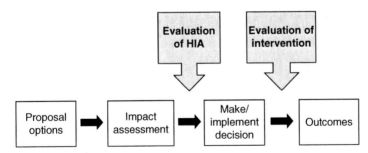

Fig. 7.1 Evaluation of HIA.

If the decision maker did not consider the HIA then it is difficult to see how the HIA could be said to be in any way effective (although it may have influenced people other than the decision maker). Even if for some other reason the decision is modified in an appropriate direction no credit for this can be given to the HIA unless the decision maker has considered the HIA. Sometimes an HIA is not considered because its report was never sent to the decision maker or sent too late or the decision maker was unaware that an HIA was being undertaken. No HIA for which any of these was true could claim to be effective. The assessors need to do everything in their power to improve the chances of the HIA being considered by the decision maker.

The HIA has been directly effective if after considering the HIA the decision maker modifies his or her decision as a result of that HIA or concludes that no modification is needed because the HIA supports the decision taken in all respects. However, if as often happens the decision maker, having considered the HIA and having reflected upon, it does not modify the decision, the HIA can still be considered effective because it will have left behind it an increased awareness and understanding of health issues. It may be that future decisions will be influenced by the consideration of the previous HIA. The ways in which HIA findings can influence a decision maker's thinking are further discussed in Chapter 8, page 83.

Table 7.1 The effectiveness of HIA

		Was the decision modified?	
		Yes	**No**
Was the HIA considered by the decision maker?	Yes	Directly effective	Indirectly effective
	No	Happy accident	Ineffective

Source: Data from Wismar M, Blau J, Ernst K. Is HIA effective? A synthesis of concepts, methodologies and results. Available at http://www.euro.who.int/__data/assets/pdf_file/0003/98283/E90794.pdf.

Effectiveness of HIA

The European Observatory of Health Systems and Policies[2] collected case studies of the effectiveness of 17 selected HIA in different countries. Three of these were not clearly linked to a specific decision and so their effectiveness in influencing a decision process cannot be assessed. In 13 of the remaining 14 there was evidence that the HIA had beneficially affected the decision or the decision-making process. In some cases recommendations from the HIA as to how the decision should be implemented were taken up, in others the HIA resulted in community views being taken into account in the decision-making process, and in others the awareness of health issues by decision makers was increased.

A study by the York Health Economics Consortium more ambitiously aimed to make a cost–benefit analysis of selected HIAs in England.[3] They studied 15 HIAs and although their methods of valuing benefits are open to question they concluded that in each case there were benefits whose value exceeded the cost of the HIA.

Evaluating HIA

Evaluation may focus on outcome or process. HIA claims to assist decision makers, to predict the future consequences of implementing different options to make recommendations for mitigation and enhancement of impacts, and, with participative HIA, to involve stakeholders in the decision-making process. An outcome evaluation would thus examine if decision makers were assisted, if predictions made were correct, how useful the recommendations were, and if stakeholders felt more involved in the decision. A process evaluation would examine the way in which the HIA was conducted to see if it was carried out in a way that was likely to produce these outcomes.[4]

Evaluating usefulness to decision makers

Outcome evaluation asking the question of whether the decision makers were assisted by the HIA would involve asking the decision makers whether the HIA helped to shape their decision making, and examination of documents and minutes of meetings to see if material from the HIA had been used in reaching the decision. Process evaluation of this area would examine the communication between the decision maker and the HIA. Were the decision makers engaged with the HIA and involved in its scoping? Was the decision maker's agenda acknowledged and addressed by the HIA? Were the findings of the HIA communicated in an appropriate and timely manner to the decision maker? An evaluation of the HIA of London draft mayoral strategies[5] concluded that the HIA had been effective in influencing strategy but it is a weakness of this study that its conclusions seem to be mostly based on interviews with assessors and stakeholders rather than with the policy makers. Elliott and Francis[6] noted the difficulty of unpicking influences on decision makers but concluded that decision makers had been influenced by the HIA.

Evaluating (validating) predictions

Outcome evaluation of predictions made in HIA involves their validation (i.e. showing that they occur in reality) and this is rarely possible. HIA requires predictions for each option considered and predictions relating to the options that were not implemented (counterfactuals) cannot be validated. Even for the predictions relating to the chosen option it is often impossible to determine if the forecast consequences were correct since the option may not be implemented exactly as assumed or other events may change the health outcomes. Furthermore, it may be necessary to wait years or decades before the predicted impacts can be observed.

One rare attempt to validate the predictions of an HIA was made by Petticrew,[7] who first of all invited his students to perform an HIA on the effects of opening a new supermarket and then attempted to assess how the nutrition of people in the neighbourhood had been affected. The HIA suggested that the nutrition of some residents would be worsened while a small survey after the opening of the supermarket suggested that nutrition had been improved. On this basis Petticrew questioned the ability of any HIA to predict. This conclusion was undoubtedly much weightier than the evidence could support. The methods used to assess nutrition after the opening of the supermarket were not robust and even if they had been they showed no more than that the predictions of that particular HIA were mistaken. Nonetheless efforts to validate predictions are rare and much more work of this type would be valuable.

Process validation of predictions is easier and involves examining the robustness of the methods used to make them. Were all relevant causal pathways identified? Were the relevant populations affected identified? Were reasons given for selecting which pathways to examine in detail? Were the right questions asked of technical experts? Was the literature search focused on the right topics and thoroughly done? How rigorously was the evidence applied to the particular context of the HIA?

Evaluating participation

Outcome evaluation of participation involves asking whether the various stakeholders felt that they were offered a proper opportunity to be involved in the HIA and whether they feel their views were adequately taken into account. This can be determined by interviewing the stakeholders to ascertain their views.

Process evaluation of participation is undertaken by examining the steps taken to obtain participation. How were the stakeholders identified? How were the stakeholders invited to participate? Were any stakeholders excluded? How were the stakeholders given the opportunity to participate? Did the timing and organization of participation make it difficult for stakeholders to participate? How was information given to them and was it given in a way that was easy for them to understand?

Case study and reflection

Apart from formal evaluation assessors can learn a great deal by reflecting on completed HIAs and identifying things which went well and contributed to success as well as things which went less well and might be done differently next time. Publication of these reflections either in the HIA report or in a separate document is extremely helpful for others trying to improve their HIA practice. Equally, case studies of HIA can be helpful in determining whether or not the HIA was effective and learning how future HIAs should be improved. The New Zealand HIA support unit has published a very useful selection of case studies.[8]

Quality assurance of HIA

Increasingly it is being realized that HIA needs a quality assurance process. Practice standards have been published for North America.[9] Birley,[10] discussing the quality of HIA, noted that 'many reports contain too much information about the tools used, too much unused factual material and too little analysis' and that too many presented evidence without inferring conclusions from it. Many HIAs are now using external peer review to assure their quality. This involves getting someone independent from the HIA team to review the reports and the way in which the HIA was conducted in order to identify any weaknesses and suggest ways in which the HIA might be improved. This procedure obviously introduces a further quality check to the work but it is very dependent on the skills and understanding of the peer reviewer.

One valuable method of quality assurance is to require that all HIA reports are put in the public domain, where they can be scrutinized by people of all opinions. Many reports are now published (see Box 1.1) on the web. One unfortunate aspect of the growth of commercial HIA is that the HIA report is owned by whoever paid for it and in many cases they are reluctant to make the report public.

Another approach to quality assurance is the use of checklists. These can be used by the assessors to ensure that they have done the task thoroughly or by the decision makers to assess the quality of an HIA presented to them.

Checklists for HIA

Checklists have been developed for assessing the quality of EIA reports,[11] and Ben Cave and colleagues have adapted this idea for evaluating HIA reports.[12] Their checklist is undoubtedly a very useful aid to quality assurance and identifies many items that should be covered in a satisfactory report. It is particularly suitable for HIA reports that are presented to planning committees.

A more generalized checklist is presented in Box 7.1.

Box 7.1 A checklist for HIA reports

Context

1. Are the options for the decision maker (including the do nothing options) clearly described and is the aim of the proposal clear? For an infrastructure proposal this would include description of the infrastructure and probably a map.

2. Are the relevant background policies and constraints described?

3. Is it clear who the HIA is intended to inform?

Baseline

4. Are relevant baselines of factors, including current use of land, socioeconomic situation, and health state that will be affected by the proposal, adequately described (including how they will evolve under the do nothing option)?

5. Are baselines for relevant subgroups (especially vulnerable groups) described?

Appraisal

6. Are the causal pathways identified and if only some are investigated is it explained why those pathways have been selected?

7. How have changes in intermediate factors been assessed? Has relevant expertise been used in assessing these?

8. How have causal links been researched?

9. Where links are not researched has this been justified?

10. Where researched by literature search has this been adequately done and are the sources clearly referenced?

Box 7.1 A checklist for HIA reports *(continued)*

11. Have appropriate key informants been identified and have they been asked the right questions?

12. If standards (e.g. air quality, noise) have been used are these appropriate and properly sourced?

13. Are impacts for the construction, operational, and decommissioning phases discussed where relevant?

Participation

14. Have the relevant stakeholders been identified?

15. Has the HIA explained how and why those who participated were selected and why those who did not participate were not selected?

16. Could those who participated be deemed to be representative?

17. What process was used to involve stakeholders and how have their views influenced the HIA conclusions?

Impacts

18. Is the nature and direction of impacts described?

19. Is the magnitude of impacts described (probability of impact, number affected)?

20. Does the HIA describe who is impacted? Are differential impacts described?

21. Does the HIA discuss uncertainty?

Recommendations

22. Does the HIA make recommendations for all options?

23. Are recommendations for mitigation of negative impacts and enhancement of positive impacts reasonable and justified?

24. Are suggestions made for monitoring after implementation?

Communication

25. Was the person/committee it was intended to inform notified that the HIA was being done? Were they given opportunity to be involved?

26. Has the HIA report been sent to this person/committee? Was it sent at an appropriate time and in an appropriate form?

27. Was there an executive summary?

28. Have other stakeholders been communicated with about the conclusions of the HIA in an appropriate fashion?

Box 7.1 A checklist for HIA reports *(continued)*

Quality assurance

29. Has the HIA report been quality assured by peer review or in some other way?

Scoring the checklist

A simple way of scoring this checklist is to rate each item as:

A. Well done

B. Barely adequate

C. Not done/badly done

D. Not relevant

One might suggest that the HIA should be rejected if more than three items are scored C or more than a third of relevant items are scored B or C.

Of course much more elaborate scoring systems are possible. More scale points could be included in the scoring and different weights could be allocated to different items.

The scoring should be related to the size and nature of the report. If it is only 25 pages long then no more than a short paragraph can be allocated to each item. If, on the other hand, it is a 200-page report one would expect all items to be discussed at length.

Source: Data from Fredsgaard MW, Cave B, Bond A. A review package for Health Impact Assessment of development projects Leeds, Ben Cave Associates 2009. Available at http://www.bcahealth.co.uk/pdf/hia_review_package.pdf. Accessed 22/3/12.

References

1. Wismar M, Blau J, Ernst K. Is HIA effective? A synthesis of concepts, methodologies and results, in Wismar M, Blau J, Ernst K, Figueras J. (eds), The effectiveness of health impact assessment: Scope and limitations of supporting decision making in Europe. Brussels: European Observatory on Health Systems and Policies, 2007.

2. Wismar M, Blau J, Ernst K, Figueras J. (eds). The effectiveness of health impact assessment: Scope and limitations of supporting decision making in Europe. Brussels: European Observatory on Health Systems and Policies, 2007.

3. York Health Economic Consortium. Cost Benefit Analysis of Health Impact Assessment: Final Report. Department of Health, 2006. Available at http://www.apho.org.uk/resource/item.aspx?RID=44796. Accessed 22 March 2012.

4. Parry JM, Kemm JR. Criteria for use in the evaluation of health impact assessments. Public Health 2005; 111: 1122–29.

5. London Health Commission. Evaluation of the health impact assessment on the draft mayoral strategies for London. London: London Health Commission, 2003. Available at http://www.londonshealth.gov.uk/pdf/hiaeval_sum.pdf. Accessed 22 March 2012.

6. Elliott E, Francis S. Making effective links to decision making: Key challenges for health impact assessment. Environmental Impact Assessment Review 2005; 25: 747–57.

7. Petticrew M, Cummins S, Sparks L, Findlay A. Validating health impact assessment: Prediction is difficult (especially about the future). Environment Impact Assessment Review 2007; 27: 101–107.

8. New Zealand Ministry of Health. Health Impact Assessment in New Zealand—HIA Case studies and case study guide. Available at http://www.health.govt.nz/our-work/health-impact-assessment/evaluation-health-impact-assessment/hia-case-studies-and-guide. Accessed 22 March 2012.

9. North American HIA Practice Standards Working Group. Minimum Elements and Practice Standards for HIA, Version 2. Oakland, CA: North American HIA Practice Standards Working Group, 2010. Available at http://www.humanimpact.org/doc-lib/finish/11/9. Accessed 22 March 2012.

10. Birley M. Health impact assessment, integration and critical appraisal. Impact Assessment and Project Appraisal 2003; 21: 313–21.

11. Glasson J, Therivel R, Chadwick A. Introduction to Environmental Impact Assessment, 3rd edn. London: Rourledge, 2005.

12. Fredsgaard MW, Cave B, Bond A. A review package for health impact assessment of development projects. Leeds: Ben Cave Associates, 2009. Available at http://www.bcahealth.co.uk/pdf/hia_review_package.pdf. Accessed 22 March 2012.

Chapter 8

Health impact assessment of policy

John Kemm

Health impact assessment claims to be applicable to projects, programmes, and policies yet most of the early applications were to projects. Policy is the process by which governments seek to achieve their goals and translate their political vision into programmes and actions to deliver 'outcomes'—desired changes in the real world.[1] Policy may be clearly enunciated and laid out in legislation or official documents, or it may consist merely of inherent leanings and attitudes. It may result in programmes or it may be manifested by inaction.

Policy is made at all levels: supranational, national, regional, municipal, local, and organizational. While HIA of local policy may not be very different from HIA of local projects, as one moves up the scale one encounters different problems, and what is possible and appropriate changes. This chapter is primarily concerned with HIA of national policy and dealing with national government. The distinction between HIA of policy and project is not always clear and large-scale projects (such as the construction of airports, major transport systems, or generating plant) have influence and consequences far beyond their immediate content, and may shape and constrain decisions in many policy areas.

Early impact assessments such as that of US policy on Cuba in the 1980s[2] or the European Common Agricultural Policy[3] were probably intended as critiques addressed to academic audiences rather than to influence policy makers. More recently, as thought has been given to how HIA can be applied to policy[4] it has become clear that this poses rather different problems to HIA applied to projects and programmes, and needs different solutions.

Health in all policies

From its earliest days the World Health Organization has urged the importance of policies that support health. The Alma Ata conference of 1978 urged that governments should 'have responsibility for the health of their people which can be fulfilled only by the provision of adequate health and social measures' and this was reiterated in WHO's global strategy Health For All by the year 2000.[5] In 1986 the Ottawa charter on health promotion called for 'health supporting policies'.[6] The European Region of WHO further developed the strategy in its European targets for Health for All by the Year 2000 (HFA2000).[7] As the year 2000 approached WHO continued the same policy with 10 global health targets[8] while WHO European region interpreted these for Europe with 21 targets for 2020.[9] Most recently the aim of improving health through policy has been framed as Health in All Policies (HiAP), introduced during the Finnish EU presidency and continued as a theme in the Portuguese EU presidency.

The HiAP approach is based on a recognition that population health is largely determined by living conditions and other social and economic factors, and is therefore often best influenced by policies and actions beyond the health sector.[10,11] Further investment in health is good for economic development.[12,13] HiAP is a logical corollary of article 7 of the EU Lisbon treaty,[14] which calls for consistency (joined-up policy making) between policies and activities. Policy consistency has much in common with the notion of the triple bottom line[15] used in the context of corporate social responsibility and sustainability, meaning that costs and benefits have to be considered not only in economic terms but also in terms of environmental capital and human capital (health).

The idea of HiAP only makes sense if it is possible to forecast how a policy will affect health and other matters. HIA or a similar process is thus an essential preliminary for HiAP.

Evidence and policy

Policy making may be considered to follow a series of steps:

- Identify the problem
- Identify the options
- Assess each option
- Choose policy

It is advised that the process of identifying and assessing options should be guided by use of evidence and consultation.[1,16] Translation of knowledge from research to policy is difficult[17,18] and policy solutions can rarely be simply plucked from the research literature. Instead, research if it informs policy does so by an 'enlightenment' process in which ideas from the research community filter through to influence the way policy problems are framed. Policy makers and researchers learn from each other.[19,20] HIA can be thought of as a tool for translating research knowledge into a form that is useful for policy makers interrogating the research base in order to predict the consequences of different policy choices.

Policy makers' expectations of HIA

If HIA is to support policy making then those carrying out the HIA must understand the policy-making process and produce an HIA that is relevant to the policy maker's needs.[21] The HIA has to be produced in time to match the 'windows of opportunity' into which policy making often has to fit. The evidence underpinning the HIA may come from several different disciplines but it must be presented in a way that convinces the policy maker and 'tells a good story'. It has to consider those impacts that are of most concern to the policy maker, although the HIA may well go beyond the immediate concerns of the policy maker. HIA of policy works best when it is done in close collaboration with the policy maker. Often policy makers find impacts more impressive if they can be quantified.[22]

The HIA must admit the uncertainty that is attached to predictions but the uncertainty message should not drown the best judgement message. Confidence intervals and similar measures of uncertainty may not be helpful for policy makers. In the end an HIA report is always based on incomplete evidence and best judgement, and it is unhelpful to pretend that the predictions are certain.

Confidentiality and policy making

Although in published documents governments stress their desire to involve others in policy development, most still wish to control how much of the policy-making process is shared with those they govern. The guidance given to UK civil servants is 'Advice to ministers is confidential. Civil servants advise, ministers decide' and when minsters have decided they expect civil servants to support their decision.[23] Accordingly, governments will only wish to make public the advice they have received after they have made their decision and only if it supports that decision. One also has to question whether policy making by government would be possible if all discussions took place in the open. This is difficult to reconcile with the value of openness often considered an HIA value (Chapter 6, page 67).

Participation and policy consultation

Consultation is usually considered an essential part of good policy making and it is likely that before selecting a policy option government will have carried out some form of consultation. In policy consultation the process is usually moderately controlled, with the questions framed by the policy makers so as to constrain the possible responses. Participation as advised in HIA is rather different from consultation in policy making. Consultation is fairly low on the ladder of citizen participation (Chapter 4, page 39) but it is unusual for policy makers to be willing to pass responsibility for consultation from themselves to an HIA assessor. One has to ask if HIA-style participation with stakeholders would be possible for national policy since every citizen could be considered to be a stakeholder. It is probably not appropriate to have both consultation organized by the policy maker and participation organized for the HIA. The best solution is to use the consultation process to inform both the policy maker and the HIA.

HIA of policy in England

British governments have repeatedly expressed their intention to apply HIA in England to their own policy making and have urged local government to do likewise. HIA is supposed to take place as part of the process in which an impact assessment has to be submitted to the Better Regulation Executive in the Department for Business Innovation and Skills for all new policies and regulations.[24] Impact assessments have to be published at four stages in policy making: after consultation, when the final proposal is made, after the legislation implementing the proposal has been passed (if it has been changed from the final proposal), and three to five years after implementation (post-implementation review) (Figure 8.1). At each stage the minister responsible for the proposal has to certify that the impact assessment gives a fair and reasonable view of the costs, benefits, and impacts of the policy and the assessment has to be submitted to a subcommittee of the Better Regulation Executive.

This impact assessment is primarily concerned with regulatory burdens and financial costs, but the guidance mentions a series of 22 specific impact tests, among them social well-being and health inequalities, safety at work and risk of accidents, human rights, statutory equality duties, greenhouse gases, and air and water quality.[25] The most recent response template does not prompt for any of these specific impact tests but a template used earlier was slightly better in that it required a statement (Yes/No) as to whether specific impact tests (including health and well-being) had been applied. For those who choose to include mention of health in their assessment the Department of Health has published guidance[26] and tools.[27] The Department of Health suggests that there should be a full HIA if the answer to two or more of their three screening questions (Box 8.1) is positive.

Although it is possible to include health and well-being impact assessment in the integrated impact assessment there is little encouragement to do so.

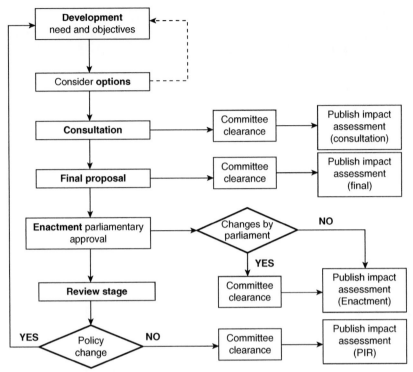

Fig. 8.1 Policy impact assessment flowchart used in England.

Box 8.1 Department of Health screening questions for HIA PIR, post-implementation review

1. Will your policy have a significant impact on human health by virtue of its effects on the following wider determinants of health?

Income

Crime

Environment

Transport

Housing

Education

Employment

Agriculture

Social cohesion

Box 8.1 Department of Health screening questions for HIA PIR, post-implementation review *(continued)*

Consider the potential to have a health impact.

2. Will there be a significant impact on any of the following lifestyle-related variables?

Physical activity

Diet

Smoking, drugs, or alcohol use

Sexual behaviour

Accidents and stress at home or work

Consider risk factors that influence the probability of an individual becoming more or less healthy.

3. Is there likely to be a significant demand on any of the following health and social care services?

Primary care

Community services

Hospital care

Need for medicines

Accident or emergency attendances

Social services

Health protection and preparedness response

Consider the likely contacts with health and social service provision.

If the answer to two or more of these questions is YES then you will need to carry out a full health impact assessment.

Reproduced from the Department of Health Screening questions for HIA. Last modified 10 November 2010. © Crown copyright 2011. Available from http://www.dh.gov.uk/en/Publicationsandstatistics/Legislation/Healthassessment/DH_4093617.

Even under the previous system when inclusion of health was theoretically mandatory an examination of impact assessments published showed that in most cases the impact assessment simply declared that there were no health impacts.[28] Under the present form of integrated impact assessment it is unusual to find that health impacts have been considered at all.

HIA in European Union

A similar process to that used in England is used in the European Union (EU) and has now become mandatory. An impact assessment unit has been established within each directorate general. In 2002 guidance was issued on integrated impact assessment.[29] Later a separate guide on HIA was issued[30] and HIAs of the European Employment Strategy were undertaken to pilot the use of HIA. Later the guidance on integrated impact assessment was reissued.[31] Health (impacts on 'health' and 'safety') is mentioned in a long paragraph headed 'Social impacts'. There are concerns that as currently practiced by the EU integrated impact assessment does not give sufficient weight to health and a survey of 137 assessments carried out in 2005/2006 found that less than half even mentioned health.[32] The current practice of impact assessment has been further criticized as giving too much weight to economic considerations and too much influence to commercial and business interests.[33] The lesson to be drawn from experience in the EU is that at the moment, as in England, health is not being adequately considered in integrated impact assessment.

Conclusion

There is reason to think that soon HIA will be able to fulfil its promise of being a valuable aid for policy makers, but if this promise is to be realized health will need to be higher on policy makers' agendas and health impact assessors will have to develop a greater understanding of policy making and government. Often health impacts are supposedly considered as part of an integrated impact assessment, but at the moment this is too often a recipe for ignoring health. However, if consideration of health was done conscientiously integrated impact assessment could be an efficient way of covering health issues in policy.

References

1. UK Cabinet Office. Modernising Government. London: The Stationery Office, 1999. Available at http://www.archive.official-documents.co.uk/document/cm43/4310/4310.htm. Accessed 22 March 2012.
2. Garfield R, Santana S. The impact of the economic crisis and US embargo on health in Cuba. American Journal of Public Health 1997; 87: 15–20.
3. Dahlgren G, Nordgren P, Whitehead M. Health impact assessment of the EU Common Agricultural Policy. Stockholm: Swedish National Institute of Public Health, 1996.
4. Lee K, Ingram A, Lock K, McInnes C. Bridging health and foreign policy: the role of health impact assessments. Bulletin of the World Health Organization 2007; 85: 207–11.
5. World Health Organization. Global health strategy for all by the year 2000. Geneva: World Health Organization, 1981.

6. World Health Organization. Ottawa Charter for Health Promotion. Health Promotion 1986; 1 (4): iii–v.

7. World Health Organization. Targets for health for all. Targets in support of the European regional strategy for health for all. Copenhagen: WHO Regional Office for Europe, 1985.

8. World Health Organization. Health for all in the 21st century, Document WHA 51/5. Geneva: World Health Organization, 1998.

9. World Health Organization. European region European Health for All Series No 6. Health21: The health for all framework for the WHO European region. Copenhagen: World Health Organization, 1999. Available at http://www.euro.who.int/__data/assets/pdf_file/0010/98398/wa540ga199heeng.pdf. Accessed 22 March 2012.

10. Sihto M, Olila E, Koivusalo M. Principles and challenges of Health in All Policies, in Stahl T, Wismar M, Ollila E, Lahtinen E, Leppo K (eds), Health in all polices: Prospects and potentials. Helsinki: Ministry of Social Affairs and Health, 2006.

11. Joffe M, Mindell J. A tentative step towards healthy public policy. Journal of Epidemiology and Community Health 2004; 58: 966–68.

12. Commission on macroeconomic and health chaired by Sachs J. Macroeconomics and health: Investing in health for economic development. Geneva: Commission on Macroeconomics, 2001. Available at http://whqlibdoc.who.int/publications/2001/924154550x.pdf. Accessed 22 March 2012.

13. Suhrcke M, McKee M, Arce RS, Tsolova S, Mortensen J. The contribution of health to the economy in the European Union. Brussels: European Commission, 2005. Available at http://ec.europa.eu/health/ph_overview/Documents/health_economy_en.pdf. Accessed 22 March 2012.

14. Consolidated version of the treaty on the functioning of the European Union, Article 7. Available at http://eur-lex.europa.eu/LexUriServ/LexUriServ.do?uri=OJ:C:2008:115:0047:0199:EN:PDF. Accessed 22 March 2012.

15. Elkington J. Cannibals with forks: triple bottom line of 21st century business. Oxford: Capstone Publishing, 1997.

16. Hallsworth M, Rutter J. Making Policy Better: Improving Whitehall's core business. London: Institute for Government, 2011. Available at http://www.instituteforgovernment.org.uk/publications/making-policy-better. Accessed 22 March 2012.

17. Kemm J. The limitations of evidence based public health. Journal of Evaluation in Clinical Practice 2006; 12: 319–24.

18. Brownson RC, Royer C, Ewing R, McBride TD. Researchers and Policymakers: Travellers in parallel universes. American Journal of Preventive Medicine 2006; 30: 164–72.

19. Davis P, Howden-Chapman P. Translating research findings into health policy. Social Sciences and Medicine 1996; 43: 865–72.

20. Innvaer S, Vist G, Trommald M, Oxman A. Health policy makers perceptions of their use of evidence: a systematic review. Journal of Health Services Research and Policy 2002; 7: 239–44.

21. Petticrew M, Whitehead M, MacIntyre S, Graham H, Egan M. Evidence for public policy on inequalities: 1: The reality according to policymakers. Journal of Epidemiology and Community Health 2004; 58: 811–16.

22. Mindell J, Hansell A, Morrison D, Douglas M, Joffe M. What do we need for robust quantitative health impact assessment? Journal of Public Health Medicine 2001; 23: 173–78.

23. Stanley M. Integrity, honest, impartiality and objectivity, in How to be a civil servant (undated). Available at http://www.civilservant.org.uk/c21.pdf. Accessed 22 March 2012.

24. Department for Business Innovation and Skills. Impact Assessment Guidance: When to do an impact assessment. London: BIS 2011. Available at http://www.bis.gov.uk/ia-guidance. Accessed 22 March 2012.

25. Department of Business Innovation and Skills. IA Toolkit—How to do an impact assessment. London: BIS 2011. Available at http://www.bis.gov.uk/assets/biscore/better-regulation/docs/i/11-1112-impact-assessment-toolkit.pdf. Accessed 22 March 2012.

26. Department of Health. Health Impact Assessment of Government Policy: A guide to carrying out a health impact assessment of new policy as part of the impact assessment process. London: Department of Health, 2010. Available at http://www.dh.gov.uk/prod_consum_dh/groups/dh_digitalassets/documents/digitalasset/dh_120110.pdf. Accessed 22 March 2012.

27. Department of Health. Health Impact Assessment Tools: Simple tools for recording the result of Health Impact Assessment. London: Department of Health, 2010. Available at http://www.dh.gov.uk/prod_consum_dh/groups/dh_digitalassets/documents/digitalasset/dh_120106.pdf. Accessed 22 March 2012.

28. Department of Health/Institute of Occupational Medicine. Putting health in the policy picture: review of how health impact assessment is carried out by government departments. London: Department of Health, 2010. Available at http://www.dh.gov.uk/prod_consum_dh/groups/dh_digitalassets/@dh/@en/@ps/documents/digitalasset/dh_113193.pdf. Accessed 22 March 2012.

29. Commission of the European Community. Communication from the Commission on impact assessment COM 2002/276. Available at http://eur-lex.europa.eu/LexUriServ/LexUriServ.do?uri=COM:2002:0276:FIN:EN:PDF. Accessed 22 March 2012.

30. Abrahams D, Pennington A, Scott-Samuel A, Doyle C, Metcalfe O, den Broeder L, Haigh F, Mekel O, Fehr R. European policy health impact assessment: A guide. Brussels: Health and Consumer Protection Directorate General of the European Commission, 2004. Available at http://www.liv.ac.uk/ihia/IMPACT%20Reports/EPHIA_A_Guide.pdf. Accessed 22 March 2012.

31. European Commission. Impact Assessment Guidelines 2009. Available at http://ec.europa.eu/governance/impact/commission_guidelines/docs/iag_2009_en.pdf. Accessed 22 March 2012.

32. Salay R, Lincoln P. Health impact assessment in the European Union. Lancet 2008; 372: 860–61.

33. Smith KE, Fooks G, Collin J, Weishaar H, Gilmore AB. Is the increasing policy use of impact assessment in Europe likely to undermine efforts to achieve health public policy? Journal of Epidemiology and Community Health 2010; 64: 478–87.

Chapter 9

Health in other impact assessments

John Kemm

HIA is only one of wide family of impact assessments. Projects and policies may be assessed for:

+ environmental impact (EIA), including impact on climate change
+ sustainability appraisal
+ social impact
+ economic impact, including impact on business
+ human rights impact
+ gender impact
+ law and order impact
+ equality impact
+ rural proofing
+ impact on specific groups.

To undertake all these impact assessments separately would be a considerable burden and most of them have areas in common. There is therefore a strong case for looking to see if assessments can be integrated.

Environmental impact assessment

The USA was one of the first countries to require EIA under the terms of the National Environmental Policy Act,[1] which stated:

'The purposes of this act are: To declare a national policy which will encourage productive and enjoyable harmony between man and his environment: to promote efforts which will prevent or eliminate damage to the environment and the biosphere *and stimulate health and welfare of man*; to enrich the understanding of the ecological systems and natural resources important to the Nation.' (italics added)

The English guidance on EIA[2] says that the environmental statement that is the end product of an EIA should consider 'effects on human beings, buildings and man-made features including:

- change in population arising from the development and consequential environment effects
- visual effects of the development on the surrounding area and landscape
- levels and effects of emissions from the development during normal operation
- level and effects of noise from the development
- effect of the development on local roads and transport
- effects of the development on buildings, the architectural and historic heritage, archaeological features and other human artefacts.'

Most of the countries discussed in part 2 of this book have also gone someway to specify that health should be covered in EIA. Unfortunately, experience in England, the USA and many other countries shows that despite a stated requirement for health in EIA, coverage of health is usually inadequate or absent. In many ways the demand for HIA could be seen as a response to this failure of EIA to cover health properly.

There are two logical responses to poor coverage of health in EIA:

- reform EIA practice so it adequately covers health
- develop HIA to complement EIA.

Most of the paths considered in EIA would also figure in a causal diagram for HIA (for example pollution, noise, traffic, amenity). Where an EIA has been done there is no sense in duplicating assessment of these intermediate variables—it is merely a question of further considering how changes in these factors will impact on human health and well-being. In addition to the paths usually considered in EIA an HIA would also consider impacts consequent on changes in employment, income, and community cohesion.

With large projects it is becoming increasingly common to commission both an EIA and an HIA, and to require that the findings of the EIA are used to inform the HIA. Where there is no EIA it is sensible to consider any substantial impact on flora or fauna in the HIA. The biophilia hypothesis[3,4] reminds us that the health and well-being of humans is linked to that of other living systems. In summary, health impacts and environmental impacts should always be considered together, although whether this is best done in a single impact assessment or in two separate but closely coordinated impact assessments depends on the circumstances.

Strategic environmental assessment

Strategic environmental assessment (SEA) originated from concern that EIA did not adequately cover all situations where consideration of the environment was needed. It was first formulated in the SEA protocol to the Espoo convention on EIA in transboundary contexts. Several countries have introduced legislation on SEA and the directive on Strategic Environmental Assessment 2001/42/EC required all countries of the EU to implement SEA through their own national legislation. While SEA was being introduced people interested in public health saw this as a golden opportunity to improve coverage of health issues and lobbied for this to be included in the new SEA legislation. The EU directive was translated into UK law (different for each country of the UK) in 2005.[5]

The SEA directive requires assessment of the plan or programme's 'likely significant effects on the environment, including on issues such as biodiversity, population, human health, fauna, flora, soil, water, air, climatic factors, material assets, cultural heritage and landscape, and the interrelationship between them.' (Annex 1 f).

The UK government was determined that in England there should be no 'gold plating' of the European directive (i.e. inclusion of additional requirements) and although the Department of Health issued a consultation document 'Draft guidance on health in SEA'[6] there has been pressure to limit the coverage of health in SEA. The situation in Scotland is similar.

There are five stages required in an SEA, all of which might be expected to involve health:

◆ Stage A Setting the context

◆ Stage B Alternatives and assessment

◆ Stage C Prepare the environmental report

◆ Stage D Consult and make decision

◆ Stage E Monitor implementation

At various stages there has to be consultation with statutory consultation bodies. In England these are currently Natural England, English Heritage, and the Environment Agency. At the moment the consultation body which deals with health is the Environment Agency and government has not approved proposals to change this. In Scotland, Wales, and Northern Ireland the consultation bodies are the corresponding agencies. There is encouragement to consult other bodies, including health authorities, but no statutory requirement to do so.

Stage A Setting the context: This includes collecting baseline data, which should include data on the health of the population, identifying environmental problems, which should include health problems, and developing objectives, which should include health objectives. The objectives developed in this stage could include a physical environment that supports health, promotion of healthy living choices, reduced risk of injury, reduced crime and fear of crime, decreasing noise, better air quality, fewer people in poverty, fewer people living in bad housing, and reduced unemployment.

Stage B Alternatives and assessment: These should include testing the plan against SEA objectives, evaluating the effect of the plan and alternatives, proposals for mitigation of adverse effects and monitoring measures, all of which should involve health elements.

Stages C, D, and E: These should cover the health issues identified in the earlier stages.

SEA could be a vehicle for institutionalizing consideration of health[7] but despite the numerous opportunities to ensure that health is adequately covered in SEA the reality is usually disappointing. A typical SEA report might contain one or two hundred pages, of which two or three might deal with health. Fisher and colleagues[8] found with difficulty some SEAs that 'did more than simply mention health' but of these most dealt only with biophysical aspects and ignored socioeconomic aspects.

Authorities needing to produce an SEA may commission a commercial firm to do this after competitive tender or decide to use their own staff. Pressures to keep down costs of SEA are an important reason for inadequate coverage of health. The commissioners of SEA do not require proper coverage in their brief and providers of SEA do not offer adequate coverage of health in their tender. Firms bidding for SEA work want to keep their costs as low as possible so that they can win the contract to do the SEA so they are unlikely to include any work that is not mentioned in the brief. Furthermore, coverage of health is deemed to be expensive since most firms have little experience in this area and consider that more senior (more expensive) staff are needed to cover health in the SEA.

Social impact assessment

Social impact assessment (SIA) is defined as 'analysing monitoring and managing the social consequences of development'.[9] The term 'social impact' is defined as encompassing health and well-being, way of life, community and environment. Reading a description of the principles of SIA[10] one is struck that if the word 'health' were substituted throughout for the word 'social' it could not be faulted as a description of HIA. One has to conclude that the objectives of and methods of HIA and SIA are very similar and the chief difference is the discipline of those carrying out the assessment. However, it is undoubtedly true that many HIAs would benefit from the skills and insights of a sociologist into social interaction.

Integrated impact assessment

Integrated impact assessment is used when two or more different forms of impact assessment are covered together. For example, the combination of SEA and sustainability appraisal is commonly described as an integrated impact assessment. In this chapter we will restrict the term to impact assessments that combine HIA with one or more other types of impact assessment. The experience of combining impact assessment by the UK government in England and the EU was described in Chapter 8. While integrated impact assessment offers a framework that could be used to ensure that health is properly considered in policy making and legislation, the way it has been implemented in most cases has not achieved this. The environmental, social, and health impact assessment (ESHIA) usually demanded by the World Finance Corporation for projects that it funds is an example of an integrated assessment. Birley[11] has discussed the difficulties of budgeting and project managing these ESHIAs.

Northern Ireland (Chapter 14) have developed an integrated impact assessment tool intended to be used with most policies to help departments and other public sector bodies take forward in one exercise a range of policy proofing processes, including equality impact assessment, rural proofing, HIA, and EIA.[12] The use of integrated impact assessment in Scotland is discussed in Chapter 13.

Several local authorities have developed integrated assessment tools. Often equality impact assessment is prominent within these integrated assessments since the Equality Act 2009 lays a clear statutory duty on local authorities to consider equality aspects in their decisions and they are open to legal challenge if they fail to do so.

Objections to integrated impact assessment

Some feel that including assessment of health impacts as part of other impact assessments is not the best course. The chief objection is that those who are not focused on health cannot be trusted to cover health issues adequately. It has to be admitted that much experience with EIA and SEA suggests that these fears are not without foundation. As Kirkpatrick and Lee[13] noted, the separate forms of impact assessment (including HIA) developed because the impacts with which they were concerned were not being adequately considered in existing impact assessment arrangements. It has to be asked if consideration of health is now sufficiently mature and well established that it can be integrated without the old deficiencies re-emerging. It must also be noted that many of those concerned about specific impacts other than health have the same concern about inclusion of their topic in an integrated assessment.

Those who argue against integrated impact assessment usually imply that a separate HIA is an alternative to an integrated assessment. However, in many busy organizations the reality is that the choice is between inclusion of health in an integrated impact assessment or no consideration of health at all. If an official is going to spend no more that 30 minutes thinking about health then one has to think how to make the best use of that 30 minutes rather than urging the official to devote three days to the topic.

The case for integrated impact assessment

HIA integrated within an EIA process has been described as 'an ideal platform to assess the potential health impacts of development actions', especially in low- and middle-income countries.[14] It encourages people to look at impacts of developments and policies as a whole rather than think in their professional silos. It avoids the need for staff to answer the same questions in several separate impact assessments and reduces the risk of 'impact assessment fatigue'. It ensures that consistent assumptions and methods are used for all types of assessment. It allows health staff to make alliances with those interested in other types of impact rather than competing with them for priority. Finally, it allows the decisions which do not raise major health issues to be rapidly dealt with while the few where health impacts are a major issue can be identified. Effort can then be concentrated on assessing the health impacts of these decisions (and perhaps undertaking a separate HIA). The case for integrated impact assessment is further argued in Chapter 13 (page 133). Although many examples of integrated impact assessment in the past have not given adequate consideration to health there is still a strong case for developing an integrated assessment that deals properly with health, rather than always demanding a separate HIA.

References

1. Executive office of the President of the United States National Environmental Policy Act. The NEPA Statute 1970. Available at http://ceq.hss.doe.gov/laws_and_executive_orders/the_nepa_statute.html. Accessed 22 March 2012.
2. Department of Communities and Local Government. Environmental Impact Assessment: Guide to procedures. London: Department of Communities and Local Government, 2000. Available at http://www.communities.gov.uk/documents/planningandbuilding/pdf/157989.pdf. Accessed 22 March 2012.
3. Grinde B, Patil GG. Biophilia: does visual contact with nature impact on health and well-being? International Journal of Environmental Research and Public Health 2009; 6: 2332–43.
4. Leger LS. Health and nature—new challenges for health promotion. Health Promotion International 2003; 18: 173–75.

5. Office of the Deputy Prime Minister. A practical guide to the Strategic Environmental Assessment. London: ODPM Publications, 2004. Available at http://www. communities.gov.uk/documents/planningandbuilding/pdf/practicalguidesea.pdf. Accessed 22 March 2012.

6. Department of Health. Draft guidance on the coverage of health in strategic environmental assessment. London: Department of Health, 2007. Available at http://www.dh.gov.uk/prod_consum_dh/groups/dh_digitalassets/documents/ digitalasset/dh_073262.pdf. Accessed 22 March 2012.

7. Wright J, Parry J, Scully E. Institutionalising policy level health impact assessment in Europe: Is coupling health impact assessment with strategic environmental assessment the next step forward? Bulletin of the World Health Organization 2005; 83: 472–77.

8. Fischer TB, Martuzzi M, Nowacki J. The consideration of health in strategic environmental assessment (SEA). Environmental Impact Assessment Review 2009; 30: 200–210.

9. Vanclay F. International principles for social impact assessment. Impact Assessment and Project Appraisal 2003; 21: 5–11.

10. Vanclay F. International principles for social impact assessment. Impact Assessment and Project Appraisal 2003; 21: 5–11.

11. Birley M. Health impact assessment: Principles and practice. London: Earthscan, 2011.

12. Northern Ireland Policy Innovation Unit. Effective Policy Making—A Practical Guide to Impact Assessment (undated). Available at http://www.ofmdfmni.gov.uk/ workbook4plusannexes.pdf. Accessed 22 March 2012.

13. Kirkpatrick C, Lee N. Special Issue: Integrated appraisal and decision making. Environmental Impact Assessment Review 1997; 19: 227–32.

14. Ahmad BS. Integrating health into impact assessment: challenges and opportunities. Impact Assessment and Project Appraisal 2004; 22: 2–4.

Chapter 10

Application of health impact assessment to various topics

John Kemm

This chapter considers some of the topics to which HIA has been applied. Each topic would merit a book in its own right, but in this chapter it is only possible to identify a few key points.

Spatial planning

In developed countries development is only allowed if planning permission is received. Planning authorities are usually departments of local government. They attempt to ensure that all new developments (residential, retail, commercial, industrial, leisure, and transport links) contribute to the physical, mental, and cultural well-being of the community. Their work impacts on health in many ways. Many planners are well aware of this[1] and are starting to use HIA as a tool to help them.

Transport

There are many HIAs of transport projects such as roads, bridges, and railway lines. The main negative impacts that are most often associated with these projects are vehicle emissions, noise, road traffic injuries, and community severance. The positive impacts are ease of travel and economic benefit.

The main emissions from cars are nitrogen oxides (NOx), particulates, carbon monoxide, and volatile organic compounds (VOC). The amount of emissions depends on the type of engine, the maintenance of the vehicle, including the exhaust system, and the speed at which it is driven. Diesel engines emit more particulates and less NOx than petrol engines. The air quality around the road depends on what is being emitted, the buildings and topography around the road, and the weather. Winds will disperse pollutants while tall buildings (urban canyons) will hold pollutants and slow dispersion. When lead was added to fuels as an anti-knock agent lead levels around roads could be high. A European study suggested that traffic-related pollution might be responsible for as much as 6% of total mortality.[2]

Vehicles travelling on roads also produce noise and vibration, which may damage structures. Once again the disturbance depends on the type of vehicle and the characteristics of the road and its surroundings. Road traffic injuries are another important impact. The likelihood of injuries depends on the speed and number of vehicles and their state as well as the volume of pedestrian and cycle traffic and the effectiveness of measures to separate pedestrian and vehicular traffic. Figures have been published for the frequency of vehicular and pedestrian injuries in UK on different types of road broken down by time, year, weather conditions, and other factors.[3]

Community severance refers to the problem of roads dividing communities and preventing journeys across them. It also refers to loss of road space for community use. In quiet residential streets a lot of communication between neighbours takes place in the street and this is lost if the streets become heavily trafficked. New roads may also cause loss of amenity. The effect of a new road on active travel (walking and cycling), which is generally good for health, has to be considered and if a new road discourages active travel that is a negative impact.

In order to predict the impact of a new road one has to predict the changes in traffic flows. Usually some of the traffic comes from pre-existing roads, thus reducing the negative impacts of traffic in those places. The net impact of a bypass could be positive if it reduces the negative impacts of traffic in a congested town centre or other places. Some of the traffic on new roads will be new journeys that would not have been made if the road had not been constructed.

New roads also bring benefits, making it easier (for those with access to cars) to travel to services, visit friends and relatives, and make leisure trips. They may also benefit businesses by making it easier to transport raw materials and finished products, and so increase opportunities for employment and income.

The UK Highways Agency has great experience and a sophisticated process for exploring and assessing the probability and the magnitude of these impacts. There are various reviews of the health impacts of transport.[4]

For railways the main negative impacts to consider are noise, severance, and loss of amenity. If railway lines are not reliably fenced then there is also a danger of injury to people and animals straying onto the line.

Airports

Airports or extensions to airports are often the subject of HIA. The main issues are usually noise, emissions, surface transport, and safety. Figure 10.1 shows a causal diagram for an airport extension.

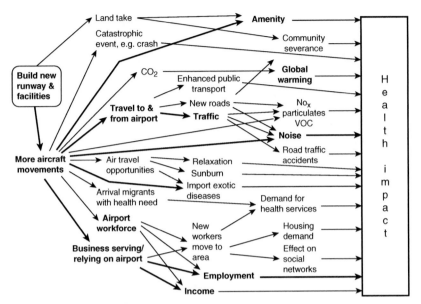

Fig. 10.1 Airport expansion.

Aircraft noise is often a cause for concern because of annoyance, disturbed sleep, impaired mental health, impaired learning and cognitive performance, and possibly effects on the cardiovascular system. There is no doubt that aircraft taking off and landing create high noise levels and this may be more damaging because it is intermittent rather than continuous. Noise at night is particularly disturbing. While technical developments are producing less noisy aircraft engines aircraft are still very noisy. The degree of noise experienced depends on the number of aircraft movements, type of aircraft, flight paths, and wind direction. The noise levels at different points on the ground can be mapped with a considerable degree of accuracy. Very high noise levels cause hearing damage but this does not occur at normal environmental noise levels. Dose–response curves for annoyance against a measure of noise (for example L_{Aeq} 16 hr dB) have been published, but the relationship between noise and annoyance is complex.[5] Studies of the effect of night-time noise on sleep have been carried out in both field and laboratory-based studies. The effect on sleep appears to be less than might have been expected. With a noise level of 90 dBA SEL the chances of the average person being wakened are about 1 in 75. Individuals varied considerably in their sensitivity to night-time noise.[6,7] This paragraph is no more than an indication of the very large literature that exists on the effect of aircraft noise on annoyance and sleep.

The effect of noise on children's learning is another matter of concern. It has been hypothesized that environmental noise impairs learning as indicated by reading age because of its effect on attention, concentration, auditory discrimination, and memory.[8] A study of children in boroughs around London Heathrow airport showed that children in schools with higher noise exposure had slightly poorer academic performance but this effect disappeared when adjusted for socioeconomic status.[9] A large study of children around three airports (RANCH) suggested that an increase in exposure of 5 dB aircraft noise was associated with between 1 and 2 months' delay in children's reading age.[10]

Chronic noise exposure has also been suggested to be associated with raised blood pressure and increased risk of myocardial infarction. The evidence regarding cardiovascular effects is fragmentary, although a recent review concluded that there was a positive relationship between aircraft noise and blood pressure,[11] but there was insufficient evidence to construct a dose–response curve.

Aircraft engines emit nitrogen oxides (NO_x) and particulates (PM_{10}, $PM_{2.5}$). The effect of these pollutants was discussed in the previous section on transport. Aircraft engines also emit carbon dioxide and water, which contribute to global warming. Airports also require surface transport links and increased road and rail traffic will also cause impacts.

Housing

Housing is an important aspect of the environment that influences people's health, and housing developments are often the subject of HIA. Damp cold housing increases the risk of asthma, respiratory infections, and other illness as well as requiring the occupants to spend more on heating and so less on other aspects of well-being. Poor security makes households vulnerable to crime and damages mental health. Overcrowding and lack of space is bad for mental health, and thin walls with sound intrusion can make this worse. Lack of maintenance and bad lighting increase the risk of accident injuries, especially for the very young and very old. When considering housing one not only has to think of the house but also its surroundings. Lack of play areas and green space, proximity to heavily trafficked streets, and air pollution may all have negative impacts on health. Projects that improve people's housing conditions may be expected to have a positive impact on health.[12–14]

However, improving the physical condition of housing is not without problems. Construction and remediation works, even if they do not involve temporary or permanent moving from home, will cause disturbance. Improvement of housing may be associated with increase in rents and so impact negatively on occupants by reducing the money they have for other purposes. Homes are very much more than buildings and housing improvement may involve disrupting established communities, with consequent harm to mental health.

Power generation

All populations need power and the means for generating electricity are frequently subject to HIA. Pre-industrial methods of heating such as open fires, especially when used inside homes, are associated with negative impacts, including injuries and indoor air pollution causing eye and respiratory disease. Developments that decrease the use of these forms of heating may have beneficial impacts on health. Power may be generated by burning fossil fuels (coal, oil, gas, peat etc) or biofuels (wood, grass etc.), by nuclear power stations, by hydroelectric schemes, by wind turbines, or in other ways. When looking at the impacts of power generation one has to consider who benefits. Often the benefit goes to the more prosperous while the negative impacts fall on the most disadvantaged members of society.

Generation of electricity by burning fossil fuels involves the consideration of emissions (chiefly SO_2, NOx, and particulates) as well as CO_2, with its implications for climate change. Additionally, there are all the impacts associated with extraction and transport of the fuel. The negative impacts in terms of death, ill-health, and injury associated with these operations are by no means negligible. Production of biofuels although carbon neutral systems (the CO_2 released in combustion is no more than the CO_2 fixed by the plants) also has appreciable impacts, including the use of land that otherwise might have been used for food production.

Hydroelectric schemes are often part of dam projects that have their own negative impacts. Tidal energy schemes may have negative impacts for coastal and fishing communities. Wind farms are often unpopular with those who live near them (noise, loss of amenity) and offshore wind farms may cause problems for shipping and fisheries.

Extractive industries

Coal and minerals may be mined by deep mine or opencast methods. Deep mining requires major construction and industrial-scale operations. Opencast mining can be very disruptive, with displacement of communities, dust, dirt, noise, and disruption of agricultural and animal husbandry. With any form of mining there will be construction of roads, with consequent increased traffic and injuries. There is likely to be a large number of employment opportunities, some of which will be taken by the existing community and many of which will be taken by workers moving into the area. In addition to employment by the mining project there will be a great deal of independent commercial activity to supply the needs of the workforce and their families. All this may be associated with many forms of ill-health (HIV, other sexually transmitted diseases, diseases associated with poor living conditions, unsafe water, and lack of sanitation).[15,16]

Extraction of oil and gas by drilling equally involves major construction work and industrial development.

Dams

Many parts of the world are short of water and dam construction is likely to be necessary for development in many places. While dams can have positive impacts, badly planned and operated dams can be the cause of numerous negative impacts, some of which have been described with passion by Jobin.[17] First there are the impacts of a large-scale construction project. Communities whose homes and land are flooded will suffer displacement, and the consequences of this are discussed later in this chapter. Communities downstream may be disrupted due to changes in flow patterns. Creation of water habitats in irrigation channels and other places may change the distribution of disease vectors (mosquito—malaria, snails—bilharzia). In addition to the populations displaced by the dam there are likely to be other population movements, with people coming in to take commercial opportunities that the displaced population may be unable to take. For discussion of dam construction in Ghana see Chapter 30.

Waste

Disposal of waste represents an ever-increasing problem for modern societies.[18,19] Some forms of waste pose particular threats and require special disposal (toxic waste, clinical waste) but all forms have to be disposed of safely. Waste management policies follow a hierarchy of methods:

- reduce waste production
- reuse
- recycle/compost
- energy recovery (incineration, pyrolysis, biogas)
- disposal (landfill).

Policies that reduce waste production (for example using less packaging) have obvious positive impacts, although there may also be negative impacts such as deterioration of contents or contamination of food and other products. A strategy of reuse also has positive impacts, although there may be negative impacts associated with handling, storing, transporting and cleaning objects for reuse.

Recycling involves the recovery of materials for reprocessing (for example glass, aluminium, copper, ferrous metals, clothing materials, paper, and cardboard). Positive impacts are conservation of materials and a reduced need for primary extraction. However, recycling often also has negative impacts. Waste transfer and waste-sorting stations may be noisy and reduce the amenity of an area. Composting on an industrial scale releases a number of spores and bio-materials that may cause disease.

Energy from waste involves combustion or some other form of thermal degradation such as pyrolysis. Low-temperature incineration releases various toxic products, including dioxins resulting from partial breakdown of materials. Modern incineration processes are far cleaner and measures that hold flue gases at high temperature for a period ensure near-complete degradation of most toxic products. Although the volume of waste material is greatly reduced there is a residue of bottom ash that has to be disposed of and also fly ash, which is considered to be a toxic waste because of the materials it contains (heavy metals etc.). Additionally, there are the impacts associated with heavy transport bringing the waste for destruction and removing bottom and fly ash. The heat produced can be used to produce electricity or even more efficiently used in combined heat and power schemes. Popular concerns about incinerators tend to be greater than 'expert' opinion considers warranted but perception of risk is a vital consideration.

Landfill is deprecated on environmental grounds and sites for landfill are becoming very scarce. Additionally, the tax on landfill makes it expensive and it will become even more so. The health impacts of landfill include attraction of vermin (especially seagulls), odours, and seepage into ground water. Later production of methane may be a problem. In developing countries landfill sites may attract people who make their living by scavenging materials from the waste and may make their homes very close to it. This lifestyle has many hazards.

Health services

Initially health services were usually considered beyond the scope of HIA but now HIA is being increasingly applied to developments of health service and health infrastructure. In part such HIAs are concerned with care pathways, clinical outcomes, and access of disadvantaged groups to care. However, health services impact on the health of populations in many ways beside the clinical activity. Health services are often the largest employers and trainers in the area. They are major purchasers and economic players, users of services, producers of waste, users of energy, and generators of traffic. Often the impact of all these activities on the health of the community is more important than the impact of clinical activity. HIA applied to health services can help to enhance the positive impacts and minimize the negative impacts.

Displacement

Large infrastructure developments may well involve displacing people from their homes and land. They may suffer disruption of their social networks and a loss of mental well-being even if they receive financial compensation for their enforced removal.[20] In developing countries large-scale displacement, which would be politically impossible in developed countries, is less rare. Whole communities may well be required to move, with loss of home, livelihood linked to the land, and cultural associations, including sacred and burial sites. The International Finance Corporation has laid down conditions that must be observed in projects funded by it that involve displacement. However, even if these are observed they may not adequately mitigate the major negative impact of enforced displacement.

Employment and income

Employment or increased income for local trades people is a positive impact of many developments. While some forms of employment are health damaging, employed people and their dependents generally enjoy better health than the unemployed. Increased income, workplace friendship, improved self-image, and structure for the day may all contribute to this. Equally, increased income is usually associated with better health. At the same time one has to look carefully at who gets employment and increased income, and whether a new development decreases the income of others or makes them unemployed (for example a new retail development may result in other retailers losing business or becoming unemployed).

Climate change

Power generation from fossil fuels, most forms of surface transport, air transport, most industrial processes, and numerous other activities involve the production of carbon dioxide, while raising cattle and other stock produces methane. Both carbon dioxide and methane contribute to climate change, which will have massive negative impacts on health: rising sea levels and flooding of coastal areas, more extreme weather events, decreased rainfall in major food-producing areas, increased rainfall and flooding in other parts. It is difficult to imagine any greater impacts and the UK will not be immune to them.[21]

However, many HIAs ignore this issue on the grounds that the contribution to climate change of the development with which they are concerned is negligible. This is true but if all developments take this view then many negligible impacts add up to an overwhelming negative impact and the problem is insoluble. HIA must learn to 'think global and act local' and consider emissions of greenhouse gases as an important negative impact on a global scale even if they are individually negligible.[22]

References

1. Planning Advisory Serivce. Prevention is still better than cure: planning for healthy outcomes. London: Planning Advisory Services, 2008. Available at http://www.pas.gov. uk/pas/aio/92315. Accessed 22 March 2012.

2. Kunzli N, Kaiser R, Medina S, Studnicka M, Chanel O, Filiger P, Herry M, Horak F, Puybonnieux-Texier V, Quenel P, Schneider J, Seethaler R, Vergnaud J-C, Sommer H. Public health impact of outdoor and traffic related pollution: a European assessment. Lancet 2000; 358: 795–801.

3. Department of Transport. Reported Road Casualties in Great Britain: 2010 Annual Report. Available at http://assets.dft.gov.uk/statistics/releases/road-accidents-and-safety-annual-report-2010/rrcgb2010-00.pdf. Accessed 22 March 2012.

4. Douglas M, Murie J, Higgins M Health Impact Assessment of Transport Initiatives: A guide. Edinburgh: Health Scotland, 2007.

5. European Commission. Position paper on dose response relationship between transport noise and annoyance. 2002. Available at http://ec.europa.eu/environment/noise/pdf/noise_expert_network.pdf. Accessed 22 March 2012.

6. Porter ND, Kershaw AD, Ollerhead JB. Adverse effects of night time aircraft noise. London: National Air Traffic Services. 2000. Available at http://www.caa.co.uk/docs/33/ERCD9964.PDF. Accessed 22 March 2012.

7. Michaud D, Fidell S, Pearsons K, Campbell KC, Keith S. Review of field studies of aircraft noise induced sleep disturbance. Journal of the Accoustical Society of America 2007; 121: 32–41.

8. Stansfeld S, Matheson MP. Noise pollution: non-auditory effects on health. British Medical Bulletin 2003; 58: 243–57.

9. Haines MM, Stansfeld SA, Head J, Job RFS. Multilevel modelling of aircraft noise on performance tests in schools around Heathrow Airport London. Journal of Epidemiology and Community Health 2002; 56: 138–44.

10. Stansfeld S, Berglund B, Clark C, RANCH study team. Aircraft and road traffic noise and children's cognition and health: a cross national study. Lancet 2005; 365: 1942–49.

11. Van Kempen E. Cardiovascular effects of environmental noise: Research in the Netherlands. Noise and Health 2011; 13: 221–28.

12. BMA Board of Science and Education. Housing and health—Building for the future. London: British Medical Association, 2003. Available at http://www.bma.org.uk/images/Housinghealth_tcm41-146809.pdf. Accessed 22 March 2012.

13. Wilkinson D Poor housing and ill-health—a summary of research evidence. Edinburgh: Scottish Office Central Research Unit, 1999. Available at http://www.scotland.gov.uk/Resource/Doc/156479/0042008.pdf. Accessed 22 March 2012.

14. Taske N, Taylot L, Mulvihill, Doyle N. Housing and public health—a review of reviews of interventions for improving health. London: National Institute for Health and Clinical Excellence, 2005. Available at http://www.nice.org.uk/niceMedia/pdf/housing_MAIN%20FINAL.pdf. Accessed 22 March 2012.

15. Gordon RL Breaking new ground: Mining, minerals and sustainable development. London: Earthscan, 2002.

16. Farrel L, Sampat P, Sarin R, Slack K. Dirty metals: Mining, communities and environment. Washington, DC: Oxfam America, Earthworks, 2004.

17. Jobin W. Dams and disease—Ecological design and health impacts of large dams, canals and irrigation systems. London & NewYork: E&FN Spon, 1999.

18. Williams PT. Waste Treatment and Disposal (2nd edn). Chichester: Wiley, 2005.

19. Bond A, Fawell J, Harrison R, and 11 others. Health impact assessment of waste management methodological aspects and information sources. Science report P6-011/1/SR1. Bristol: Environment Agency, 2005.

20. Downing TE. Avoiding new poverty: Mining induced, displacement and resettlement. Report No 58. London: International Institute for Environment and Development, 2002.

21. Kovats S. Health Effects of Climate Change in the UK 2008: An update of the Department of Health Report 2001/2002. London: Health Protection Agency, 2008. Available at http://www.dh.gov.uk/prod_consum_dh/groups/dh_digitalassets/@dh/@en/documents/digitalasset/dh_082836.pdf. Accessed 22 March 12.

22. Burdge RJ. The focus of impact assessment (and IAIA) must now shift to global climate change. Environmental Impact Assessment Review 2008; 28: 618–22.

Chapter 11

Making health impact assessment happen

John Kemm

It is clear that HIA is being used in many countries and many contexts. It is also clear that there are many situations where HIA could assist decision making but it is not being used. This chapter considers what steps might be taken to increase the use and usefulness of HIA.

Who will do an HIA?

At the moment many HIAs are undertaken by enthusiasts in public health or local authority departments for whom HIA is only a small fraction of their duties. There is a large commercial sector offering EIA and increasingly some companies are also offering to undertake HIA or include health alongside the EIA. However, if HIA is to be more widely used there must be many more people who are willing and able to undertake them.

If more HIAs are to be done then decision makers who want HIA must either pay others to do it (a commercial firm or possibly a university or similar institution) or they must do it themselves. It is unlikely that the organizations making decisions will want to employ extra staff to undertake an HIA so they will have to require their existing staff to do it. Staff may be reluctant to take on this task because they feel that they do not have the relevant knowledge or the skills.

The skills required for HIA

There is debate within the HIA community as to what extent special training is needed before one can undertake an HIA. It has to be remembered that the vast majority of HIA practitioners had no special training (because none was available when they started) and simply learnt by doing. While training by experienced practitioners can undoubtedly speed the learning process the doing element of learning HIA will always be important.

HIA is an eclectic activity and requires numerous skills.[1] Project management skills are required to identify the various elements in the process, to decide the order and timescale in which they will be undertaken, and to ensure timely completion to the quality required. Negotiation skills are required to ensure that the agenda of the assessment team fits that of the decision makers. Leadership and team working are needed to draw together the contributions of experts in different disciplines and from the stakeholders. Community skills with an ability to listen actively and draw out meaning from the many inputs are needed to engage with those affected by the proposal and to facilitate participation. Research skills are required to assist the collection and understanding of data on the current health state of the relevant populations and to obtain literature searches to gather information on the different causal paths. Advice and help from experts in different disciplines will usually be required to analyse how the proposed options will affect intermediate variables such as employment, income, traffic, exposure to pollutants, and so on.

The key requirements are robust common sense, an ability to synthesize disparate elements in order to form a big picture, and a capacity to persuade different people to work together. These skills are not the preserve of public health specialists and many people working in other posts have them. A basic understanding of public health and the determinants of health is required but just as a requirement to observe budgets does not mean that everyone has to be an economics expert, a requirement to recognize the determinants of health does not mean that everyone doing an HIA has to be a public health expert.

Training for HIA and networks

At the moment very little training for HIA is available. Some university public health courses include modules on HIA and some university courses on EIA include consideration of health. In the UK several organizations provide one-day introduction to HIA courses and a few offer three- to five-day courses. The arrangements made in several other countries are described in the chapters in the second half of this book. Birley has described different levels of HIA competence and devised courses to build HIA capacity in a major oil company[2] and in countries where major developments are being planned.[3]

Sharing experience and mutual support is an important way of increasing HIA skills. Many countries have developed HIA networks for this purpose, as described in the later chapters of this book.

Accreditation for HIA

Anyone can claim competency in HIA and the only way in which someone wishing to assess their competency can do so is by examining their track record. This situation has drawbacks and some have argued that health impact assessors, like most other professionals, should have some type of formal accreditation. The Institute of Environmental Management and Assessment is one organization that assesses competency in EIA and requires practitioners to demonstrate appropriate training and experience before granting accreditation.[4] There are, however, problems with introducing such a system for HIA. First there would have to be an accrediting body and currently no suitable organization appears willing to take on this role. Furthermore, considerable work would have to be done to determine the criteria against which applications would be judged (for example what constitutes appropriate training). One hopes that at some time when HIA is better developed an internationally recognized accreditation scheme will be implemented but that stage has not yet been reached.

Paying for HIA

HIAs have a cost and if they are to be widely used then one has to decide who will pay for them. The costs of HIA were discussed on page 22. In the early days this question was largely avoided. Individuals employed by organizations such as health authorities or local authorities used their time on the HIA and incidental expenses were lost in the accounts of their employing organization. This of course does not mean that the HIA had no costs only that no one worked out what these were. As the number of HIAs put out to tender increases the cost will become clearer. In the USA (Chapter 23) health departments have sometimes charged the cost of doing an HIA to the permitting authorities, who then recouped this in permit fees.[5]

Where an HIA is required in order to consider a development proposal it would seem reasonable that the developer should bear the cost of the HIA. Where the planning authority requires an EIA to inform its decision it is the responsibility of the developer to commission the EIA and pay for it. It has been suggested that a similar process should apply to HIAs. This arrangement raises the difficult question of for whom the assessor is working. In an ideal world they would be seeking to give impartial advice to the decision maker (planning authority) but the developer may well raise issues with the assessor and suggest changes of emphasis before passing the assessment to the decision-making authority. It is not suggested that improper conduct occurs but the situation creates a conflict of interest (Birley[3] refers to this as 'bias'). It would be far better if when an HIA was required the decision-making authority were responsible for commissioning it so it was clear that the assessors were working for them. The developer should then be required to pay the cost of the assessment with suitable arrangements to ensure that they were not overcharged.

Governance of HIA and regulatory authorities

Whoever does the HIA and whoever pays for it, it is necessary to be sure of its quality. This becomes even more necessary as more commercial firms offer to undertake HIA. Organizations undertaking HIA and those who commission HIA may set up their own quality-control procedures, as described in Chapter 7 (page 76). In HIA of policy ministerial sign-off may be required (see page 84). At an international level the World Bank and other lending institutions exercise some governance since a satisfactory HIA is often a condition for a loan but it is not clear that this power is effective. If accreditation of HIA practitioners were to be introduced then those responsible for accreditation would exercise some governance. However, the best protection against flawed HIA is openness. If HIA reports are available for scrutiny by all, weak and badly performed HIA will be revealed.

Making HIA mandatory

At the moment, in most countries in most situations HIA is not mandatory and whether it is carried out or not depends on the interests of the decision makers and those who seek to advise them. Some have suggested that HIA should be mandatory, either being part of the standard working procedures of the department or institution or even being required by legislation (as is EIA in many situations). The danger of following this route is that unless staff are committed to thinking seriously about health issues the HIA degenerates into a mere tick box exercise. Before HIA is made mandatory it is essential that those expected to do the HIA feel confident in their knowledge and understand the importance of considering health.

The term 'institutionalizing' HIA is often used to mean making HIA part of the normal practice and ways of working of an organization. Making HIA mandatory is one way of 'institutionalizing' HIA but there are also other ways of doing this.

Increasing interest of government in HIA

There is no doubt that governments have the power to encourage the use of HIA both for their own policies and by lower layers of government under their jurisdiction. There are now several examples of how HIA use has flourished under one administration then withered when it has been replaced by an administration less interested in HIA. An early example was British Columbia (Canada), which was a leader in HIA and then withdrew its support under a different administration.[6] Similarly, a considerable capacity for HIA was developed in the Netherlands, but then dropped back when the administration changed. Support for the application of HIA to English policy that had been built up under one administration appears to have withered under the next (see page 84).

Future developments of HIA

HIA has made considerable progress and been widely adopted but if HIA and the consideration of health in decision making is to become even more widespread then HIA must become better and more available, and decision makers must become more ready to use it.

Making HIA better

There are several ways in which the practice of HIA could and should become better:

- understanding causal links
- describing the magnitude of impacts
- using models to estimate impacts
- describing the distribution of impacts.

One main claim of HIA is to predict the health consequences of implementing different options. Too often the causal links between proposals, intermediate variables, and health impacts are poorly understood. Epidemiology and other disciplines are continually adding to the knowledge base available to HIA. Understanding is extending beyond physicochemical exposures to socioeconomic factors such as employment, income, and aspects of social capital. Assembling knowledge of determinants and their links to health in an easily accessible form will help HIA to make better predictions.

Better understanding of how aspects of the environment (physical and social) cause impacts will allow progress with quantifying impacts. At the same time better understanding of the relationships will allow the building of models that deal with many more variables and impacts than the current rather restricted models.

HIA also aspires to describe the distribution of impacts between different groups, indicating which groups in the population will benefit and which will be harmed or at least benefit less. At the moment most HIAs only do this in the vaguest terms. As HIA improves, rather than indicate overall impacts it will more clearly identify the different impacts experienced by separate groups in the population.

Making HIA more available

If HIA were to be requested for every situation where it could be useful then the demand could not currently be met. Capacity to do HIA could be increased by:

- training HIA specialists
- developing accreditation for HIA specialists
- increasing the pool willing and able to undertake HIA
- making more use of integrated impact assessment.

If more HIAs are to be done them more people need to be trained in how to do them. There need to be more short courses (one to seven days) introducing people to HIA and giving them a basic understanding of the topic, more modules in courses for public health specialists, planners, environmentalists, and political scientists on HIA, and perhaps some degree courses devoted purely to HIA. Didactic teaching is no substitute for experience but such courses will allow practitioners to build a sound theoretical base and also encourage HIA to develop as a discipline.

Parallel with the development of academic courses and awards for HIA the development of a discipline would be stimulated by accreditation. The several barriers that need to be overcome before accreditation can be established have been discussed earlier in this chapter but a robust accreditation scheme would not only make it easier for those who wish to commission HIAs but also encourage HIA practitioners to attain and maintain levels of competence.

Courses and accreditation are steps to building a profession for HIA specialists but to make HIA the exclusive preserve of specialists would be counterproductive. If the use of HIA is to be widespread then most HIAs will have to be done by people whose main occupation is something other than HIA. The main task of HIA specialists will be to undertake the most complicated HIAs and to support non-specialists to undertake other HIAs.

Furthermore, the task of thinking through health consequences must be made as easy as possible. The same decision makers who would be required to consider health impacts are not only fully occupied but also expected to consider many other types of impact. The case for integrated impact assessment was made in Chapter 9. It must be admitted that in many cases so far integrated impact has failed to give proper consideration to health but it is surely worth persisting and introducing an integrated impact assessment that gives proper attention to health.

Making decision makers more ready to use HIA

Decision makers would become more likely to use HIA if the following steps were taken:

- Undertake more evaluation of HIA.
- Make decision makers more aware of HIA.
- Improve understanding of policy making by HIA practitioners.

There is still some scepticism among some decision makers as to how useful HIA really is. There is need for a great deal more evaluation of HIA to demonstrate that its predictions are well founded in evidence, that it helps people to understand why decisions that affect them are taken, and that it informs the decisions. Chapter 7 reviewed some of the ways that this could be done. The HIA community needs to devote much more effort to the evaluation of HIA and communicating these findings to decision makers.

There are many decision makers (including ministers and policy makers) who do not use HIA because they are unaware of the possible health impacts of their decisions or that HIA could help them. Further efforts need to be made to ensure that all who could be helped by HIA are aware of it. In addition to personal advocacy this might be done by organizing short seminars and workshops within organizations, and by circulating short papers describing how HIA could be useful.

Lastly, if HIA is to be made useful to policy and decision makers HIA practitioners must understand policy makers' concerns and ways of working. Too often HIA practitioners do not appreciate how organizations such as ministries and local authorities work. Interchange between these two worlds is invaluable. For HIA practitioners, experience of doing the jobs of civil servants and local authority officers will give insights as to how to make HIA more useful. Equally, when civil servants and local authority officers work with HIA teams they bring invaluable insights to the HIA.

References

1. Kemm J. What is HIA and why might it be useful?, in Wismar M, Blau J, Ernst K, Figuras J. (eds), The effectiveness of health impact assessment: Scope and limitations of supporting decision making in Europe. Brussels: WHO European Observatory on Health Systems and Policies, 2007.
2. Birley M. Health impact assessment in the Royal Dutch Shell Group. *Environmental Impact Assessment Review* 2005; 25: 702–13.
3. Birley M. Health Impact Assessment: Principles and practice. London: Earthscan, 2011.

4. Institute of Environmental Management and Assessment. IEMAs individual EIA practitioner registration scheme (latest information booklet dated 2011),. Available at http://www.iema.net/registers/eiapractitioners#howapply.
5. Wernham A. Health impact assessments are needed in decision making about environmental and land use policy. Health Affairs 2011; 30: 947–56. Available at http://www.healthcare.gov/prevention/nphpphc/advisorygrp/wernhan-health-affairs-paper-10032011.pdf.
6. Banken R. Strategies for institutionalising HIA ECHP Health Impact Assessment. Discussion Papers Number 1. Brussels: WHO European Centre for Health Policy, 2001. Available at http://www.euro.who.int/__data/assets/pdf_file/0010/101620/E75552.pdf.

Part 2

HIA across the world

Chapter 12

Devolution, evolution, and expectation: health impact assessment in Wales

Eva Elliott, Gareth Williams,
Chloe Chadderton, and Liz Green

Introduction

This chapter describes the Wales Health Impact Assessment Support Unit (WHIASU) and the evolution of HIA in the context of Wales as a devolved nation with its particular approach to public health. The character of WHIASU, as of any organization, can only properly be understood in terms of its history and the wider social, policy, and political context of which it is a part. WHIASU's emphasis on involving people potentially affected by a proposal in HIA mirrors the stress in Welsh policy documents on citizen engagement as a mechanism for policy and service development. This was intended to contrast markedly with individual choice as the driver for change in England[1] as well as resonating with a sociological theory of knowledge that supports the value of deliberative processes that involve lay people in dialogue with professionals.[2]

The history of HIA and public health structures in Wales

In 1999 Wales became a devolved administration within the UK and the National Assembly of Wales acquired limited but significantly enhanced decision-making powers in a number of policy areas, of which health was one. In preparation for the new administration, the Welsh Office published 'Better Health, Better Wales',[3] which prepared the way for a distinctively Welsh approach to health policy with an aspiration to address social class and geographical inequalities in health within Wales.[4] It noted the legacy of ill-health and social disadvantage in Wales since the decline throughout the twentieth century of its traditional industries, deep coal mining and steel making.

It emphasized the need for all areas of government, as well as the health service (NHS), to address the wider social determinants of health as a means of reducing health inequalities. The first minister for Health and Social Services, Jane Hutt, was both applauded and condemned for focusing on public and preventative health rather than on secondary healthcare services.

'Better Health, Better Wales' proposed HIA as a mechanism for action across policy areas, to facilitate policy decisions to create long-term, sustainable health gains. The creation of WHIASU confirmed a strong commitment to a long-term strategy for health improvement and addressing health inequalities.

Soon after this a national guidance document, 'Developing Health Impact Assessment in Wales',[1] prepared the way for an HIA development programme. Initially the Assembly commissioned a number of pilot projects to test the process and its usefulness for informing decisions. These included two desk-based HIAs, one described as a preliminary HIA on Objective One (European Structural Funding) in Wales[5] and one on the impact of the Home Energy Efficiency Scheme.[6] Both of these were led by civil servants within the Welsh Assembly. Cardiff University's School of Social Sciences was commissioned to undertake a third HIA of housing regeneration options in a post-industrial former coal-mining community in one of the South Wales valleys.[7] This HIA was used directly to inform local municipality decisions about how to address poor housing in the village in ways that would maximize opportunities to improve health and minimize any harm. Feedback on the process was also provided and formed the basis for theorizing the role of HIA in developing what the authors called 'civic intelligence'.[2]

The Wales Health Impact Assessment Support Unit

WHIASU was created in 2001 and is as an academic collaboration between the School of Social Sciences and the Department of Epidemiology and Public Health of the University of Wales College of Medicine. It was funded for two years with two half-time researchers/HIA development workers and managed directly by the National Assembly. The purpose of the unit was to develop the capacity of local government and other organizations to undertake HIA. This was largely achieved through training, often using real HIAs as a training opportunity, and providing a web-based resource.[8] The Unit also had a remit to respond to members of the public or community groups who might be interested in the use of HIA in relation to developments that affected them.

From the outset research skills in WHIASU have improved the evidence-gathering components of HIA, and case studies have been used as a way of reflecting on and evaluating different kinds of HIA as well as theorizing the contribution of HIA to health knowledge more broadly. HIAs on housing regeneration and opencast mining have yielded papers in environmental, health, and sociological books and journals. In 2005 a study was funded to assess the impact of HIAs undertaken in Wales on the development of individual and organizational health knowledge and skills as well as their impact on decision making.[9] Research has also been used to develop guidance on public engagement[10] and for conducting HIAs on opencast mining and waste-processing applications, both of which have been a focus of public and professional concern in Wales.[11]

WHIASU's history should also be understood in terms of devolution in Wales, where the distinctive approach to policy, including health policy, has been characterized as 'new localism',[12] and a 'strategy which shifts resources and power away from central control and towards front-line managers, local democratic structures and local communities, within an agreed framework of national minimum standards and policy priorities'.[13] In 2003, the five health authorities were abolished and replaced with 22 local health boards (LHBs), coterminous with local authorities, which were set up to plan and commission local services.[14] LHBs and local authorities had a duty to jointly undertake a local health needs assessment and develop a health, social care and well-being strategy and delivery plan for their area. This local focus and partnership provided an ideal mechanism through which to build HIA and was seen as a vehicle for operationalizing joint responsibility for local health.

Another important change in 2003 which affected WHIASU and the positioning of HIA was the creation of two national public health bodies. The National Public Health Service for Wales (NPHS) is a national service but also employs local public health directors who work within each LHB and lead a local public health team. The Wales Centre for Health (WCfH) has a statutory remit 'to develop and make information about the protection and improvement of health available to the public, to undertake and commission research into such matters and to contribute to the development and provision of training.' WHIASU was re-commissioned with an initial three-year rolling contract managed by WCfH and an additional full-time HIA development worker was funded. The WHIASU work programme is co-directed by two academics in the School of Social Sciences. This was the first step to WHIASU becoming an academic/public service partnership and an integral part of the public health structure rather than a pilot project.

Wider partnerships also contributed to recognition of the value and importance of HIA. On the national level WHIASU worked closely with the NPHS and the Welsh Local Government Association (WLGA), with whom the unit published practical guidance on HIA,[15] and the Chartered Institute of Environmental Health. All these partners promoted awareness and training to a wide range of audiences in the health and local government sectors. The WLGA also published 'The Route to Health Improvement', which provided a framework for local authorities to maximize their health improvement role[16] and highlighted HIA as one approach they could use to ensure that decision-making processes maximize health and consider inequalities.

In 2009 further restructuring of the NHS and reorganization of public health has required WHIASU to redirect its efforts to new partners at the local and national level. A new body, Public Health Wales, unified public health organizations working at a national level while the 22 LHBs were abolished and replaced by seven health boards, coterminous with the hospital trusts, which employ their own directors of public health. At the same time the WLGA health improvement policy division, which had been the link between public health and local authorities, was disbanded so WHIASU had to change the way in which it directed its support and rebuild relationships with the public health directors and their public health teams. However, HIA and WHIASU are still mentioned as key to delivering public health goals in strategic policy documents.[17] In addition, the necessity for WHIASU to work with the Welsh Government at the policy level in developing more equity-focused HIA is mentioned. This may strengthen HIA at the national level, in line with European Union efforts to support member states in developing a framework for equity-focused HIA.

Changing patterns of HIA in Wales

Beside shifts in structures, developments in other sectors have meant that the types of HIA and who does them have changed through time. In addition, as the number of assessments has increased, there has been a shift from supporting organizations and their partners to undertake HIA to assessing the quality of externally funded HIAs.

In the early years of WHIASU, HIA was felt to be a way of building health literacy into the decision-making processes of non-health organizations. The challenge was to demonstrate how all sectors within local government could play a role in health improvement and show that the task of reducing health inequalities was 'everyone's business'.[18] At the same time, as elsewhere in the UK, the links between planning and health were becoming more explicit. HIA is referred to in a number of Welsh Government policy and guidance documents in a wide range of areas, including road and rail transport, minerals, waste and land use planning (see Box 12.1).

However, with this increase in the promotion and use of HIA have come some major challenges. WHIASU moved away from developing the capacity

Box 12.1 Timeline of HIA in planning in Wales

- 2002: Welsh Assembly Government Technical Advice Note—Waste (TAN 21) for waste states that HIAs be conducted for the Wales Waste Strategy and its associated Plans.

- 2005: Development of a Strategic Impact Assessment policy Gateway Screening Tool to assess the implications for a wide range of determinants, including health.

- 2006: Welsh Assembly Government Draft Ministerial Interim Position Statement—Planning Policy Wales (DMIPPS 02/06) supports a consideration of health and well-being at a local level and is supplementary guidance to Planning Policy Wales for large planning applications and Local Development Plans.

- 2007: 'One Wales'[29] included a commitment to require all opencast mining proposals and developments in Wales to be subject to a HIA with community participation. This became reality with the publication of Welsh Assembly Government Minerals Technical Advice Note (MTAN 2) for minerals and opencast mining in early 2009.

- 2008: Welsh Assembly Government Welsh Transport Appraisal Guidance for transport requires an HIA to be undertaken.

- 2010: Our Healthy Future[17]—further recognition of the important role that HIA can have in health improvement. Its sister paper 'Fairer Outcomes for all'[30] promotes the use of HIA in planning and with communities.

- 2011: National Spatial Improvement Programme for the rail network in Wales.

- 2011: Wales Waste Sector Action Plans, include promotion of HIA as best practice in all local and national waste management proposals and developments.

of sectors to incorporate health into their decision-making process to keeping a watchful eye on the proliferation of commercial HIAs undertaken by private consultants, many of whom had little or no experience of health or HIA. Commercial developers pay for HIAs alongside their statutory obligation to conduct an EIA. The linkage of these HIAs to commercial interests and mistrust of their quality and scope has led to an increased use of review tools.

Furthermore, the perception of local communities that HIA was a protest tool that could be used to campaign against a particular development had to be managed. Whereas initially HIA was promoted as a mechanism to build the knowledge that citizens hold about the potential health impact of developments on their communities, HIA is now used by communities to highlight their lack of a voice in the planning processes.

More recently there appears to be another change in production of HIAs, with a shift towards positive citizen involvement in regeneration and housing development. In addition the Equity Action programme, which focuses on developing capability across European Member States to include equity in policy level HIA, may mean that more HIAs will be conducted at the Welsh Government level with WHIASU support. Discussions are also taking place regarding quantification in HIA. WHIASU is gradually building a training strategy fit for the needs of the new teams and partnerships in local government and public health structures. However, a resource unit in HIA needs to do more than improve generic training resources to improve a set of public health competencies. It must also attend to the changes in the social, political, and policy landscape, and spot opportunities to empower those who could best use the resources to make a different to the health of people in Wales.

Definitions, passions, and progress

HIA, as practiced in Wales, has evolved from the traditional definition outlined in the Gothenberg consensus.[19] Although useful, this definition reduces HIA to a linear process and brackets out the complexities of knowledge production in different kinds of contexts, exaggerates the role of prediction at the expense of more productive forms of understanding and imagination, and obscures the multiplicity of agendas, interests, and competing values that are always brought to bear in any HIA. HIA sets up a process of dialogue and opens up a knowledge space[2] that involves policy makers, scientific experts, and, increasingly, members of relevant publics to engage collectively in the analysis and discussion of evidence and theory.[20] A more nuanced sociological, and our preferred, definition is this:

> '...a process through which evidence (of different kinds), interests, values and meanings are brought into dialogue between relevant stakeholders (politicians, professionals and citizens) in order imaginatively to understand and anticipate the effects of change on health and health inequalities in a given population.'[21]

The value of bringing a sociological understanding to HIA is that it foregrounds the complexity of the social in the labour of producing an HIA. Sociological theory, as it has done in thinking about the nature of social capital and social cohesion for instance, can coexist alongside public health and epidemiology, and can contribute to a more fine-grained, textured theory of change in particular contexts.

However, our key argument about the nature of knowledge in HIA is that what is sometimes referred to as 'lay knowledge' needs to be seen as something more than knowledgeable opinion or belief. Elsewhere we have maintained that HIA can help to facilitate and improve professional/citizen alliances similar to what is described as popular epidemiology. While this 'lay knowledge' is often used to refer to 'common misconceptions',[22] it is more useful to view such knowledge as data rather than as a barrier to knowledge about potential environmental hazards. It not only brings potentially useful insights into how new developments might impact on a particular place but also offers alternative forms of reasoning.[23] For instance, in the case of contested land use developments, underlying disputes may focus on technical questions such as safe thresholds, whereas the issue for local residents may not just be about avoiding the risk of increased cancer levels but assaults on their ability to live well in their home environments.[24–28]

This does not mean that lay claims about health and well-being impact should be taken at face value. HIA provides a framework through which different views of evidence and health can both be made explicit and scrutinized. It acknowledges that there are different kinds of knowledge, some of which is the contextual knowledge that communities have of the places in which they wish to live. It does require a different attention to the meaning and significance of different claims. If, for instance, an opencast mine threatens to raise levels of dust that might not threaten respiratory health or mortality rates, but will prevent people from enjoying, and children from playing in, the open air or if it impacts on everyday activities such as keeping a house clean, then these are impacts that can more clearly be considered and acted upon.

HIA provides a sometimes emotionally charged deliberative space through which to contest and debate the validity and salience of the impacts within a particular local or national context. Whilst some people, keen to see HIA as a predictive evidence-based tool, may be horrified at this debasement of scientific knowledge, we argue that such deliberative spaces are the critical conscience of scientific progress. For public health, regulatory bodies, policy, and people HIA provides an opportunity to identify, debate, and build a healthy future.

References

1. National Assembly for Wales. Developing health impact assessment in Wales 1999. Available at http://www.hiaconnect.edu.au/files/Developing_HIA_in_Wales.pdf. Accessed 30 January 2012.

2. Elliott E, Williams GH Developing a Public Sociology: From Lay Knowledge to Civic Intelligence in Health Impact Assessment. Journal of Applied Social Science 2008; 2: 14–28.

3. Welsh Office. Better Health, Better Wales. Cardiff: Welsh Office, 1998.

4. Williams G.H. History is what you live: understanding health inequalities in Wales, in Michael P, Webster C, (eds) Health and Society in Twentieth Century Wales. Cardiff: University of Wales Press, 2006.

5. Breeze C, Kemm J. The health potential of the Objective 1 programme for West Wales and the Valleys: A preliminary health impact assessment. Available at http://www.wales.nhs.uk/sites3/Documents/522/Objective1_full_hia.pdf. Accessed 2 February 2012.

6. Kemm J, Ballard S, Harmer M. Health impact assessment of the new home energy efficiency scheme. Cardiff: National Assembly for Wales, 2000. Available at http://wales.gov.uk/topics/health/improvement/index/energy/?lang=en. Accessed 2 February 2012.

7. Elliott E, Williams G. Housing, health and wellbeing in Llangeinor, Garw Valley: A health impact assessment. Available at http://www.wales.nhs.uk/sites3/Documents/522/English.pdf. Accessed 2 February 2012.

8. Wales Health Impact Assessment Support Unit. www.wales.nhs.uk/sites3/home.cfm?OrgID=522. Accessed 6 February 2012.

9. Francis S, Elliott E. Health Impact Assessment in Wales: Its impact on skills, knowledge and action. Cardiff: Cardiff University, 2005.

10. Chadderton C, Elliott E, Williams G. Involving the public in HIA: An evaluation of current practice in Wales. Cardiff: Wales HIA Support Unit, 2008. Available at http://www.wales.nhs.uk/sites3/page.cfm?orgid=522&pid=10101. Accessed 30 January 2012.

11. Chadderton C, Elliott E, Williams G. A guide to assessing the health and wellbeing impacts of opencast mining. Cardiff: Wales HIA Support Unit, 2011. Available at http://www.wales.nhs.uk/sites3/Documents/522/OpencastguidanceFinal.pdf. Accessed 2 February 2012.

12. Greer S. Four way bet—How devolution has led to four different models for the NHS. London: The Constitution Unit, 2004.

13. Stoker G. New localism, progressive politics and democracy. The Political Quarterly 2004; 75, Supplement 1: 117–29.

14. Smith T, Babbington E. Devolution: a map of divergence in the NHS. Health Policy Review 2006; 1: 9–40.

15. Welsh Assembly Government. Improving Health and Reducing Inequalities: A practical guide to health impact assessment. Cardiff: Welsh Assembly Government, 2004.

16. Welsh Local Government Association. The Route to Health Improvement: An organisational development package to build capacity for local authorities. Cardiff: Welsh Local Government Association, 2006.

17. Welsh Government. Our Healthy Future. Cardiff: Welsh Assembly Government, 2010.

18. Wanless D. The Review of Health and Social Care in Wales. Report of Project Team. London: Department of Health, 2003.

19. European Centre for Health Policy. Health impact assessment: main concepts and suggested approach. Gothenburg consensus paper. Brussels: WHO Regional Office for Europe, 1999. Available at http://www.apho.org.uk/resource/item.aspx?RID=44163.

20. Kemm J, Parry J. What is HIA? Introduction and overview, in Kemm J, Parry J, Palmer, S (eds), Health Impact Assessment. Oxford: Oxford University Press, 2004, pp 1–14.

21. Elliott E, Williams G. Developing a civic intelligence: local involvement in HIA. Environmental Impact Assessment Review 2004; 24: 231–43.

22. Moffatt S, Phillamore P, Bhopal R, Foy C. If this is what it's doing to our washing, what is it doing to our lungs? Industrial pollution and public understanding in north-east England. Social Science and Medicine 1995; 41: 883–91.

23. Alaszewski A, Horlick-Jones T. Risk and health: review of current research and identification of areas for further research. Available at http://www.kent.ac.uk/chss/docs/riskandhealth.PDF. Accessed 2 February 2012.

24. Elliott E, Harrop E, Williams GH. Contesting the science: public health knowledge and action in controversial land-use developments, in Bennett P, Calman K, Curtis S, Fischbacher-Smith D (eds), Risk Communication and Public Health, 2nd edn. Oxford: Oxford University Press, 2010.

25. Williams G, Elliott E. Exploring social inequalities in health: the importance of thinking qualitatively, in Bourgeault L, DeVries R, Dingwal R (eds), Handbook on Qualitative Health Research. London: Sage, 2010.

26. Moffatt S, Pless-Mullolli T. It wasn't the plague we expected. Parents' perceptions of the health and environmental impact of opencast mining. Social Science and Medicine 2003; 57: 437–51.

27. Pless-Mulloli T, Howel D, King A, Stone I, Merefield J, Bessell J, Darnell R. Living near opencast coal mining sites and children's respiratory health. Occupational and Environmental Medicine 2000; 57: 145–51.

28. Wakefield S, Elliott S, Eyles J, Cole D. Taking Environmental Action: The Role of Local Composition, Context, and Collective. Environmental Management 2005; 37: 40–53.

29. Welsh Assembly Government. One Wales—A progressive agenda for the government of Wales. Cardiff: Welsh Assembly Government, 2007.

30. Welsh Assembly Government. Fairer Health Outcomes for All. Technical Working Paper. Cardiff: Welsh Assembly Government, 2011.

Chapter 13

Health impact assessment in Scotland

Margaret Douglas and Martin Higgins

In 2002, HIA in Scotland was described as 'still on the runway' following a survey of HIA activity that found few examples of completed HIAs and confusion about what it is and how it should be done.[1] This chapter describes how since then HIA has slowly taken off, although there is still some way to go before it is considered to be a mainstream public health activity.

A nation within a nation

Scotland is a country of 5.2 million people that forms part of the UK but has had its own parliament since 1999. The Scottish Parliament has responsibility for devolved matters, including health, education, housing, planning, and a range of other policy areas. The UK parliament retains responsibility for reserved matters, such as foreign policy and some important health determinants such as employment policy and fiscal policy. Health services accounted for one-third of the total Scottish Government draft budget in 2011–12 and this can focus attention on health services at the expense of other policy areas that also influence health.

Most of the public health workforce is based in 14 territorial NHS Boards, which are responsible for health service delivery. There are 32 local authorities, which have a statutory responsibility to work in partnership with other organizations, including NHS Boards. Multiple partnership groups are responsible for different areas of work as part of community planning. Public health professionals are involved in some of these, such as children's services partnerships and health improvement partnerships addressing specific health topics, but it is unusual to see public health involvement in wider issues like planning, housing, and transport, which are often seen as not relevant to health.

Scotland shares language and popular media with England, and is strongly influenced by ideas from over the border—English policies are commonly 'tartanized' for Scottish use. Yet Scotland's values and political allegiances can differ significantly from England and the rest of the UK. In the 2010 UK election the Conservative party won 36% of the seats overall but only one of the 59 Scottish seats. The Scottish Parliament has been led by a Scottish National Party (SNP) administration since 2007, which is in favour of Scottish independence from the UK and describes itself as 'moderate left-of-centre'.[2]

An early action of the SNP government was to establish a ministerial inquiry into health inequalities, which culminated in the publication of 'Equally Well'[3] in 2008. This took a cross-government approach and identified actions across sectors to reduce health inequalities. However, some determinants of health inequalities lie outside the jurisdiction of the Scottish Government. 'Equally Well' notes the impact of poverty and the benefits system on health, but as financial benefits are a reserved matter the recommendations in 'Equally Well' are limited to providing benefits advice services. The government's anti-poverty policy 'Achieving our Potential'[4] goes further, stating an intention to 'press the UK Government to transfer responsibility for personal taxation and benefits to Scotland, to allow the development of an approach to equity and boosting economic activity that fits with Scottish circumstances'. Although 'Equally Well' takes an inter-sectoral approach to health inequalities, Health in All Policies (page 81) is not talked about in Scotland.

The SNP identifies its top priority as sustainable economic growth, and has established a performance management system with seven targets that are intended to contribute to sustainable economic growth. One of the targets is healthy life expectancy, which is deemed to contribute to sustainable economic growth through a contribution to population growth. The performance framework also includes a set of 15 national outcomes, which include 'we live longer healthier lives' and 'we have tackled the significant inequalities in Scottish society'. Local government funding in Scotland is no longer ring-fenced for specific purposes, so local authorities have greater autonomy to decide how their budget is prioritized. In return, local authorities produce a single outcome agreement that details for each national outcome the indicators that they will use to measure progress and the actions being taken to achieve them.

The explicit priority given to economic growth can limit efforts aimed at other issues, like health. HIA can be seen as simply an added bureaucratic burden and a restriction on growth. An example is spatial planning policy. Scottish planning policy identifies a 'properly functioning planning system' as being 'essential to achieving its central purpose of increasing sustainable economic growth'.[5] It states that 'constraints and requirements … should be necessary and proportionate'. The Chief Planner wrote to all heads of planning in 2008 highlighting concerns that HIA could 'add to the challenge' of implementing the planning system and stating that Scottish Government had 'no intention of placing HIA on a statutory footing'.[6]

Battle of the impact assessments

As in other countries, other forms of impact assessment are better established than HIA. European legislation requires SEA for policies in selected sectors, but Scottish legislation goes further, requiring SEA for all sectors. However, the scope of SEA in Scotland is intentionally restricted to impacts on the physical environment. Thus the Scottish SEA guidance states, 'the definition of health in the context of SEA should… be considered in the context of the other issues outlined in Schedule 3(6) of the Act, thereby focusing on environmentally-related health issues such as significant health effects arising from the quality of air, water or soil'.[7] SEAs in Scotland will therefore not include all relevant health impacts.[8] This is a matter of dismay for the public health community but a position guarded by environmentalists who fear that if the scope were widened, social issues would outweigh environmental concerns.

UK equalities legislation encourages the use of Equality Impact Assessments (EQIAs) of public policies. EQIAs assess whether a policy may directly or indirectly discriminate against certain groups of people, and promote equal opportunities and good relations between groups. These impacts are considered in relation to selected 'protected characteristics', including age, gender, ethnicity, and others but excluding socioeconomic status. EQIAs may therefore miss differential impacts for people who are socioeconomically disadvantaged and do not routinely consider wider determinants. However, the focus on differential impacts borne by different population groups is useful to assess equity. Some organizations have successfully widened the scope of EQIA to include other vulnerable populations and health determinants.

There are many other forms of impact assessment that are required to varying degrees. Scottish Government requires Business and Regulatory Impact Assessment (an assessment of impacts on businesses and voluntary organizations) for new legislation. Transport developments must be assessed using Scottish Transport Appraisal Guidance. The Scottish Commissioner for Children and Young People promotes Children's Rights Impact Assessments. Human Rights Impact Assessments are also now being promoted as a way to ensure Scottish Government does not breach human rights legislation.

To a policy maker, the impact assessment landscape is cluttered if not overwhelming. Recognizing this, 'Equally Well'[3] recommended the development of integrated impact assessment with a strong focus on health inequalities. This is challenging because each form of impact assessment uses a different process and has proponents who fear that integrating with other assessments may dilute proper consideration of 'their' issue. Implementation of the 'Equally Well' recommendation is discussed below.

Networking on a shoestring

The Scottish Health Impact Assessment Network (SHIAN) set up in 2001 to promote and support HIA in Scotland is now hosted by the national health improvement organisztion NHS Health Scotland. The network coordinator (one of the authors) is funded for one day a week on secondment. The network has no other dedicated resource but relies on support and goodwill from its members and partnerships with other organizations, for example it has worked with the Medical Research Council Social and Public Health Sciences Unit, Greenspace Scotland, the Glasgow Centre for Population Health and the Institute for Occupational Medicine. The chair (the other author) is a public health consultant in NHS Lothian and members of the network are professionals in NHS boards, local authorities, and other organizations.

Over the years SHIAN has produced and updated generic guidance on HIA and has produced topic-specific guides with substantial evidence reviews on the health impacts of housing,[9] transport,[10] greenspace,[11] and (forthcoming) the built environment. It has also produced an e-learning course on HIA[12] and provides ad hoc face-to-face training. It holds national networking meetings usually twice a year, and provides informal support and advice for those doing HIA in Scotland.

SHIAN promotes a two-tier approach to HIA. The first tier is widespread use of screening/scoping exercises—often termed rapid impact assessment—that involve a group of stakeholders using a checklist to identify affected populations and health determinants. These have proved a quick and cost-effective way to identify impacts and inform changes. The second tier involves more detailed appraisal and is reserved for proposals with more significant health impacts and the potential to influence change. Both tiers include explicit consideration of affected populations and differential impacts, as this is a core principle of HIA. SHIAN also supports integration of health into other impact assessments as a way to ensure health issues are considered while reducing the assessment burden.

SHIAN continues to survive as a fairly loose support network that is open to anyone in Scotland interested in HIA. At times it has fitted rather uneasily within Health Scotland, whose primary role is to implement public health programmes and support NHS boards to meet government targets. SHIAN's focus on influencing wider health determinants through impact assessment may seem a direct challenge to this function, but there is a tradition of similar public health networks in Scotland which have demonstrated the value of this way of working. It continues to be supported by Health Scotland and, most importantly, by SHIAN members.

Different approaches

The development of HIA in Scotland has not been led by government policy but has grown organically as individuals have used HIA in their own work. As a result, different approaches have been tried in different parts of the country. This may lack consistency but has allowed experience to be built up, different approaches to be tried, and local guidance to be adapted to suit particular organizational or local contexts. HIA now has 'roots' in different organizations across the country where there is expertise and experience of using it to inform policies and improve health.

In Glasgow, Scotland's largest city, several detailed HIAs have been carried out of significant policies such as planning proposals, housing policy, and the Commonwealth Games. One stimulus was involvement in the WHO Healthy Cities movement, which had healthy urban planning and HIA as key themes between 2003 and 2008. Glasgow has a Joint Director of Public Health between the city council and the NHS board, and a corporate health policy team with the skills to lead HIAs and influence council policy. Together with other public health organizations in Glasgow they produced an HIA of the 2014 Commonwealth Games, which involved a high-profile scoping event, systematic literature review, extensive community consultation, and a bespoke survey.[13] The recommendations were incorporated into the Games Legacy Plan and continue to be monitored.

Following a well-received HIA of the draft spatial strategy for the East End of Glasgow,[14] Glasgow planners developed the Healthy Sustainable Neighbourhood Model as a spatial planning tool to identify relevant impacts. This is now being tested formally as part of a Scottish Government funded 'Equally Well' test site.

In Edinburgh and the Lothians there has also been significant HIA activity largely because the HIA network chair and coordinator both work in the Lothian NHS Board. Both detailed and rapid HIAs have been done in Lothian. There has been joint work with the City of Edinburgh Council, West Lothian Council and East Lothian Council on several detailed HIAs, particularly of planning and housing proposals. West Lothian Council now has supplementary planning guidance requiring HIA of some planned developments. Some recent work has produced health technical reports rather than HIA reports, as a response to the known caution about HIA of the Chief Planner.

Lothian also makes extensive use of a rapid HIA approach, which uses a screening/scoping checklist (see Box 13.1) with a group of stakeholders to identify affected populations and impacts, and to agree recommendations. This has been adapted to meet the requirements for EQIA as well as considering wider

Box 13.1 Rapid impact assessment questions in Lothian

All NHS Lothian policies, plans, or strategies are subject to rapid impact assessment. Full guidance and the NHS Lothian Rapid Impact Checklist are available online at http://www.nhslothian.scot.nhs.uk/YourRights/EqualityDiversity/ImpactAssessment/Pages/default.aspx.

The checklist covers the following areas:

1. Groups of the population that may be differentially affected by the proposal.
2. Areas of health determinants. These include prompts to consider impacts on:
   - equity
   - lifestyles
   - social environment
   - physical environment
   - access to and quality of services.

populations and health determinants. Within Lothian NHS Board all new strategies and plans must be subjected to this form of rapid impact assessment. Guidance has been developed to support this and a quality assurance process is in place. Over 60 of these rapid assessments were done in 2010. The Board has also carried out some more detailed assessments of its own proposals, including new primary care out-of-hours services and a new hospital for older people. Following the HIA of the new older people's unit a set of principles were developed to inform planning of all new healthcare facilities in Lothian. These have now been integrated into the capital planning process. The intention is that this builds wider health issues—such as designs that encourage physical activity—into new facilities without requiring a detailed HIA each time.

Several other areas of Scotland have used a similar rapid impact assessment model to integrate HIA into EQIA, capitalizing on the legal requirement for EQIA. Fife has developed an integrated impact assessment process that considers equalities, health, and environmental issues.[15] This is used routinely to screen council proposals for health impacts. Aberdeen has recently developed a similar approach.

There have been several contentious renewable energy developments in rural or island communities that could have significant impacts on people's way of life and therefore health. An HIA of a wind farm in Lewis identified negative impacts on local people resulting in part from a likely influx of new workers. This development had already caused conflict between opponents and supporters on the island. The HIA was not well received by the council, which supported the development, and led to negative press coverage accusing the assessors of racism. This experience demonstrated that HIA is not a good way to resolve conflict and probably inhibited further HIA work in the Western Isles. Another HIA into plans for new wind farms off the coast of Argyll is ongoing.

Elsewhere there have been more patchy experience of HIAs. They have often been done opportunistically or because of a local professional with a specific interest. These include HIAs of local transport strategies, superpubs, and licensing policies. SHIAN has provided direct support for some. For example, following the publication of the guide to HIA of greenspace, SHIAN supported some case studies to show how the guide could be used in practice.

Within Scottish Government there was lukewarm support for HIA until the publication of 'Equally Well' recommended the use of integrated impact assessment. Two members of SHIAN worked with Scottish Government health directorates to develop and pilot a model approach. They did not attempt to integrate health into business or environmental assessments but used a model that assesses impacts on equality, health, and human rights—all impacts relating to people. The pilot included only health policies but was judged to be highly successful. Further work is underway to implement this approach more widely across Scottish Government and in NHS Boards. This is now being supported by the equalities team in Health Scotland, which has a remit to support NHS Boards to ensure their services do not discriminate. Again there is the risk that the focus remains too strongly on health services rather than wider determinants, and further work is required to show the value in other policy areas.

Progress so far

HIA has developed slowly in Scotland. In the absence of any requirement to use HIA, its development has been 'bottom up', reflecting the enthusiasm and interests of individuals. Undoubtedly there has been increased activity over the past few years, and a growing number of people now have HIA expertise and experience, but it remains patchy. SHIAN has promoted HIA as a mainstream part of public health activity, which uses similar skills and methods to other areas of public health work and should be a key mechanism to work in partnership and influence wider determinants of health. The directors of public health are supportive of HIA but it is still not seen as part of the core business of NHS Boards. Very few public health professionals have time identified for HIA. In some local authority departments HIA has been tried, found to be valuable, and is now routinely used, but others see it as potentially another bureaucratic hurdle for policy making, and in competition with other forms of impact assessment that take priority because they have a statutory basis. Overall, a strategic approach to using HIA to improve policies remains elusive. It feels as if HIA has taken off slowly and is still in low clouds.

Taking HIA forward

HIA is not an end in itself: it is a way to influence and improve policy to achieve better health outcomes. Integrating health into other assessments may be a better alternative than promoting separate HIA. Integrating with EQIA, as in the Scottish Government project, is one approach that has been successful. EQIA is a legal requirement and there is so much overlap between EQIA and HIA that it makes sense to combine them. The next steps must include using this approach in other policy areas as a way of addressing the wider determinants of health. There should also be scope to improve health coverage in SEA. Currently there is resistance to this but we will continue to argue that SEA is incomplete if human health is not fully considered. When integrating into other assessments, some fundamental HIA principles such as considering the full range of determinants of health, identifying differential impacts, particularly on vulnerable groups, and working in partnership with policy makers and affected populations need to be preserved.

There is already a lot of enthusiasm on which HIA can build. Maintaining a high profile for SHIAN and publicizing the HIAs that have been done, and the difference that they have made, can build further support. Involving a wider range of people can help strengthen the view that public health professionals in Scotland should be routinely involved with HIA. There are now many examples where HIA has made a real difference and led to better policies in Scotland. We hope that over the next few years HIA will contribute to influencing wider determinants of health and improving the health of the Scottish population.

References

1. Douglas M, Muirie J. HIA in Scotland, in Kemm J, Parry J, Palmer S. (eds), Health Impact Assessment. Oxford: Oxford University Press, 2004.
2. SNP. SNP home page. Available at http://www2.snp.org/. Accessed 25 February 2012.
3. Scottish Government. Equally Well: Report of the Ministerial Task Force on Health Inequalities. Edinburgh: The Scottish Government, 2008.
4. Scottish Government. Achieving Our Potential: A Framework to tackle poverty and income inequality in Scotland. Edinburgh: The Scottish Government, 2008.
5. Scottish Government. Scottish Planning Policy, Department of the Built Environment. Edinburgh: The Scottish Government, 2010.

6. Mackinnon JG. Health Impact Assessments, letter 08. Edinburgh: Scottish Government Department of the Built Environment, October 2008.

7. Scottish Executive. Strategic Environmental Assessment Toolkit, SEA Gateway. Edinburgh: Scottish Executive, 2006.

8. Douglas MJ, Carver H, Katikireddi SV. How well do strategic environmental assessments in Scotland consider human health? Public Health 2011: 125: 585–91.

9. Douglas M, Thomson H, Gaughan M. Health impact assessment of housing improvements: a guide. Glasgow: Scottish Health Impact Assessment Network, 2003.

10. Douglas M, Thomson H, Jepson R, Hurley F, Higgins M, Muirie J, Gorman D. Health Impact Assessment of Transport Initiatives: A Guide, Edinburgh: NHS Health Scotland, 2007.

11. Health Scotland, Greenspace Scotland, Scotland National Heritage and Institute of Occupational Medicine. Health impact assessment of greenspace: a guide. Scottish HIA Network guides. Stirling: Greenspace Scotland, 2008.

12. NHS Health Scotland. Health Scotland Virtual Learning Environment. Available at http://elearning.healthscotland.com/mod/scorm/view.php?id=47. Accessed 10 February 2012.

13. Glasgow Corporate Policy Health Team l, NHS Glasgow and Clyde and others. 2014 Commonwealth Games Health Impact Report: Planning for legacy. Available at http://www.glasgow.gov.uk/NR/rdonlyres/13B2AA3B-B065-4006-A2B8-23E0847485B4/0/CWGHIAFullReport.pdf. Accessed 10 February 2012.

14. Ison E. Health impact assessment (HIA) of the draft East End Local Development Strategy, Changing Places: Changing Lives. Glasgow: Glasgow Centre for Population Health, 2007. Available at http://www.gcph.co.uk/assets/0000/0444/HIAofEELDS_Final_Dec07.pdf.

15. Fife Rights Forum—Fife Integrated Impact Assessment Tool. Available at http://www.fiferights.org/information-resources-and-training/fife-integrated-impact-assessment-healthandwellbeing-138. Accessed 10 February 2012.

Chapter 14

Health impact assessment in the island of Ireland

Owen Metcalfe, Claire Higgins, and Teresa Lavin

Introduction

This chapter considers the development of HIA across the island of Ireland over the past decade. It explores factors affecting the implementation and conduct of HIA and identifies opportunities for future progress. A case study is provided of an HIA conducted on a cross-border project, highlighting HIA's potential as a tool to enhance partnership working at many levels.

Background

HIA has been developing across the island of Ireland since 2001 as a way to progress healthy public policy. A baseline report published in that year concluded that while knowledge of HIA and HIA activity were relatively limited, there was strong support for its development.[1] HIA has developed significantly across Ireland since then.[2] A follow-up review of HIA conducted in 2009 found that a range of agencies across the island had a firm knowledge base on HIA as well as the tools and support to enable them to carry out HIA. However, it also identified difficulties with implementing HIA at both strategic and operational levels.[3]

Legislative context and government support for HIA

HIA is not a statutory requirement in either Northern Ireland (NI) or the Republic of Ireland (RoI), mirroring the broader European picture. Policy commitments and objectives for HIA are included in the RoI health strategy 'Quality and Fairness: A health system for you' (2001),[4] while in NI the public health strategy 'Investing for Health' (2002)[5] devotes a chapter to the adoption of HIA as a way to progress healthier public policy. The Ministerial Group on Public Health in NI is tasked with assessing the public health implications of government policy through the development and implementation of 'Investing for Health'.[5] New public health policy frameworks will be published in both NI and the RoI in 2012. Alongside this the health services in both jurisdictions have recently produced policy documents on tackling health inequalities which recognize the need to work in partnership with a range of organizations within and outside the health sector.[6,7]

The role of local government does not extend to the provision of health services in either jurisdiction. However, as the majority of HIAs conducted across the island of Ireland are at the local level, local government support for HIA is vital. A study of HIA at this level found 'an appetite and willingness to engage in factors affecting health and wellbeing of their local populations'.[2] While there is no formal recognition of HIA at this level, one mechanism facilitating a 'health lens' is Healthy Cities. Currently five cities across the island (Belfast, Derry, Galway, Cork, and Waterford) have World Health Organization Healthy Cities status. Belfast Healthy Cities led the HIA sub-network in phase IV of the WHO programme (2003–2008).

HIA has been referred to as a deductive process with an understanding of how the world works underpinning conclusions of how health will be impacted by a given policy, programme, or initiative under consideration. The HIA process therefore takes into account that not everything can be measured in an objective and scientific way but this can be challenging to convey to decision-makers, who are often under pressure to measure, monitor, and evaluate. As recognized by O'Mullane and Quinlivian,[2] 'legislation is not enough for HIA to operate effectively in a State and action to promote HIA must also relate to organisational and community practice in both jurisdictions'. Elsewhere, it has been suggested that 'a paradigm change is required' to address the current policy-action gap and bring about more extensive use of HIA.[8]

The consideration of health in other impact assessments

As Chapter 9 notes, HIA as a part of other impact assessment processes can be useful and the acronym HIA is not essential as long as health is properly considered. However, integration must be mindful of becoming diluted.[9] The integrated impact assessment (IIA) or policy toolkit in NI outlines 13 assessments, including health, as part of the policy-making process, which presents a plethora of issues to be considered for decision makers. EIA and SEA are mandatory processes and both present opportunities for the consideration of health. A recent study examining health in SEAs conducted across the island found that this opportunity has not been realized and health is not considered in many SEAs.[10]

Republic of Ireland and Northern Ireland working together on HIA

The Institute of Public Health in Ireland (IPH) is an all-island body with three core areas of work: to strengthen public health intelligence, to build public health capacity, and to develop and evaluate policies and programmes. The IPH is funded by the Department of Health and Social Services and Public Safety (DHSSPS) in NI and the Department of Health in the RoI. Since its inception, the IPH way of thinking has developed within an understood framework of the social determinants of health and has developed HIA as a key component of its work throughout the island of Ireland.

Institute of Public Health in Ireland work in HIA

The IPH has played a key role in developing capacity and skills for HIA across the island of Ireland over the last decade. Building capacity for HIA is framed within the wider context of increasing capacity for an HiAP approach and building a value base which supports action on health inequities. Increasing awareness of the need for a cross-government approach to health and health inequities requires working at multiple levels but one practical way in which this is being achieved is through the development of briefing papers[11] that show the impacts of policy from other sectors (such as housing, transport, and education) on the health of the population and on vulnerable groups.

The IPH provides support and guidance for organizations who wish to conduct HIAs on their own or external policies and projects. This includes the development of tools and resources for HIA, the delivery of introductory and comprehensive HIA courses and advice, and input to HIAs being undertaken. In addition, two to three HIA forums are held each year, originally as a network for those who had attended a comprehensive course to meet and discuss their HIA work, but these now have evolved into a mechanism that facilitates the discussion of pertinent issues of local or national interest.[12]

Case study—growing health: an HIA on a community allotment/garden proposal

This case study demonstrates the added value of conducting an HIA on a cross-border programme of work to develop community allotments/gardens and an associated training programme in five local government districts.

The project was initiated by the North West Cross Border group, who identified community allotments/gardens as a mechanism to enhance health in the region. HIA was seen as a tool to support the community allotment/garden programme to maximize its health outcomes. Specifically it was anticipated that the HIA would:

- provide a baseline of health status in the North West area
- review international evidence on the health impacts of community allotments/gardens
- engage potential future users to determine the local health impact
- develop recommendations to support the funding application and implementation.

The aim of the HIA was to enhance the health impacts of the proposal and focus on actions to reach vulnerable groups and encourage sustainable use of the project. HIA guidance developed by the IPH was used to guide the HIA, which followed recognized international methodology.[13] This involved developing a community profile, scanning government policy, reviewing literature, and engaging both statutory and community stakeholders in each of the five local areas. Thus evidence from a wide range of sources was used to inform the recommendations.

Due to the timing of this HIA, it is too soon to comment on outcomes as the funding application has not been assessed. It is possible, however, to consider how HIA can build capacity, promote engagement, and enhance the role of local government in a health agenda.

The project involved a range of partners, including four local government districts in NI and one in the RoI, the Public Health Agency (NI) and the Health Service Executive (RoI). Gaining support for HIA from all the partners was important to enable it to proceed. Other agencies who became involved through the HIA included environmental agencies and community/voluntary groups with experience in allotment projects.

Local government had a central role to play in this HIA, which reflects recent research highlighting the importance of this level of government in influencing health.[2] The HIA was undertaken to build capacity and empower local government officers to participate fully in the HIA and coordinate the gathering of required information at a local level, e.g. identifying relevant policies and organizing stakeholder meetings. A two-day training programme was delivered to all partners and screening took place at this stage. Collective engagement from across the areas showed clear enthusiasm for HIA as a mechanism to strengthen the proposal.

Local community allotment/garden projects are exceptionally effective in providing people with opportunities to take responsibility for and improve their own health and well-being.[14] Health inequalities across the island of Ireland are well documented and it is evident that health is not equally distributed, particularly in the North West of the region. The HIA provided a health equity focus to determine which groups would require additional support to access and use the demonstration sites. The equity dimension of the proposal focused on setting up demonstration sites in areas of disadvantage. The HIA re-tuned this focus on equity to give consideration as to who should be targeted within each area. This particularly highlights the well-documented importance of community input and community development approaches to the HIA process.[15]

The HIA was undertaken to support a funding proposal but its outputs go beyond this. It increased awareness of local factors contributing to health and provided a stimulus for local people to become more engaged in managing their environment and appreciate the benefits of producing food locally. It enhanced partnerships across sectors and across borders, and provides a template for future working in a broad range of issues relevant to health.

Conclusion

While HIA is recognized as a tool to support decision makers to address both potential health impacts and health inequalities in proposals, putting HIA into practice remains a challenge. With no legislative basis for HIA in either jurisdiction there needs to be discussion about how appropriate legislation could be drawn up to make HIA a legal obligation. However, it is recognized that legislation does not always result in practice and effort would still be required to ensure HIAs were done.

For HIA to succeed and be recognized as a viable tool to support HiAP, a collection of facilitating factors and driving forces need to be in place. These include identifying and empowering champions such as the health agencies in both jurisdictions to be real advocates for the need to ensure multiagency working to improve health. An understanding across government of the social, economic, and environmental determinants of health needs to be developed and the linkage between government departmental portfolios and health needs to be recognized. Building on this, skills are required to engage in a process to identify how policies and projects (including those developed by local government) impact on health.

Across the island of Ireland the new public health policy frameworks present a great opportunity to enhance the health of the population. However, this comes with a caveat. Without the champions, skills development and a greater understanding of the need for an HiAP approach, HIA will remain an ad hoc tool rather than the systematic support mechanism that it has the potential to be.

References

1. Institute of Public Health in Ireland. Health Impact Assessment: a baseline report for Ireland and Northern Ireland. Dublin: Institute of Public Health in Ireland, 2001.
2. O'Mullane M, Quinlivan A. Health Impact Assessment (HIA) in Ireland and the role of local government. Environmental Impact Assessment Review 2011, 2012; 32: 181–186.
3. Gillespie N, McIldoon N. Review of Health Impact Assessment for the Institute of Public Health in Ireland. Dublin: Institute of Public Health in Ireland, 2009.
4. Department of Health and Children. Quality and Fairness—a Health System for You. Dublin: Department of Health and Children, 2001.
5. Department of Health, Social Services and Public Safety. Investing for Health. Belfast: Department of Health, Social Services and Public Safety, 2002.
6. Health Service Executive. Health Inequalities Framework 2010–2012. Dublin: Health Service Executive, 2010.
7. Public Health Agency. Business Plan 2010–2011. Available at http://www.publichealth.hscni.net/.
8. Kearns N, Pursell L. Time for a paradigm change? Tracing the institutionalisation of health impact assessment in the Republic of Ireland across health and environmental sectors. Public Health 2011; 99: 91–96.
9. Metcalfe O, Higgins C. Healthy Public Policy—is health impact assessment the cornerstone? Public Health 2009; 123: 296–301.
10. Lavin T, Higgins C, Metcalfe O, Moore S. Consideration of health in SEA on the island of Ireland. Dublin: Institute of Public Health in Ireland, 2011.
11. Institute of Public Health in Ireland HIA resources (see HIA evidence reviews). Available at http://www.publichealth.ie/ireland/hiaresources. Accessed 27 February 2012.
12. Institute of Public Health in Ireland—HIA Forum 2011 (also links to other years). Available at http://www.publichealth.ie/ireland/hiaforum/hiaforum2011. Accessed 27 February 2012.
13. Institute of Public Health in Ireland. Health Impact Assessment Guidance. Dublin: Institute of Public Health in Ireland, 2009.
14. Institute of Public Health in Ireland. Snippet of Growing Health, 2011. Available at http://www.publichealth.ie/.
15. O'Mullane M. Prioritising health in policy and project appraisal: Are HIAs used for policy in Ireland? Recommendations for HIA in Practice, PhD Thesis, University College Cork, 2009.

Chapter 15

Development of health impact assessment in the Netherlands

Lea den Broeder and Brigit Staatsen

HIA in the Netherlands began in the early 1990s and developed along two different lines: one shaped by the public health approach and the other stemming from the environmental field.

Public health based HIA

Public health based HIA evolved according to the paradigm presented by the Lalonde model of health. The development of public health based HIA in the Netherlands has been described by Roscam Abbing[1] and was initially strongly focused at national level. In the policy paper 'Safe and Sound. Framework for the national health policy 1995–1998'[2] the Minister of Health announced that her Ministry would give practical support for the development of HIA (see Box 15.1). A two-step system, with a screening procedure that helped identify possible health-relevant policies and an HIA commissioning and assessment procedure, was developed. The HIAs produced mainly concerned national policies and addressed a variety of policy fields, ranging from tobacco discouragement and health insurance policy to national housing policy and the high-speed rail link. The HIA work was supported by a small Intersectoral Policy Office located at the Netherlands School of Public Health. However, in 2003 the Ministry of Health decided to discontinue this unit, and since then the focus has been on local HIA applications.

Environmental health impact assessment

The second line of development in HIA emerged from the environmental field. Most EIAs in the 1990s paid only limited attention to health, merely testing whether legal limit values for air pollution or noise, for example, would be exceeded when plans or projects were implemented. Most limit values are a trade-off between public health and economic interests, and exposure to air pollution levels below these limit values is still associated with considerable

Box 15.1 An interview with Professor Ernst Roscam Abbing, the founding father of Dutch HIA

In 1992 Ernst Roscam Abbing was Director of the Municipal Public Health Service in the city of Rotterdam. He published an article in a national newspaper stating that the extension of the local airport would harm the population's health and wondering why EIA, but no HIA was undertaken. The city Aldermen were not supportive, but after reading a report on the topic the Minister of Health decided to set up a national HIA support unit.

Why was the HIA unit initially successful and why was it disbanded after a number of years?

At first, the Minister of Health was highly involved and ensured that the unit was financially supported. More recently economic development came to be more highly valued than health.

Why was there no HIA legislation developed?

We were hesitant to pursue legislation and preferred to rely on administrative agreements. There were already so many legal requirements in place that statutory HIA might turn into a tick-box exercise. Also, high-ranking civil servants were opposed to the idea of an HIA law.

What were the highlights of those early years?

Firstly, a multi-step approach with a rapid screening procedure to identify policies potentially relevant to health. We developed word-search software to screen policies. In those days it was ahead of its time but nowadays Google could do the job! Secondly, we managed to get some consensus with those working in other policy fields regarding the definition of health and health determinants. We made less progress with the development of quantification in HIA. Presently this is being accomplished, for example through societal cost–benefit analysis. Even though health should—at the end of the day—not be expressed in financial terms, quantification does ensure that other sectors recognize health interests as 'real'. HIA makes dilemmas visible.

health risks. In addition, positive health impacts and impacts on lifestyle are not considered in EIA. After 2000 a number of international and national developments, such as the EU guideline 2001/42/EG for SEA and the National Action Programme for Health and Environment 2002–2006,[3] promoted the integration of health in local environmental, traffic, or spatial policies and the importance of EIA for this purpose.

In 2009 the Commission of EIA experts recommended that assessment of health impacts should be undertaken for large infrastructural industrial projects and airports near residential areas and that health should be considered when designing residential areas and in those projects where people were worried about potential health risks (e.g. intensive farming or the impacts of exposure to electromagnetic fields near high-voltage power lines). Alternatives that could prevent or limit negative health impacts, such as positioning dwellings and schools so that the health effects of noise, air pollution, and other risks were minimal and access to green spaces and opportunities for cycling and walking optimal, should be considered in EIA.[4] In practice, however, most EIAs focus on preventing environmentally related health risks and do not consider health in a broader sense. There is no legal obligation for EIA to consider health impacts outside the environmental scope. If a first screening of the planned activity points to large health impacts or many concerns about potential health effects, a more detailed quantitative health impact assessment should be carried out.

Two streams merging

Over the past few years the two streams in HIA have started to come together. Environmental HIA has expanded its approach from a focus on 'classical' environmental factors to aspects such as lifestyle, social cohesion, and access to facilities, while public health authorities in municipalities show greater interest in spatial planning. The risk-based approach (as used in the environmental field) is being joined with a health promotion approach, which seeks opportunities to enhance population health. It has been suggested that EIA should focus more on developing a 'healthy' alternative rather than the most 'environmental friendly 'alternative. In government policies the Ministry of Health, Welfare and Sport advocates an HiAP approach, as described in 'Being Healthy, Staying Healthy',[5] which emphasizes both health enhancement and reduction of health risk.

Legal position of HIA in the Netherlands

There are currently several legal frameworks in place that potentially promote the application of HIA in the Netherlands. The Public Health Act requires that municipalities examine the health consequences of local policies, but gives no guidance about how this should be done and does not mention HIA. The Inspectorate for Health Care has concluded that municipalities do not live up to this legal requirement and the HIA tools that have been developed for the local situation are little used. The City and Environment Act regulates infrastructural planning in environmentally vulnerable sites. The law defines the conditions under which development is permitted and requires an assessment of the impacts on population health. The Act led to the development of the HIA for City and Environment tool described in a later section (page 145).

In decision making on national policies consideration of health is more a process of attaining mutual consent than the application of a single HIA method. New policies are discussed in the Ministerial Board, where the Minister of Health, Welfare and Sport can raise concerns about the health impacts of other minister's policies. Here the focus of the Ministry of Health is on identifying and using parallel interests in different policy fields. Health in general, and HIA in particular, are not high on the agenda of other ministries, as illustrated by the lack of attention to HIA in the new national policy on spatial planning.[6]

Several publications have highlighted the limited or absent health focus in EIA and SEA.[7] Although legislation on EIA and SEA includes an obligation to consider health impacts, this is formulated in a generic way and gives no specific details of recommended procedures, tools, or indicators. The only exception to this was the recommendation by the Minister of Transport in 2010 that the HIA City and Environment tool and the DALY method should be used in EIAs of road infrastructure. The pressure to effectively translate the generic obligations into real practice comes not so much from policy makers as from professionals working in the environmental and health field who are exploring methods and procedures to include health in environmental assessments.

Meanwhile, the National Action Plan for Environment and Health 2008–2012, a joint initiative of five Ministries,[8] underlines the importance of assessing the health and environmental aspects of policy decisions. The plan mentions the need to develop tools and methods for HIA. The 2011 progress report of the Action Plan mentions that the Ministry of Infrastructure and Environment applies HIA as a way to avoid health risks due to environmental or infrastructural measures.

Methods for HIA in the Netherlands

There are many HIA instruments and methods available for different purposes, situations, and applications in the Netherlands. Some methods focus on qualitative assessments, others on quantification of health impacts. Which method is needed depends on the type, location, and scale of the initiative as well as the perception of the health risks associated with it. In 2009, an online HIA database was established that provided an overview of available instruments.[9]

Many practitioners would like a 'roadmap' of qualitative and quantitative HIA methods, describing when and how they should be applied. In 2011, a working group of experts compiled an advisory letter on the available HIA methodology for EIA, describing situations in which the different methods could be used best and how.[10] The main conclusion was that exposure-oriented methods could easily be used but that more health-oriented approaches, such as disease burden calculations, although complex to use, should be applied in situations where screening indicated large health impacts or uncertainty about potential health effects.

In 2005 the National Institute for Public Health and the Environment (RIVM) published general guidance on HIA containing a step-by-step approach as well as an HIA checklist. Much attention was paid to the process approach in HIA that promotes health sensitivity in other policy fields. An HiAp approach, including a generic framework for HIA, for local policy development, is the basis of the Guide for Healthy Municipalities. This online guidance provides practical advice about intersectoral cooperation to prevent smoking, obesity, depression, alcohol abuse, and injury, and to promote sexual health. This includes process guidance regarding such cooperation, such as how to create support in other sectors and how to involve different stakeholders.

Spatial planning tools

The Ministry of Environment and Infrastructure supported the development of the HIA City and Environment method. This method can be used to assess the potential impacts of spatial plans (e.g. infrastructural, traffic circulation plans) on environmental exposures relevant for health. Population-based exposure concentrations are calculated based on limit values and available exposure response functions—each exposure category receives a health impact score and label (good/insufficient/bad) and is visualized in contour maps. The method has been used in EIAs and local spatial planning. A handbook with background information on the calculations is available.[11] An evaluation by users and decision makers in 2010 showed that the tool had been applied successfully in more than 90 projects and gave a good overview of environmentally related health risks. However, because of the broad exposure categories used, it was not always sensitive enough to compare plan alternatives and did not give a picture of cumulative and non-environmental health risk.

An online health in spatial planning checklist has been developed by RIVM for planners and decision makers at the start of the spatial planning process.[12] The checklist looks at changes in social and lifestyle factors as well as environmental determinants, and links to the most recent background information on specific determinants and their health effects. By answering a set of questions the planners can get a broad overview of the potential positive or negative health impacts of the planned initiative. Fifty professionals who evaluated the tool concluded that it was useful but not very often used and that it needed to be expanded with information and recommendations on the general HIA process and other determinants.

Quantitative methods

The Dutch approach to HIA emphasizes the need for quantification of health effects whenever possible. The advantages of quantification are discussed in Chapter 3 (page 25). Integrated health measures combining different health impacts such as mortality and morbidity allow evaluation of plans with various health outcomes.

Integrated metrics such as the burden of disease metric can be used for:[13]

◆ comparative evaluations of plan alternatives ('How bad is it?')

◆ evaluation of the effectiveness of policies (largest reduction of disease burden)

◆ estimation of the accumulation of health risks

◆ communication of health risks.

Dutch institutions played an important part in the development of quantitative HIA models and tools through their contribution to the EU projects DYNAMO and INTARESE (discussed in Chapter 17, page 163). These models are usually difficult for non-health experts to apply and often the data needed for quantification of health impacts are difficult to obtain or lacking, especially at the local level. Studies on the health impacts of Schiphol airport are briefly described in Box 15.2.

Box 15.2 Expansion of Amsterdam Schiphol Airport

An HIA and epidemiological studies have been carried out to assess the (potential) health impacts of the expansion of Schiphol Airport. RIVM carried out a monitoring programme during the period 2002–2008 to keep a close watch on the ongoing impacts of the expansion on health.

The results of this monitoring programme confirmed most health impacts as predicted in the HIA studies of the 1990s. The main impacts observed were annoyance, sleep disturbance, impacts on school performance (in children), and high blood pressure in relation to increased noise levels. A special commission of stakeholders was installed to safeguard the quality of the living environment. Based on the monitoring programme results the municipal health service of Amsterdam advised that public health should be part of future decision making on Schiphol.

Research on HIA in the Netherlands

Very little research has yet been carried out regarding HIA implementation in the Netherlands. The published research focuses mostly on the effectiveness of HIA, and in particular the effectiveness of HIA as a process. Bekker[14] has evaluated four cases of HIA. She describes how a 'technocratic' focus in HIA, excluding non-expert stakeholders, leads to a politicization of knowledge instead of a rationalization of policy, making the HIA less effective. Additionally, studies were performed regarding HiAP, which may be viewed as the broader framework for HIA.[15] These studies have provided knowledge regarding the conditions necessary to carry out HiAP effectively. They also show the importance of closer proximity to other policy fields—intersectoral cooperation is generally easier when carried out with 'soft' sectors (education, social services, etc.) than with sectors like spatial planning. Knol evaluated some methods and tools for integrated environmental HIA, recommending a general procedure including a practical expert elicitation to deal with uncertainties.[16]

Barriers to the use of HIA

There are several barriers to the use of HIA in the Netherlands:

- There is no comprehensive legislation for HIA in the Netherlands. In part this because of the current economic crisis, which leads to pressure to limit the EIA process strictly to legislative requirements.

- Public health professionals and agencies lack knowledge on the most effective way to address the potential health benefits or negative impacts at an early stage of policy or plan development. Moreover, there is no national or central support or education programme.

- There is method 'overload'. Several methods and tools are available in the Netherlands for the assessment of health impacts, including qualitative and quantitative methods and process directions. Public health and/or environmental practitioners lack knowledge about when to apply which HIA methodology. A road map providing guidance could be useful.

- It is difficult to assess the quantitative health impacts of complex projects and plans. Models and methods in the area of environmental HIA have been developed but are still hard for non-experts to apply. In addition, relevant input data is often lacking at local level, as well as consensus about attributable risks and weight factors.

The direction and future of HIA in the Netherlands depends on progress in overcoming these barriers. Different stakeholders, on a national and local level, will contribute to this but economic, cultural, and social developments will also be important.

Conclusions

Expertise, methods, and knowledge for HIA are available in the Netherlands. Much attention has been paid to HIA at the local level and many interesting developments have occurred during the last decade. Health experts participate more often in the EIA process and the Commission for EIA provides information to consultants on HIA methodology. The national government advocates the application of HiAP, which provides a background for HIA, but implementation proceeds slowly. Even though in several cities (e.g. The Hague, Rotterdam, and Amsterdam) there is a close collaboration between the municipal health service and city planners, there is no systematic approach and many municipalities do not carry out HIAs of their local policies.

Acknowledgements

We thank Professor Roscam Abbing for his valuable comments.

References

1. Roscam Abbing E. HIA and national policy in the Netherlands, in Kemm J, Parry J, Palmer S. (eds), Health Impact Assessment: Concepts, theory, technique and applications. Oxford: Oxford University Press, 2004.
2. Ministry of Health, Welfare and Sports. Gezond en Wel. Kader voor het volksgezondheisbeleid 1995-1998 [Safe and sound. Framework for the national policy 1995–1998]. Parliamentary document 24126, No 3. The Hague: Ministry of Health, Welfare and Sports, 1995.
3. Ministry of Housing, Spatial Planning and the Environment. Actieprogramma Gezondheid en Milieu. Uitwerking van een beleidsversterking [Action programme for health and environment: Development of a policy reinforcement]. Parliamentary document 28 089, No 2. The Hague: Ministry of Housing, Spatial Planning and the Environment, 2002.
4. National Council for Environmental Assessment. Factsheet no 13. Health in EIA. Available at www.eia.nl. Accessed 26 March 2012.
5. Ministry of Health, Welfare and Sport. Being Healthy, Staying Healthy. A vision of health and prevention in The Netherlands. Ministry of Health, Welfare, and Sports: The Hague, 2007. Available at http://www.rivm.nl/vtv/object_binary/o5512_fo_being_ healthy.pdf. Accessed 26 March 2012.
6. Vries de L. Letter to the Minister on national policy infrastructure & space. Utrecht: National Health Services, 2011.
7. Alphen T van, L den Broeder, I Storm. More attention for health in EIA [in Dutch]. Bilthoven: RIVM, 2008.

8. Ministry of Infrastructure and Environment. National Approach Environment and Health 2008–2012. Ministry of Housing, Spatial Planning and the Environment: The Hague, 2008.

9. RIVM. HIA database. Available at http://gezondeplannen.ibase.info/. Accessed 26 March 2012.

10. Fast T, wekkeboom JK, Zwerver C. Methods for health in EIA and planning [in Dutch].Fastadvies, 2012. Available at http://www.ggdkennisnet.nl/thema/organisatie-medisch-milieukundige-zorg/publicaties/publicatie/4026. Accessed 26 March 2012.

11. Fast T, Weerdt RVD. Manual for HIA City & Environment. Available at http://www. rijksoverheid.nl/documenten-en-publicaties/brochures/2010/07/01/handboek-gezondheidseffectscreening-stad-milieu-voor-de-inrichting-van-een-gezonde-leefomgeving.html. Accessed 26 March 2012.

12. RIVM. Guide to spatial planning. Available at http://www.gezondheidinmer.nl/isurvey/default.aspx. Accessed 26 March 2012.

13. Knol AB, Staatsen BAM. Trends in the environmental burden of disease in the Netherlands 1980-2020. Bilthoven: RIVM, 2005. Available at http://www.rivm.nl/bibliotheek/rapporten/500029001.html. Accessed 26 March 2012.

14. Bekker M. The politics of healthy policies. Redesigning Health Impact Assessment to integrate health in public policy. Rotterdam: Eburon, 2007.

15. Storm I, Jansen J, Schuit A. Effects of policy measures outside public health domain on health. An explorative study [in Dutch]. Bilthoven: RIVM, 2009. Available at http://www.rivm.nl/bibliotheek/rapporten/270304001.html. Accessed 26 March 2012.

16. Knol AB. Health and the environment: assessing the impacts, addressing the uncertainties. Thesis, Utrecht University, 2010.

Chapter 16

Health impact assessment in Spain

Elena Aldosoro, Carlos Artundo, and Ana Rivadeneyra

Legal and policy context

The Spanish state is currently made up of a central administration and 17 highly decentralized regions or autonomous communities (ACs), with their own governments and parliaments. The development of HIA reflects this political structure. Health competences have been transferred to the ACs and their health departments hold primary responsibility for healthcare policy, planning, and regulation within their territory. The national Ministry of Health, Social Policy and Equity (MHSPE) is accountable for strategic functioning and coordination of the National Health Service, including the provision of a general framework for public health policy and basic enabling legislation.

As with other countries with a decentralized administration, drivers for the development and practice of HIA have mainly evolved at the regional level, where the health authorities are increasingly engaging with the health determinants agenda. Within this framework, health policy documents and strategies issued in the last decade have paid more attention to health equity and the determinants of health. Likewise, the health plans formulated by the regional administrations increasingly include explicit reference to HIA as a way of implementing HiAP and improving public policy formulation. Interest in HIA has also grown at a national level in line with the MHSPE's focus on the surveillance of the social determinants of health and the reduction of health inequalities. These were among the main priorities of the Spanish presidency of the EU in 2010. A commission of experts, appointed in 2008 to design a national strategy to reduce social inequalities in health, recommended use of HIA in policy formulation and the development of research and capacity building for HIA across Spain.[1]

Until very recently there was no statutory requirement for HIA in Spain. HIA practice has developed in accordance with WHO recommendations and the above-mentioned policy framework. The situation is currently evolving in the context of a wider process of public health reforms launched by the central and regional health administrations in the last few years. As part of the reforms, a new generation of public health laws is being introduced to support the modernization, reorganization, and strengthening of public health. While differing in approaches and degree of formality, some of the new laws already approved or under discussion include provisions that pave the way for developing a legal context favourable to HIA in Spain.

Normative reform has already been achieved in a number of ACs, including Valencia, Catalonia, the Balearic Islands, Castilla-León, Extremadura, and Andalucia. The new public health Acts introduced in Catalonia[2] in 2009 and the Balearic Islands[3] in 2010, while not establishing an explicit legal mandate for HIA, include services to be provided by the public health departments. In addition, the Catalonian Act lists HIA delivery among the functions assigned to the Public Health Agency of Catalonia. In Andalucia a new Act passed in 2011[4] requires HIA on public policies and programmes that significantly affect health, as well as on general urban planning schemes and a predefined group of projects and activities subjected to EIA. In the Basque Country a bill under discussion portrays HIA as a governance tool to advance HiAP and introduces an obligation to perform HIA on policies, programmes, projects, and regulations that are likely to have a significant effect on health.

In addition to this legislation by ACs, the approval of the Spanish General Public Health Act[5] by the national parliament in September 2011 represented a milestone in the development of HIA in Spain. Driven by the HiAP approach, health equity, and the wider determinants of health, it explicitly introduces HIA as an effective tool to promote healthy public policies. Furthermore, it creates a legal mandate for HIA, stating that 'the public administrations will have to carry out HIAs on regulations, plans, programmes and projects being selected for significantly impacting on health'. In addition, in order to provide a general framework for future enabling regulations at national, regional, and local levels, this Act establishes a new statutory obligation that will certainly help the development and institutionalization of HIA across Spain.

History of HIA and examples of HIAs undertaken in Spain

The first initiative supporting HIA practice in Spain was the publication of a guidance manual in Spanish in 2005.[6] Most HIAs documented so far have been conducted at the regional or local level and led by proactive health administrations. In the Basque Country in 2006, the Department of Health performed an HIA of a regeneration project in a disadvantaged neighbourhood in

Bilbao.[7] This pioneering experience was followed by the development and validation of a screening tool for regional public policies in 2009–2010.[8] Currently another HIA is being conducted on two components of the regeneration plan of Pasaia Bay, the new fish market and the renewal of an urban area called La Herrera.

HIA practice in other ACs is more recent. In Andalusia in 2009, the General Direction of Public Health launched a research project to develop new tools and capabilities for HIA. Two pilot HIAs have resulted from this project: a prospective HIA of an urban renewal project in the city of Alcalá de Guadaira[9] and the validation of a screening procedure and tools on a regional intersectoral plan by means of a participative workshop with relevant stakeholders. In the Balearic Islands in 2009, the Public Health Department developed a new tool to support the HIA process and take account of the health needs and involvement of key stakeholders. This tool, a web platform created as a common space for sharing knowledge, is currently being validated through its application to a housing regeneration project at Palma de Mallorca beach. In Catalonia, the Public Health Agency of Barcelona has taken the lead in developing HIA-related tools and methods by applying an HIA to a set of planned rehabilitation measures in a deprived neighbourhood in inner city Barcelona.[10]

Other HIAs documented in Spain include a study on the health impacts of the construction of a subway in the city of Granada conducted in 2005 in the context of a public health master's degree for the Andalusian School of Public Health. The municipality of Vitoria-Gasteiz, a member of the Spanish Network of Healthy Cities, has also used an HIA to assess the health effects of a major project that involved burying the current railroad running through the city centre, re-utilizing the space released, and constructing a new transport hub.[11]

In addition to these experiences, framed around the WHO Gothenburg Consensus Statement, HIA implementation in Spain includes other initiatives with a strong focus on quantification and risk assessment methods and tools. Some examples include the HIA procedures implemented as part of research projects APHEIS,[12] ENHIS-II,[13] APHEKOM,[14] and CERCA,[15] which are providing valuable evidence on the health impacts of air pollution across Spain.

Capacity building and awareness for HIA development and practice

Over the last few years a number of training sessions and workshops on basic concepts and methods of HIA have taken place in Spain, led by national HIA practitioners and some international experts. These activities have primarily targeted public health professionals, health policy planners, and, to a lesser extent, technical staff from the municipalities and regional administrations. Most of this training has been organized in those ACs more familiar with HIA. Some training has also been provided in ACs with no practical experience of HIA as a first step to raise awareness and to create new capacities. In addition, a basic HIA training module has been included in the education programme of the Andalusian School of Public Health as well as in the public health master's degree offered at the University of the Basque Country. The Spanish Network of Healthy Cities has also led some training sessions targeting the municipalities included in the network.

Other formal activities to raise HIA awareness have included an international policy dialogue jointly organized in 2008 in Seville by the European Observatory of Health Systems and Policies the General Direction of Public Health of the Andalusian Health Department. In addition, two meetings of international experts took place in the cities of Mahon and San Sebastian in 2010. Furthermore, HIA has been included among the topics discussed at the annual convention of Public Health Directors held since 2008 at the Summer School of Public Health in Mahon and organized by the Health Department of the Balearic Islands.

HIA-related networking activities have also been organized over the last few years at the national and regional levels. Communities of practice bringing together HIA practitioners, other key stakeholders, public health institutions, and scientific societies have been created in the Basque country, Andalucia, the Balearic Islands, and Catalonia. In addition, the General Directorate of Public Health at the MHSPE announced a project in 2012 to create a national network of public health experts to develop a strategic approach to HIA implementation across Spain. Although political changes have delayed the formal constitution of the network, it has already paved the way for proactive collaboration among public health institutions and professionals interested in HIA. In the field of EIA, the Spanish Society of Environmental Health is leading initiatives to develop methodological guidelines to promote the systematic consideration of health in EIA processes.

Other recent developments that have contributed to new alliances and increasing HIA awareness and capacity in Spain are the creation of the Spanish Association of Health Impact Assessment in 2010 and the celebration of the XI HIA International Conference in April 2011 in Granada, which was attended by delegates from 25 countries and discussed cutting-edge HIA theory and practice from around the world. The Andalusian School of Public Health has also launched CREIS,[16] a new website that gives access to HIA materials and information in Spanish.

Conclusion

HIA in Spain is still in the earlier stages of development. Practice of HIA remains unevenly distributed across regions and is usually on projects. It is often conducted as a pilot in research settings and as a test of new tools and methods. However, as this chapter has shown, significant advances have been made in the last few years in line with policy makers' growing interest in health equity, health determinants, and, more recently, HiAP. The new public health Acts being formulated at national and regional levels are providing new opportunities to undertake HIA across Spain and, more importantly, to promote its contribution to decision-making processes. Nevertheless, experience in other countries has shown that further capacity building and resources in the form of guidelines, tools, and evidence will be needed to develop the use of HIA. Strong political commitment from policy makers and stewardship from public health professionals is also critical to raise awareness of HIA and to engage non-health sectors in the process. The experience of those ACs that have made progress with HIA is raising interest in other ACs and will serve as a lever for future action to promote the development and practice of HIA in Spain.

Acknowledgements

The assistance of the following with this chapter is gratefully acknowledged:

Bacigalupe Amaia,[A] Boldo Elena,[B] Cabeza Elena,[C] Colom Toni,[D] Esnaola Santiago,[A] Fernandez Alberto,[E] Gómez Francisco,[F] Martin Piedad,[E] Morteruel Maite,[G] Angelina González de Viana,[H] and Vargas Francisco.[I]

References

1. Comisión para Reducir las Desigualdades Sociales en Salud en España. Avanzando hacia la equidad Propuesta de políticas e intervenciones para reducir las desigualdades sociales en salud en España. Ministerio de Sanidad y Política Social: Madrid, 2010. Available at http://www.mspsi.gob.es/profesionales/saludPublica/prevPromocion/promocion/desigualdadSalud/docs/Propuesta_Politicas_Reducir_Desigualdades.pdf. Accessed 28 February 2012.

[A] Health Studies and Research Department, Basque Health Government

[B] Health Institute Carlos III-CIBERESP

[C] Public Health General Directorate, Balearic Islands Health Department

[D] Balearic Islands Health Department

[E] Andalusian School of Public Health, Andalusian Health Department

[F] Health and Consumers Affairs Department, Vitoria-Gasteiz City Council

[G] Public Health Agency of Barcelona-CIBERESP

[H] Catalonian Health Department

[I] Public Health Directorate, Spanish Ministry of Health, Social Policies and Equity

2. Llei 18/2009, de 22 d'octubre, de salut pública. Available at http://www.boe.es/boe/dias/2009/11/16/pdfs/BOE-A-2009-18178.pdf. Accessed 28 February 2012.

3. Ley 16/2010, de 28 de diciembre, de salud pública de las Illes Balears. Available at http://www.boe.es/boe/dias/2011/02/04/pdfs/BOE-A-2011-2108.pdf. Accessed 28 February 2012.

4. Ley de salud publica de Andalucia. Available at http://www.parlamentodeandalucia.es/webdinamica/portal-web-parlamento/pdf.do?tipodoc=bopa&id=65373. Accessed 28 February 2012.

5. Ley 33/2011, de 4 de octubre, General de Salud Pública. Available at http://www.boe.es/boe/dias/2011/10/05/pdfs/BOE-A-2011-15623.pdf. Accessed 28 February 2012.

6. Rueda JR. Guía para la evaluación del impacto en la salud y en el bienestar de proyectos, programas o políticas extrasanitarias. Gobierno Vasco, Vitoria-Gasteiz: Departamento de Sanidad, 2005. Available at http://www9.euskadi.net/sanidad/osteba/datos/d_05-04_guia_evaluacion_impacto_salud.pdf. Accessed 28 February 2012.

7. Bacigalupe A, Esnaola S, Calderon C, Zuazagoitia J, Aldasoro E. Health impact assessment of an urban regeneration project: opportunities and challenges in the context of a southern European city. Journal of Epidemiology and Community Health 2010; 64: 950–55.

8. Aldasoro E, Sanz E, Bacigalupe A, Esnaola S, Calderon C, Cambra K, Zuazogoitia J. Avanzando en la evaluación del impacto en la salud: análisis de las políticas públicas sectoriales del Gobierno Vasco como paso previo a la fase de cribado sistemático. Gac Sanitaria 2012; 26: 83–90.

9. Venegas J, Artundo C, Bolívar J, López LA, Rivadeneyra A. HIA of an urban regeneration project in Alcalá de Guadaíra: a pilot experience in Andalucía. XI International Health Impact Assessment Book of Abstracts 2011 available at http://si.easp.es/eis2011/wp-content/uploads/2011/04/HIA11_book_of_abstracts.pdf

10. Morteruel M, Díez E. Health impact assessment of buildings rehabilitation measures in a neighbourhood of Barcelona. XI International Health Impact Assessment Book of Abstracts 2011 available at http://si.easp.es/eis2011/wp-content/uploads/2011/04/HIA11_book_of_abstracts.pdf

11. Gómez F, Estibalez JJ. Health impact assessment of the tunnelling of the railroad in Vitoria-Gasteiz, Spain. XI International Health Impact Assessment Book of Abstracts 2011 available at http://si.easp.es/eis2011/wp-content/uploads/2011/04/HIA11_book_of_abstracts.pdf

12. APHEIS monitoring the effects of air pollution on health in Europe. Available at http://www.apheis.org/. Accessed 28 February 2012.

13. Environment and Health Information System, WHO. Available at http://www.euro.who.int/en/what-we-do/data-and-evidence/environment-and-health-information-system-enhis. Accessed 28 February 2012.

14. Aphekom. Improving knowledge and communication for decision making on air pollution and health in Europe. Available at http://www.aphekom.org. Accessed 28 February 2012.

15. Boldo E, Linares C, Lumbreras J, Borge R, Narros A, García-Pérez J, Fernández-Navarro P, Pérez-Gómez B, Aragonés N, Ramis R, Pollán M, Moreno T, Karanasiou A, López-Abente G. *et al.* Health impact assessment of a reduction in ambient PM2.5 levels in Spain. Environment International 2011; 37: 342–48.

16. Centro de Recursos en Evaluación del Impacto en Salud, CREIS. Available at http://www.creis.es. Accessed 28 February 2012.

Chapter 17

Health impact assessment in Germany

Rainer Fehr and Odile Mekel

Evolution of HIA in Germany

The potential of HIA for health promotion and protection was recognized early in Germany; case studies of HIA projects were conducted and some infrastructure was developed. Contributions from Germany to international HIA research include an integrative view of HIA and efforts towards health impact quantification.

The first paper in German calling for HIA was published just before the German Environmental Impact Assessment (EIA) Act was passed in 1990.[1] In 1992, the Conference of German Ministers of Health approved a resolution on HIA in the context of EIA. The first German research project on HIA was conducted from 1992 to 1995, and the first German HIA workshop was held in 1993. From 1995 onwards, a research project at the University of Bielefeld on quantitative risk assessment included HIA issues.[2] In 1997, a survey on HIA training in Germany was conducted and the first (and up to now: only) book in German on HIA[3] was published. The North Rhine-Westphalian Public Health Service Act, §8 calls for HIA in local planning[4] but a survey of HIA practice in the state demonstrated the need for improvement.[5]

A paper on the German developments constituting one of the earliest published guides to HIA was presented at the 1997 WHO/ILO consultation on HIA in Geneva[6] and at the Leo Kaprio HIA Workshop in 1999. In the Gothenburg discussion paper,[7] the Bielefeld approach was presented as one of six HIA models together with an overview of computer tools and resources, organized along the 10 steps of the HIA procedure.[8]

Within the framework of the German National Environmental Health Action Plan, a national HIA workshop agreed on 10 recommendations for promoting HIA in Germany.[9] Within the North Rhine-Westphalian Environmental Health Action Plan, a discussion on health in planning stressed the need for intersectoral cooperation.[10]

HIA terminology

Terminology has always been an issue in the discussion of HIA in German. With EIA officially (and undisputedly) being translated as *Umweltverträglichkeitsprüfung*, it seemed obvious to translate HIA as *Gesundheitsverträglichkeitsprüfung*. This term, however, never became popular because it is lengthy and not a precise translation of HIA, conveying a notion of 'compatibility testing'.[7] For some, it evokes associations of 'red tape', whereas the positive vision of potential health-promoting impacts is lost. The terms *Gesundheitsfolgenabschätzung* or *Gesundheitsfolgenanalyse* are now more widely used, while the term *Gesundheitsbilanz* is being explored.

In Germany, in addition to activities with explicit reference to either HIA or roughly equivalent German terms, there are activities of similar character, for example under the heading of 'planning involvement' (*Mitwirkung an Planung*) or simply as 'expert testimony' (*Gutachten*). Much of this work exists only as 'grey' literature or is never made publicly accessible. The absence of a universally accepted terminology in Germany makes it harder to identify the status quo.

Concerning the legal basis for HIA in Germany, besides EIA and SEA there are Public Health Service Acts in several federal states, including North Rhine-Westphalia, calling for involvement in spatial planning. In one state (Sachsen-Anhalt), the Act explicitly speaks of *Gesundheitsverträglichkeitsprüfung*.[11] These Acts, however, do not seem to have induced much HIA activity.

HIA projects in Germany

The first German HIA project was conducted within the framework of the North Rhine-Westphalian Research Consortium on Public Health and funded by the Federal Ministry of Research and Technology. Predominantly rooted in environmental health, the project developed a methodology including the Bielefeld 10-step HIA procedure, produced practice examples, and conducted training workshops.[12]

HIA projects with German involvement, co-funded by the European Commission (EC), produced HIA examples, tools, and guidelines, and strengthened international cooperation. In these projects, German researchers and public health professionals took on a variety of roles, including leadership, participation, advisory board member, etc.:

♦ Environmental Health Information Management (EHIM)

♦ European Policy Health Impact Assessment (EPHIA)

♦ Promoting and Supporting Integrated Approaches for Health and Sustainable Development at the Local Level Across Europe (PHASE)

- Environment and Health Information System Supporting Policy-Making in Europe, with HIA component (ENHIS)
- Effectiveness of Health Impact Assessment (HIA Effectiveness)
- Dynamic Modelling for Health Impact Assessment (DYNAMO HIA)
- Integrated Assessment of Health Risks of Environmental Stressors in Europe/Health and Environment Integrated Methodology and Toolbox for Scenario Assessment (INTARESE-HEIMTSA)
- Risk Assessment from Policy to Impact Dimension (RAPID)
- Impact of Structural Funds on Health Gains (Healthgain.EU).

As an example, the EPHIA project produced guidelines that were simultaneously published in Dutch, English, French, and German.[13] Information on international HIA projects has been summarized and published[14] but knowledge of international HIA projects is still limited in Germany.

Examples of HIA from Germany

Based on a broad understanding of HIA, the NRW Centre for Health (LZG. NRW) and predecessor institutes produced a range of HIA examples covering a wide range of topics, as shown in Table 17.1. Some impact assessments dealt with employment strategy, housing policy, spatial planning, and demographic change, while others focused on environmental health topics, for example waste site extension, transport planning, and drinking water privatization.

Generally these HIAs used the stepwise procedure mentioned earlier. Most of them involved some quantification of selected health determinants and/or health effects, and sometimes probabilistic modelling was applied. With the exception of the housing subsidy programme, HIA participation of stakeholders or the public was weakly developed or absent.

Even in a country with no explicit HIA programme it is possible to perform HIAs. The EC co-funded projects provide an opportunity to improve HIA practice. Planning processes in Germany involve the public extensively and large numbers of institutions. The number of statements and suggestions received by planning officials can be substantial, so that the HIA may be just one among many statements. For those testifying on health it is a challenge to optimize their contribution, especially in the absence of standard procedures. For those managing the planning process, it is likewise challenging to evaluate and integrate the multitude of suggestions received, and to fully utilize the HIA input.

Integration of HIA with other assessments

Partially triggered by language concerns, an in-depth understanding of the English term HIA was sought. Interpreting the three basic components as

Table 17.1 Examples of health impact assessments from Germany

Policy/plan/project	Type	Spatial reference	Qualitative aspects	Quantitative aspects
1. European Employment Strategy (EES)[21]	Policy	Germany/Europe	◆ Policy analysis: implementation in Germany, especially flexibility of employment, literature reviews ◆ Participatory workshop: aspects of implementation of EU strategy in Germany, scenario development, prioritization	◆ Self-reported health status; absenteeism ◆ Modelling the flexibility of employments ◆ Point estimates and distributional estimates of additional and/or avoided cases of impaired health
2. Demographic change in Ruhr area[29]	Baseline for policies	Federal state and subregion	◆ Decreasing and ageing population ◆ Selection of appropriate groups of diagnoses: certain neoplasms, myocardial infarction, dementia	◆ Application of WHO methodology 'Burden of disease', using disability adjusted life Years (DALYs) ◆ Based on predicted changes of age distribution: Estimation of changes of burden of disease
3. Joint regional land utilization plan Ruhr[30]	Plan	Consortium of six cities	◆ Planning process, structure and content of regional joint plan ◆ Legal basis for human health as an item of concern ◆ Coverage of health in the text/maps/environmental report, assessment, and recommendations	(not implemented)
4. Housing subsidy program NRW[31]	Program	Federal state	◆ Analysis of components of the subsidy programme ◆ Causal web with various causal pathways ◆ Participatory workshops	◆ Modelling of selected causal pathways ◆ Point estimates of additional and/or avoided cases of disease and injury
5. Waste site extension[32]	Project	Four hamlets	◆ Structure model with seven exposure pathways ◆ Complex physicochemical processes within the waste site, range of emitted pollutants, e.g. in leachate, additional road traffic ◆ Vulnerable populations, e.g. children and teenagers	◆ Modelling for 'receptors' in several locations ◆ (Carcinogenic) emissions, pollutant levels, exposures ◆ Additional cancer risks and cancer cases ◆ Noise exposure

(continued)

Table 17.1 (Continued) Examples of health impact assessments from Germany

Policy/plan/project	Type	Spatial reference	Qualitative aspects	Quantitative aspects
6. Highway project: circular road[33]	Project	City/outskirts	◆ Various siting options ◆ Innercity traffic relief ◆ Planning areas with vulnerable populations, e.g. seniors	◆ Traffic densities; chemical emissions, pollutant levels, exposures; noise exposures, espec. at night ◆ Injuries and deaths due to traffic crashes
7. Drinking water privatization[34]	Policy	Federal state/ Europe	◆ Qualitative model: legal requirements, over-achievements vs. economic approach ◆ Identification of eight carcinogens in drinking water	◆ Additional cancer cases: point estimates and distributional estimates for lifetime risks ◆ Relative risks; additional cancer cases
8. Environmental tobacco smoke (ETS) and non-smoker protection[35]	Policy	Federal state	◆ Non-smoker protection legislation in NRW (2008) ◆ Affected by ETS: health of children (including pre-natal), of adults ◆ Range of health impacts of ETS exposure	◆ Application of WHO methodology 'Environmental burden of disease', before and after policy implementation ◆ Estimation of fractions of burden of disease (e.g. DALYs) attributable to ETS
9. Living on a contaminated site[36 37]	Baseline for clean-up projects	City quarters	◆ Discussion of quantitative risk analysis for impact assessments ◆ Sample applications: settlements on sites contaminated with (i) cadmium and (ii) dioxins and furans	◆ Quantitative exposure assessment, using personal and chemical-specific parameters ◆ Point estimates and probabilistic exposure estimates ◆ Measured (HBM) vs. modeled exposure
10. Traffic noise/children[38]	Baseline for policies	For example cities	◆ Development of guideline for this topic ◆ 'High annoyance' and 'sleep disturbance' were identified as proxy outcomes for which data were available ◆ Various scenarios of noise reduction described	◆ Calculation of attributable cases, based on modeled exposures and adjusted exposure-response functions ◆ Estimation of health gains under various scenarios

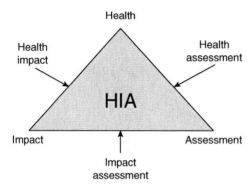

Fig. 17.1 The 'semantic triangle' of health impact assessment.

corners of a triangle, three binary components emerge (Figure 17.1). While 'health impact' identifies the key topic in HIA, the other two terms pinpoint relevant *contexts*, one being (other) 'health assessments' and the other being (other) 'impact assessments'.

This view leads to the larger issue of the science–policy interface which, in Germany, features a range of approaches, including expert opinion and testimony, hearings, and advisory councils. Formal impact assessment procedures are established in the environment sector in Germany but not yet in the health sector. Discussion of HIA is often related to the EIA 'culture'.

HIA and other health assessments

HIA can be regarded as one health assessment among others, including health needs assessment, health technology assessment (HTA), health systems performance assessment, and health-related evaluation.

Comparison of HIA with HTA is instructive. A specific strength of HTA lies in the systematic and transparent exploitation of published scientific study results. Intensive networking helps to establish high standards of HTA performance. HTA results provide the basis for healthcare decision making. Interesting features of HTA include 'horizon scanning' of emerging technological developments and early warnings/early assessments. With proper adaptations, HIA might learn lessons from HTA. On the other hand, a specific strength of HIA is the adjustable mix of methods, including stakeholder participation and modelling. HTA may benefit from adaptations of this mix. HTA professionals also noticed with interest the broad scope of HIA topics both inside and outside the healthcare system: the strong role of stakeholder and public participation.

Another line of health assessments refers to economic analyses. Again, it is useful to draw comparisons with HIA. An international survey in 2006 involving respondents from 16 countries[15] found that economic valuation was rarely done within HIAs although participants identified numerous advantages and disadvantages of such valuation.

In summary, these assessments involve comprehensive, multidisciplinary, structured procedures intended to provide evidence-based support for policy formation and decision making. For most of them, a 'parent' culture can be identified, for example technology assessment. They all face the double challenge of being scientifically rigorous while also complying with health policy rationales. The assessments are motivated by the prospect of more efficiency and improved policy impact, based partially on standardization, systematic usage of existing experiences, and benchmarking opportunities. They vary with respect to their toe-holds in the public health policy cycle, strength of relationship with respective 'parent' culture, level of implementation, and scope of practical impact.

HIA and other impact assessments

Internationally, a host of impact assessments has emerged, as described in Chapter 9, and the list of impact assessments for which names have been coined is long and growing. A smaller number of them are supported by specific 'cultures', for example legal basis, political support, legacy of experience, material infrastructure, etc.

Many of these impact assessments are at least partially related to human health, especially EIA and SEA. In Germany there are traditions of EIA and SEA engaging with health. In the city state of Hamburg in the period 1990 to 2003 about 170 projects were subjected to EIA and continuous involvement of the health sector in these led to a set of recommendations, including measures to prevent foreseeable limit value violations.[16] A recent report from the city state of Bremen focusing on environmental health examples underlines the need for improvement.[17] However, taken as a whole, coverage of health in EIA is still limited in Germany.

As for SEA, a study looking at more than 50 SEA guidelines and guidance web pages found health to be mentioned in almost all the documents but few of them indicated how to assess health, whom to consult, and when to include health experts.[18] Since 2008, a working group anchored at the German EIA Association has worked on establishing adequate coverage of health in EIA/SEA and planning procedures in general.[19]

HIA could learn lessons from other impact assessments in the 'family',[20] such as the importance of a legal basis, high-ranking support, established routines, and a focus on benefits and costs. Many of the other assessments provide inspiration and insights for HIA. It seems essential to 'think' integration and be aware of the societal, administrative, and scientific contexts, including the range of other health and impact assessments with their respective cultures. In contrast, to carry out integrated assessment is not always feasible but its advantages deserve critical debate and evaluation. Where integration is not possible, there should at least be coordination of impact assessments in order to avoid duplication of work, interferences, inconsistencies, and participation fatigue. Exchange of information and discussion between HIA, other health assessments, and other impact assessments should be continued.

Quantification of health impacts

The quantification of health impacts is moving forward rapidly. Health impact metrics play a key role in health protection, health promotion, and possibly health policy at large. Quantification has been a core issue from the early days of HIA work in Germany. From 1995 to 2001, the project 'Quantitative risk assessment' (QRA) examined cross-relations to HIA and the 1997 HIA book[3] contains a chapter on QRA. The German working group 'Probabilistic exposure and risk assessment', started in 1997, evolved into a forum for public, environmental, and occupational health professionals and consumer protection specialists, and repeatedly discusses HIA issues.

Within the EC co-funded project 'European Policy HIA' (EPHIA) 2001–2003, approaches to quantification were explored.[21] The project 'Reference values and distributions for exposure factors for the German population' (Xprob), co-funded by the German Federal Environment Agency (UBA) examined standards and models of probabilistic exposure assessment and created a database system ('RefXP') that provides highly detailed data for exposure modelling.[22] This distributional information also supports quantification in HIA.

Over the years, different approaches, models, and tools have been developed internationally for health impact quantification. To provide a forum for 'overarching' discussion, an invitational scientific expert workshop was held in Düsseldorf (Germany) in March 2010[23] and an open workshop in Granada (Andalusia) in April 2011.[24] Both workshops provided opportunities to share expertise and to propagate good practice.

Results from these workshops include quantification models intended to assist and improve science–policy interaction. Such models exist in both the environmental health and the general public health arenas. In environmental health, current 'flagship' projects—especially INTARESE and HEIMTSA—aim at 'full-chain' modelling starting from policy options and extending all the way to monetarization. In general public health modelling (e.g. the DYNAMO-HIA project), the chain tends to be limited from risk (or protective) factors to health outcomes. Up to now, there has been little cross-project debate.

In summary, health impact quantification offers a range of advantages. It may help to integrate preventive and curative efforts by providing a common metric for 'preventive' and 'treatment' results and it can facilitate comparisons of potential impacts across alternatives and scenarios. Disadvantages include the incorporation of numerous value- and model-based assumptions that are not always made explicit, risking an unwarranted patina of robust science, and de-emphasizing, or even omitting, stakeholder participation. The quantification approach seems to fit with prevalent health, environmental, and policy science paradigms but the long-term relevance of the current approaches for HIA development is difficult to assess.

Overall use of HIA

In Germany, the potential of 'explicit' HIA for health protection and promotion is under-utilized. Recently, there have been indications of a growing interest in HIA and the topic is now covered in a variety of sources,[25–27] but Germany may still be regarded as a country on the 'threshold' of HIA.

A rapid HIA related to the Ruhr Regional Land Utilisation Plan (RFNP) helped to establish the need to strengthen consideration of health and the health sector in intersectoral cooperation situations. In Germany in policy development, numerous sectors put forward specific departmental plans (*Fachpläne*) to support their interests, such as housing, sports, or nature conservancy, at local or regional level. Efforts under way to establish such plans for the health sector will create opportunities for HIA.[28]

In Germany, HIA needs to be seen as a flexible tool that can be adjusted to suit the different situations in which it may be applied. HIA offers significant opportunities to promote and protect human health. These opportunities can constitute a key element of regional and local health policy, if used systematically and efficiently. Mapping the legal basis and current practice of HIA would make a welcome contribution to further development of HIA in Germany. Being a key idea of HiAP, HIA deserves a permanent place in the public health toolbox.

References

1. Wodarg W Die Gesundheitsverträglichkeitsprüfung (GVP)—eine präventivmedizinische Aufgabe der Gesundheitsämter. Das öffentliche Gesundheitswesen 1989; 51: 692–97.
2. Mekel O, Zielke S, Fehr R Vergleichende Risikoabschätzung und Prioritätensetzung. Materialien Umwelt und Gesundheit Nr. 57, lögd NRW, 2004.
3. Kobusch AB, Fehr R, Serwe HJ (eds) Gesundheitsverträglichkeitsprüfung. Grundlagen—Konzepte—Praxiserfahrungen. Baden-Baden: Nomos Verlagsgesellschaft, 1997.

4. ÖGDG NRW/Gesetz über den öffentlichen Gesundheitsdienst des Landes Nordrhein-Westfalen (ÖGDG NRW). Available at https://recht.nrw.de/lmi/owa/br_bes_text?print=1&anw_nr=2&gld_nr=&ugl_nr=2120&val=4659. Accessed 31 January 2012.

5. Machtolf M, Barkowski D Status-Quo-Analyse zur UVP-Praxis in NRW—Abschlußbericht. Institut für Umwelt-Analyse (IFUA), Bielefeld, Januar 2000. Materialien Umwelt und Gesundheit Nr. 13, lögd NRW, 2000.

6. Fehr R Environmental health impact assessment: evaluation of a ten-step model. Epidemiology 1999; 10: 618–25.

7. Lehto J, Ritsatakis A: Health impact assessment as a tool for intersectoral health policy, in Diwan V *et al.*: (eds), Health Impact Assessment—from theory to practice. Göteborg: Nordic School of Public Health, 2000, pp. 23–87.

8. Fehr R Environmental health impact assessment: the example of transportation, in Diwan V *et al.*: (eds), Health impact assessment—from theory to practice. Göteborg: Nordic School of Public Health, 2000, pp. 213–29.

9. Welteke R, Fehr R (eds) Workshop Gesundheitsverträglichkeitsprüfung Health Impact Assessment. Available at www.apug.de/archiv/pdf/tagungsband_hia_workshop_berlin_2001.pdf Accessed 31 January 2012.

10. Bunzel A, Lorke V, Rösler C Kommunale Zusammenarbeitsstrukturen zur Berücksichtigung von Umwelt- und Gesundheitsbelangen in Planungsverfahren. Köln & Berlin: Difu, 2005.

11. Gesundheitsdienstgesetz LSA. Available at /http://st.juris.de/st/gesamt/GesDG_ST.htm. Accessed 31 January 2012.

12. Fehr R, Kobusch AB *et al.* Gesundheitsverträglichkeitsprüfung (GVP). Abschlussbericht. Materialien Umwelt und Gesundheit Nr. 23, lögd NRW, 1996/2001.

13. Abrahams D *et al.* European Policy Health Impact Assessment (EPHIA): Gesundheitsverträglichkeit Europäischer Politikentscheidungen. Empfehlung zum Vorgehen, 2004. Available at www.sag-ase.ch/doc/EPHIA.pdf. Accessed 31 January 2012.

14. Fehr R, Mekel O, Welteke R Prospektive Abschätzung von Gesundheitsverträglichkeit—europäische Impulse zum Entwicklungsfeld Health Impact Assessment. UVP-report 20, Nr. 3, 2006, pp. 96–101.

15. Nowacki J, Fehr R Economic valuation of effects on health within health impact assessments. Italian Journal of Public Health 2007; 4: 187–94.

16. Lommel A. Praktische Erfahrungen mit der UVP in Hamburg. Vignette 2.9.A, in Fehr R, Neus H, Heudorf U (eds), Gesundheit und Umwelt. Ökologische Prävention und Gesundheitsförderung. Bern: Verlag Hans Huber, 2005.

17. Kaiser B Gesundheitsbelange in UVP-Verfahren aus Sicht eines Gesundheitsamts. UVP-Report 25 (2+3), 2011, pp. 88–90.

18. Nowacki J, Martuzzi M, Fischer TB (eds) Health and strategic environmental assessment. Rome: WHO Europe, 2011.

19. von Zahn K, Berger C: Die Arbeitsgruppe 'Menschliche Gesundheit' der UVP-Gesellschaft. UMID, 2011, pp. 111–14.

20. Fehr R, Gulis G, Staatsen B, Martuzzi M. Family of health-related impact assessments—opportunities to support rational policy-making. DGSMP, DGEpi, and EUMAS, Berlin, 21—25 September 2010. Available at www.lzg.gc.nrw.de/_media/pdf/

service/vortraege/fehr_etal_english_family_dgsmp_final_2010_09_22.pdf. Accessed 31 January 2012.

21. Haigh F, Mekel O, Fehr R, Welteke R. Pilot health impact assessment of the European Employment Strategy in Germany 2004. Available at www.liv.ac.uk/ihia/ IMPACT%20Reports/HIA_of_the_EES__Germany.pdf. Accessed 31 January 2012.

22. Mekel O, Mosbach-Schulz O, Schümann M *et al.* Evaluation von Standards und Modellen zur probabilistischen Expositionsabschätzung. WaBoLu-Hefte 02/07-05/07. Berlin: Umweltbundesamt, 2007.

23. Fehr R, Mekel O. Quantifying the health impacts of policies—Principles, methods, and models. Scientific Expert Workshop, Düsseldorf, 16–17 March 2010. Bielefeld: LIGA. NRW, 2011.

24. LIGA.NRW, EMC, IOM. Health Impact Quantification 2011 Workshop, Granada, 14–15 April 2011. Available at www.lzg.gc.nrw.de/service/veranstaltungen/archiv/110413_ workshop_health_impact_quantification/index.html.

25. German Wikipedia. Available at http://de.wikipedia.org/wiki/Health_Impact_ Assessment. Accessed 31 January 2012.

26. Fehr R. Gesundheitliche Wirkungsbilanzen (Health Impact Assessment, HIA) als Beitrag zur nachhaltigen Gesundheitsförderung, in Göpel E (ed). Nachhaltige Gesundheitsförderung—Gesundheit gemeinsam gestalten, Bd. 4. Frankfurt/Main: Mabuse-Verlag., 2010.

27. Linden S, Töppich J Health Impact Assessment (HIA)/ Gesundheitsverträglichkeitsprüfung, in Blümel S *et al.* (eds), Leitbegriffe der Prävention und Gesundheitsförderung. Köln: BZgA , 2011, pp. 331–36.

28. Fehr R, Dickersbach M, Welteke R. Vorarbeiten zum lokalen Fachplan Gesundheit. Bielefeld: LZG.NRW.

29. Terschüren C, Mekel OCL, Samson R, Classen TK, Hornberg C, Fehr R. Health status of 'Ruhr-City' in 2025—predicted disease burden for the metropolitan Ruhr area in North Rhine-Westphalia. European Journal of Public Health, 2009; 19(5): 534–40.

30. Volmer M, Welteke R, Fehr R. Berücksichtigung des Schutzgutes 'Menschliche Gesundheit' im Rahmen der Aufstellung des 'Regionalen Flächennutzungsplans der Planungsgemeinschaft Städteregion Ruhr'. UVP-report Heft 1+2, 2010, pp. 54–60.

31. Mekel O, Sierig S, Fehr R. Health Impact Assessment of the North Rhine-Westphalian housing subsidy programme 2010, 3rd European Public Health Conference, 'Integrated Public Health' Amsterdam: EUPHA & ASPHER, 10—13 November 2010. Available at http://www.lzg.gc.nrw.de/_media/pdf/service/vortraege/mekel_101206_HIA_WoFP_ eupha.pdf. Accessed 6 March 2012.

32. Kobusch AB, Serwe HJ, Protoschill-Krebs G *et al.* Gesundheitsverträglichkeitsprüfung zur Erweiterung der Zentraldeponie Heinde. Bielefeld, Hildesheim: Typoskript, 1995.

33. Serwe HJ, Protoschill-Krebs G, Gesundheitsverträglichkeitsprüfung der B 9n. Bielefeld: Typoskript, 1995.

34. Fehr R, Mekel O, Lacombe M, Wolf U. Towards HIA of drinking-water privatization— the example of waterborne carcinogens in NRW. Bulletin of the World Health Organization 2003; 81: 408–14.

35. Hornberg C, Claßen T, Samson R. Burden of Disease (BoD) durch Environmental Tobacco Smoke (ETS), Working paper. Bielefeld: University of Bielefeld and NRW Institute of Health (LIGA.NRW), 2008.

36. Mekel O, Nolte E, Fehr R. Quantitative Risikoabschätzung (QRA), Möglichkeiten und Grenzen ihres Einsatzes für umweltbezogenen Gesundheitsschutz in Nordrhein-Westfalen. Exemplarische QRA: Wohnen auf einer Altlast. Materialien Umwelt und Gesundheit Nr. 52, lögd NRW, 1997.

37. Mekel O, Fehr R. Quantitative Risikoabschätzung (QRA), Möglichkeiten und Grenzen ihres Einsatzes für umweltbezogenen Gesundheitsschutz in Nordrhein-Westfalen. Expositionsmodellierung vs. Human-Biomonitoring am Beispiel von Dioxinen und Furanen. Materialien Umwelt und Gesundheit Nr. 55, lögd NRW, 2000.

38. Mekel O, Sierig S, Claßen T. Road traffic noise induced health effects on children—Feasibility study of quantifying the health impacts, 8th International HIA Conference, Dublin, 2007. Available at http://www.publichealth.ie/files/file/hiaconference/parallel/2.1.3OdileMakel.pdf. Accessed 6 March 2012.

Chapter 18

Health impact assessment in Denmark

Marie Louise Bistrup and
Henrik Brønnum-Hansen

Reporting on HIA in Denmark

Researchers in Denmark have learned and written about the development of
HIA in Europe, especially in the UK, Finland, and the Netherlands.[1] The first
report in Denmark on the subject, published in 2005, defined HIA, explained
its concepts, origins, and use, and presented information on HIAs prepared in
some other countries.[2] This report was based on a survey carried out by the
National Institute of Public Health in 2004 with the purpose of identifying
HIAs or assessments that shared characteristics with an HIA. The institute
wrote to all health departments in Denmark's 271 municipalities and 14
regions (at that time) and enquired—based on the definition of HIA in the
Gothenburg consensus paper[3]—whether the department, municipality, or
administrative region had prepared any assessments similar to HIAs. Based on
the responses from the municipalities and administrative regions, semi-
structured interviews were conducted to collect information about the HIA or
HIA-like cases identified. A similar request for information was directed
towards the relevant ministries.

Of 271 municipalities, 141 responded, of whom 21 reported having
prepared HIAs or similar assessments. Ten of 14 regions responded, of whom
five reported having prepared HIA or similar assessments. The report showed
that many municipalities and a few regions had prepared 'proper' HIAs, while
several had prepared HIA-like assessments. Several risk assessments or HIAs
prepared by national government agencies were also identified. All information was analysed and included as an annex to the publication.[2]

Origins of HIA at the municipal level

A reform of Denmark's structure of local government in 2007 reduced the
number of municipalities from 271 to 98, and transformed the 14 regions
(counties) into five administrative regions. The structural reform led to a

larger average population in each municipality and increased the municipalities' responsibility for preventing disease and promoting health.

The National Board of Health provided an incentive for developing HIA at the city or municipal level by commissioning researchers to produce a manual describing in practical terms how to produce an HIA report. Comments on the draft manual were sought from resource people in municipalities already working on or interested in producing HIAs. The goal of the publication was to inspire municipalities to start working on HIA. It focused on the screening and scoping processes, and included several references from Denmark and elsewhere and links to internet resources.[4] The development of HIA in Denmark was supported by a number of academics who have been engaged in HIA work at an international level and have thus been able to assist Danish municipalities to prepare HIAs.

Health impact assessment in the WHO Healthy Cities project

The WHO Regional Office for Europe launched the WHO Healthy Cities project in the late 1980s, and two cities in Denmark, Copenhagen and Horsens, were included in the WHO European Healthy Cities Network. These two cities then initiated the Danish Healthy Cities Network and in 2000 the Network made a study tour of healthy cities in neighbouring Sweden and Finland,[5] learning about their experience with HIA.

HIA was one of the core themes in Phase IV (2003–2008) of the Healthy Cities Project. HIA was described as a useful tool for promoting integrated planning, reducing inequity, and achieving sustainable development as well as contributing to the evidence base on and raising awareness of determinants of health. The WHO Regional Office for Europe developed and pilot-tested an HIA toolkit for European cities, invited cities to participate in training courses, and encouraged cities to use the tools.[6]

In 2010, a group from the Danish Healthy Cities Network prepared a survey on the actual and planned use of HIA in Denmark.[7] Electronic questionnaires were sent to 69 municipalities in the Danish Network, 29 municipalities outside the Danish Network and the five administrative regions in Denmark. Fifty-two (72%) members of the Danish Network, 13 (45%) non-members and all five administrative regions responded. The results indicated wide knowledge of the concept of HIA by both municipalities (89% for Danish Network members and 69% for non-members) and administrative regions (100%). Sixteen of the 98 municipalities and one of the five administrative regions reported experience of using HIA. Most of these had worked with HIA for three or less years.

The survey identified four main approaches to HIA:

- ◆ HIA as part of presenting political proposals
- ◆ HIA before presenting political proposals
- ◆ HIA within spatial planning
- ◆ HIA within the health sector.

How do cities and municipalities use HIA?

Thirteen cities or municipalities in the national Healthy Cities Network had experience with preparing HIA and of these six municipalities had established routines in some or all city departments when preparing cases for political decisions in the municipal council. The tool most frequently used is the screening tool, which is a way of assessing the potential effects on health of proposals for political decisions. Only a few cities produced 'full' HIAs but nine reported using HIA or screening tools in urban planning or environmental assessment procedures. Only nine of the 13 cities produced written reports for each HIA completed. In several cities information on completed HIAs is only available for internal use in the department(s) that prepared the HIA.

HIA is perceived as a meaningful procedure but the time and effort required present obstacles to its use. It was difficult to adapt HIA to existing patterns of work and difficult to develop methods for considering health within SEA. Most municipalities have placed the responsibility for conducting HIA in health departments but a few have placed it in departments responsible for spatial planning or the environment.

Several municipalities have asked for support from academia in undertaking HIA and advice on tools, capacity-building, getting HIA onto the agenda of government authorities, robust methods for evaluating HIA, and demonstration of the effectiveness of HIA.[7]

Take-up of HIA at national level

The survey carried out at the National Institute of Public Health in 2004 identified several assessments prepared at the national level. The presumption that HIA is primarily carried out for activities in sectors not related to health is reflected in themes for the studies such as:

- ◆ the health effects of particulate pollution and the effects of particulate filters[8]
- ◆ the health effects of ending the use of antimicrobial growth promoters in feed[9]

- the role of nutrition and physical activity in promoting health[10]
- the potential effects of preventing disease and exclusion from the labour market.[11]

The Socialist People's Party (Socialistisk Folkeparti) attempted to introduce HIA at national level and drafted a bill[12] asking Parliament to ensure that from the year 2009 the government prepare an HIA on the direct and indirect effects on health of bills put forward by the government, but this was not passed.

Health technology assessment

It can be debated whether health technology assessment (HTA) is a variation of HIA or an independent method for assessing the potential effects of health technology on health. In 2000, the basic concepts and methods of HTA were presented.[13] Like HIA, HTA may be considered as bridging the domains of decision-making and research.[14] The use of HTA is well developed in Denmark and in the rest of Europe, and the international HTA community offers courses, resources, and collaboration.

The challenges in intercountry networks are whether or not to promote similar methods of carrying out HTAs, how data can be shared, and the degree to which results from one country, region, or setting can be used in other countries, regions, and settings.

Use of quantitative methods in Denmark

Dynamic quantitative HIA tools such as PREVENT and DYNAMO-HIA, based on epidemiological evidence, have been developed and improve as increasing computer power increases the capacity to handle complex causality webs. The PREVENT model was tested by applying it to a synthetic population established by micro-simulation and shown to slightly overestimate the effect of reducing exposure, but gives results that are reasonable for realistic scenarios of health promotion.[15] The applicability of the model for estimating smoking-related mortality from various diseases was assessed based on data from Denmark.[16] Denmark was one of five countries along with The Netherlands, England, Wales, and Sweden that in the 1990s as part of a European Union concerted action produced harmonised PREVENT models.[17] Thus, PREVENT was populated with Danish data and used for studies that estimated mortality due to cigarette smoking and the effect on mortality from ischaemic heart disease of reduced prevalence of exposure to cardiovascular risk factors. Selected scenarios exemplified the health benefits of successful implementation of some of the targets in the public health policy of the Government of

Denmark.[18] PREVENT is also an important tool[19–21] in the European collaborative project Eurocadet, in which Denmark, along with at least 11 other countries, aims to contribute to the prevention of cancer in Europe.

Simulations with data on the population of Copenhagen are being established using DYNAMO-HIA in order to create scenarios of the effect of targeted health interventions among disadvantaged or vulnerable groups in Greater Copenhagen.

Since 2007, the Centre for Energy, Environment and Health has built up an integrated environmental HIA system that links various computational modules[22] to support the planning of future Danish energy systems and help policy makers optimize future energy production, taking into account the protection of the environment and human health, healthcare costs, and social costs.

HIA applied to government public health policy

The PREVENT model was used to estimate the potential health benefits of implementing some targets of the government's Public Health Programme for 1999–2008.[18] One target was to reduce the proportion of daily smokers by one-third over a 10-year period. Reaching the target was predicted to reduce the number of deaths from ischaemic heart disease by 800 annually, corresponding to a reduction of more than 5%. Mortality from ischaemic heart disease among residents of Denmark younger than 65 years would be reduced by 10% for men and 15% for women. Furthermore, there would be reduced mortality from other tobacco-related causes of death.[23]

A second target of the Public Health Programme for 1999–2008 was that adults should carry out half an hour of physical activity daily. Reaching this target would reduce mortality from ischaemic heart disease among people younger than 65 years by 3% for men and 6% for women.[23]

Gulis[24] reviewed the effectiveness of an HIA of a campaign to eat more fruits and vegetables called 'six per day'. Although the assessment was not linked to a pending decision and did not follow formal methods Gulis concluded it had been effective in raising politicians' awareness of the issues, encouraging intersectoral collaboration, and providing evidence to support arguments for health promotion and disease prevention.

HIA of noise action plan in Copenhagen

An intersectoral working group consisting of members from the Health and Care Administration and the Technology and Environment Administration collaborated to produce an HIA of the noise action plan for the City of Copenhagen.[25] The report examines the health effects of population exposure to noise and estimates the health-promoting effects of noise-reducing activities. One highly exposed area in Copenhagen, Folehaven, was used as a case because a detailed noise action plan for that area already exists. Several kinds of noise-reducing interventions were analysed for potential health benefits.

The noise levels from road traffic in Copenhagen and Folehaven were presented, and the number of dwellings and people affected by increasing noise levels calculated. The potential negative health effects of noise were annoyance, disturbed sleep, stress, increased blood pressure, and cardiovascular disease. The negative effects of road traffic noise on children's cognitive abilities (learning, memory, and ability to focus) and annoyance were also mentioned.

Based on research, the health effects of road traffic noise on population health were stated and the potential risks for the population of Copenhagen and Folehaven calculated. These data serve as a basis for calculating the potential health benefits of several noise-reducing interventions. The noise-reducing activities are: new effective windows, two kinds of noise-reducing asphalt, reducing speed, reducing heavy road traffic through residential areas, increasing the use of bicycles and public transport, and installing noise barriers along roads. Other secondary effects of road traffic on health such as air pollution, crashes, less physical activity, and the risk of exacerbating social inequity in health were described but not quantified.

The data were recent, valid and used to illustrate clear alternatives for choosing noise-reducing interventions. The potential health gains of various interventions were clearly identified. This HIA is a convincing example of an assessment with a well-defined objective that produced alternative recommendations from which politicians could choose.

Availability of data

Similar to other Nordic countries, Denmark has exceptional opportunities to carry out registry-based research. The unique personal identification number for all citizens enables individual level data to be linked between registries and between registries and surveys. Since the personal identification number was introduced in 1968, individuals can be followed up for decades. Furthermore, a business identification number and a building and housing identification number enables registry-based research that combines health, social status, occupation, and conditions in the local living area[26] Denmark's specialization for linking data between surveys and registries was used in a comprehensive study including quantification of the effects of exposure to various risk factors.[27] The availability of data should prompt a moral impetus for academia to process this data into evidence to support HIA in order to stimulate sustainable development and equitable access to equity in health.

The usefulness of HIA

The Danish Healthy Cities Network acknowledges the need for capacity building in HIA. The Danish Network will discuss and evaluate which elements from HIA work effectively in the municipal and regional settings and the role HIA should play in the municipalities and administrative regions. The Danish Network suggests that an effectiveness study could compare types of models by testing and evaluating their effect on population health, on the improvement of proposals, and on administrative and political processes. The results would give valuable information in the progress of strengthening HIA methods in Denmark. The results would also provide new knowledge for local political debate on health promotion and disease prevention.[4]

The information being used in and emerging from assessments is valuable in the policy-making process for policy makers, critics, administrators, interest groups, and stakeholders. The criticisms of impact assessments are that they are costly and take time, and impact assessment has not been accepted in Denmark as a routine part of policy and decision making.

It is not the assessments per se but the decisions made based on assessments that result in change. A good HIA provides data, information, and recommendations for various solutions among which politicians or administrators can choose. Politicians will assert their autonomy to make any decision they want regardless of the recommendation of an impact assessment. One of the good effects of a solid assessment is that all the information can be made publicly available, so a constituency can assess whether or not a decision maker made the best decision based on the impact assessment.

Conclusion

Capacity building and the development of methodological competencies—including how to use models such as PREVENT and DYNAMO-HIA to estimate effects on public health of policies in HIAs—would make the use of HIA more approachable.

The values of HIA (see Chapter 6) include democracy, described in the Gothenburg Consensus Paper as 'emphasizing the right of people to participate in a transparent process for the formulation, implementation and evaluation of policies that affect their life, both directly and through the elected political decision makers'.[3] To satisfy this value it is important to make information related to the HIA available to stakeholders and the wider the public.

References

1. Quigley R, den Broeder L, Furu P, Bond A, Cave B, Bos R. Health impact assessment: international best practice principles. Special Publication Series No. 5.Fargo, ND: International Association for Impact Assessment, 2006.

2. Bistrup ML, Kamper-Jørgensen F. Sundhedskonsekvensvurderinger: koncept, perspektiver, anvendelse i stat, amter og kommuner [Health impact assessment: concepts, perspectives, application by government, regions and municipalities]. Copenhagen: National Institute of Public Health, 2005.

3. Health impact assessment. Main concepts and suggested approach. Gothenburg consensus paper. Copenhagen: WHO Regional Office for Europe, 1999.

4. Sundhedskonsekvensvurdering—fra teori til praksis [Health impact assessment—from theory to practice]. Copenhagen: National Board of Health, 2008.

5. Sund By Netværket studietur til Sverige og Finland, 21.–26. maj 2000 [Danish Healthy Cities Network study tour to Sweden and Finland, 21–26 May 2000]. Copenhagen: Danish Healthy Cities Network, 2000.

6. WHO Urban health—Health Impact Assessment. Available at http://www.euro.who. int/en/what-we-do/health-topics/environment-and-health/urban-health/activities/ health-impact-assessment. Accessed 28 February 2012.

7. Sundhedskonsekvensvurdering i danske kommuner og regioner: anvendt og planlagt praksis for sundhedskonsekvensvurdering [Health impact assessment in municipalities and administrative regions: the use and planned practice of health impact assessment]. Copenhagen: Danish Healthy Cities Network, 2010.

8. Blands J, Hjaldsted B, Loft S, Sigsgaard T, Taudorf E, Palmgren F *et al.* Vurdering af partikelforureningens og dieselpartiklers sundhedsskadelige effekter [Assessment of the harmful health effects of particulate pollution and diesel particulate]. Copenhagen: Ministry of the Environment and Ministry of Health, 2003.

9. Impacts of antimicrobial growth promoter termination in Denmark—the WHO international review panel's evaluation of the termination of the use of growth promoters in Denmark. Foulum, Denmark, 6–9 November 2002. Geneva: World Health Organization, 2003.

10. Matthiessen J, Rasmussen JB, Andersen LB, Astrup A, Helge JW, Kjær M *et al.* Kost og fysisk aktivitet—fælles aktører i sygdomsforebyggelsen [Diet and physical activity— joint actors in preventing disease]. Søborg: Danish Veterinary and Food Administration, 2003.

11. Mossing R, Bach E, Borg V, Burr H, Fallentin N, Flyvholm MA *et al.* Den mulige gevinst af forebyggelse af sygefravær og udstødning fra arbejdsmarkedet [The potential benefits of preventing sick leave caused by disease and exclusion from the labour market]. Copenhagen: National Institute for Occupational Health, 2002.

12. Beslutningsforslag nr. B 66, af 16. december 2008: Forslag til folketingsbeslutning om vurdering af lovforslag med konsekvenser for sundheden. [Motion for a parliament resolution to assess bills that affect health].

13. Medicinsk teknologivurdering. Hvorfor? Hvad? Hvornår? Hvordan? [Health technology assessment? Why? What? When? How?]. Copenhagen: Danish Centre for Health Technology Assessment, 2000.

14. Health Technology Assessment Handbook. Copenhagen: Danish Centre for Health Technology Assessment, National Board of Health, 2007.

15. Brønnum-Hansen H. How good is the PREVENT model for estimating the health benefits of prevention? Journal of Epidemiology and Community Health 1999; 53: 300–305.

16. Brønnum-Hansen H, Juel K. Estimating mortality due to cigarette smoking: two methods, same result. Epidemiology 2000; 11: 422–26.

17. Baan C, Barendregt J, Bonneux L, Brønnum-Hansen H, Gunning-Schepers L, Kamper-Jørgensen F et al. Public health models. Tools for health policy making at national and European level. Amsterdam: Institute of Social Research, University of Amsterdam, 1999.

18. The Danish Government Programme on Public Health and Health Promotion 1999–2008. Copenhagen: Ministry of Health, 2000.

19. de Vries E, Soerjomataram I, Lemmens VEPP, Coebergh JWW, Barendregt JJ, Oenema A et al. Lifestyle changes and reduction of colon cancer incidence in Europe: a scenario study of physical activity promotion and weight reduction. European Journal of Cancer 2010; 46: 2605–16.

20. Soerjomataram I, de Vries E, Engholm G, Paludan-Müller G, Brønnum-Hansen H, Storm HH et al. Impact of a smoking and alcohol intervention program on lung cancer and breast cancer incidence in Denmark: an example of dynamic modeling with PREVENT. European Journal of Cancer 2010; 46: 2617–24.

21. Menviellea G, Soerjomataram I, de Vries E, Engholm G, Barendregt JJ, Coebergh JWW et al. Scenarios of future lung cancer incidence by educational level: modelling study in Denmark. European Journal of Cancer 2010; 46: 2625–32.

22. Centre for Environment, Energy and Health. Available at http://www.ceeh.dk/English/index.html. Accessed 29 February 2012.

23. Brønnum-Hansen H. Forventet effekt af forebyggelse. Notat til Sundhedsministeriet [Predicting the effects of disease prevention. Memorandum to the Ministry of Health]. Copenhagen: National Institute of Public Health, 2002.

24. Gulis G, Contributing to a public health culture: health and economic impacts of a health promotion campaign in Denmark, in Blau J, Wismar M, Ernst K, (eds), The effectiveness of health impact assessment. Scope and limitations of supporting decision-making in Europe. Copenhagen: WHO Regional Office for Europe, 2007, pp 247–56.

25. Sundhedskonsekvensvurdering af Københavns Kommunes støjhandlingsplan: Folehaven som case [Health impact assessment of the noise action plan for the City of Copenhagen: Folehaven as a case]. Copenhagen: City of Copenhagen, 2011.

26. Thygesen LC, Ersbøll AK (eds). Danish population-based registers for public health and health-related welfare research—a description of Danish registers and results from their application in research. Scandinavian Journal of Public Health 2011; 39(Suppl 7): 1–209.

27. Juel K, Sørensen J, Brønnum-Hansen H. Risk factors and public health in Denmark. Scandinavian Journal of Public Health 2008; 36(Suppl 1): 1–227.

Chapter 19

Health impact assessment in Switzerland

Jean Simos and Nicola Cantoreggi

Introduction

The development of HIA in Switzerland has been strongly influenced by the federal organization of the country, which is similar in many ways to that of the USA, despite the difference in size. The 26 cantons and half-cantons of the Helvetian Confederation have equivalent prerogatives to the US states, with independent governance of many public policy areas including health, except for a few matters such as communicable diseases control and health insurance, which are federal concerns. For this reason, there is no nationwide public health policy, let alone a national programme of health promotion.[1]

Legislation for HIA in Geneva

From 1991, the State of Geneva showed its determination to give more attention to the issue of health by basing its local health policy on the WHO Health for All policy and joining the WHO European Healthy Cities Network.[2] Core themes of Phase IV (2003–2008) of the Healthy Cities programme included introduction of HIA.[3] As a result of strains on the cantonal budget, the health promotion budget was reduced by 25% and public health officers hoped that HIA could save money by reducing future health problems. Similar concerns have prompted interest in HIA in other Swiss partners. Embedding HIA in the framework of the new cantonal Public Health Act, which was influenced by article 54 of the Quebec Public Health Act (see Chapter 24, page 227), further strengthened the legal basis for HIA in Geneva.

Geneva created an HIA Unit within the Health Directorate of the Department for Economic Affairs and Health with a mission to carry out pilot HIAs. The unit functions both as supervisor and as main assessor for HIA. At the end of 2007, it was transferred to the University of Geneva in order to benefit from the research and training facilities offered by an academic institution.

The first comprehensive HIA conducted by the Unit concerned a smoking ban in café-restaurants and other public places. This issue was well suited for a first HIA since it was clearly linked to health and received strong support from health experts on the steering committee. At the same time it required knowledge from many fields beside health (economic, technical, and public safety) and so stimulated cooperation with stakeholders from non-health fields. Following this, HIAs on other policies were commissioned, including the promotion of electric bicycles, banning the sale of alcohol to those aged under 18 years, the collection and management of solid waste, the use of volatile organic compounds (VOC) in paints and varnishes, and the use of pesticides in agriculture.

Geneva has also adapted SEA to include consideration of health in urban planning.[4] This approach was applied to a suburban development project (the Mon Idée et Communaux d'Ambilly (MICA) project) where it revealed difficulties in identifying which organizations were responsible for particular issues such as mobility. It also showed the need for HIAs to match the time scales of the decision process and fit the arcane processes of political and administrative institutions.[5] Geneva has also conducted HIAs related to urban planning programmes such as the Geneva metropolitan cross-border area master plan and the Bernex-Est development project. Both qualitative and quantitative approaches have been developed for HIA related to urban planning. Qualitative approaches were used to explore issues where a linear cause–effect model did not appear to be appropriate (e.g. mix of activities and housing) or could not be supported by quantitative data (e.g. health impacts of public open spaces). Quantitative approaches were used to analyse issues where there was a clear cause–effect and quantitative data were available (e.g. mobility and health, road safety, air and noise pollution).

Attempts to embed HIA in Ticino

The Canton of Ticino produced a health promotion policy firmly based on the Ottawa Charter and the determinants of health approach. A report to the cantonal Parliament advocated the use of HIA as a tool and its application to all cantonal public policies. This lead to a pilot programme to use HIA to appraise cantonal public policies in the 2003–2007 legislative programme and the creation of the Interdepartmental Health Impact Assessment Committee (HIA Committee) to oversee these activities. Steered by the cantonal Department of Health and Social Welfare, the HIA Committee framed principles for the selection of policies to be assessed and developed ad hoc tools for the pre-screening, screening, and scoping stages.

Committee members and other people involved were given access to essential documentation and training for the HIA. The intention was to anchor HIA in all public administration sectors, and promote empowerment and collaboration between departments. Following this agenda, several decisions were identified as potential topics for HIA (promotion of retail trade, supervision of prisoners outside prison, provision of medical equipment, etc.). The possibility of integrating HIA and consideration of socioeconomic determinants into EIA was also explored but could not be achieved. In the end Ticino only managed to conduct one comprehensive HIA (on a transportation plan for the Mendrisio area).

Experience in Ticino shows the importance of gaining political support for HIA and managing the anxieties of politicians and civil servants that HIA might conflict with other interests.[6] While the development of a multisectoral approach in public health policies was encouraging, further work needs to be done to integrate HIA procedures into public policy formulation.

Agenda 21 and HIA in Jura

Health promotion is the guiding principle in the canton of Jura's Agenda 21 (Juragenda 21). In 2002, the canton decided to develop HIA as a tool to support the decision-making process for the local Agenda 21. While taking a similar approach to that adopted in the Canton of Ticino, Jura developed a more extensive experimental programme with numerous case studies conducted for the canton. Moreover, Jura has created a joint monitoring group involving the local departments of health and of environment and infrastructures.

The strategy adopted aimed to devise a procedure that was suited to the Jura government's ways of working and likely to be supported at both political (heads of department) and administrative (heads of service) levels. While the HIA process has been led by the Department of Health, it has also interacted with other departments, notably through their participation in the monitoring group, which provides an opportunity to test the reaction of all participants towards HIAs. The group decided to develop the practical and operational tools at the same time as integrating with political and institutional level processes. The involvement of civil servants from non-health departments in the group has been crucial for identifying potential obstacles, finding ways to make HIA acceptable to the decision makers, speeding up the decision-making process, and keeping the scope of assessment proportional to the issue under consideration.

The first HIA concerned the development of a technology centre on the outskirts of the canton's capital Delémont but was not entirely satisfactory since the project plans were insufficiently developed and the relation of the HIA to other assessments was poorly understood. The second HIA concerned the planned rehabilitation of historic neighbourhoods promoted by the Jura government and was able to take account of the problems revealed in the first

HIA. Features that contributed to success were clarity about the architectural options under consideration, clear assessment criteria, allocation by the project monitoring group of defined tasks within the assessment, choice of a pilot site for analysis in order to identify the key issues, and formulation of recommendations precise enough to guide the decision-making process. Other HIA conducted in Jura related to developing dinosaur tracks in Cortadoux as a tourist attraction, rehabilitation of old housing in Porrentruy, and the development of a regional activity centre in Delémont.

The monitoring group is now focusing on making HIA an integral part of public policy making. It has screened about a dozen items of the 2007–2010 legislative programmes to identify those which should be subject to HIAs.

HIA in the other cantons

Apart from the cantons of Geneva, Ticino, and Jura, the other Swiss cantons up to 2010 have not completed an HIA. The cantons of Vaud, Fribourg, and Aargau have recently started HIA or expressed their intention to do so and could be categorized as 'newly starting'. The cantons of Neuchâtel and Thurgau have joined the Swiss HIA platform but not yet done an HIA. The other cantons have asked to be informed about HIA but have not made any commitment and could be categorized as 'wait and see'.

The federal level

In 2002 the Swiss Society for Public Health with the support of the Swiss Federal Office of Public Health (FOPH) published 'Targets for health in Switzerland' based on national implementation of the WHO Europe Health 21 framework.[7] Target 14 advocated the use of HIA as a tool to assess the impact of policies on health.

Following the recommendations of this document, in 2003–04 FOPH set up a series of workshops in which stakeholders from other federal departments and from cantonal health departments participated. In 2005, an internal report called 'Guidelines for a multi-dimensional health policy' identified many examples of public policies from the sectors of health, economics, education, social, family, migrants' integration, environment, urban planning, housing, agriculture, and transportation, which had impacted negatively on health and determinants of health. It strongly recommended the inclusion of HIA within any sustainability assessment.

In 2006, directly following this first report, FOPH produced a second report called 'Integrate a multi-dimensional health policy', which examined the possibility of developing an HIA tool and asked if it could be integrated in the already existing sustainability assessment tool. The report suggested that an HIA tool should:

- be as user friendly as possible
- require a minimum of time when used in other federal departments (all budgets are strained)
- be applicable to all kinds of federal activities (laws, strategies, programmes, projects, concepts)
- produce assessments within reasonable deadlines
- be helpful in clearly identifying the effect on health of policies made by any department or office
- lead to optimization of political goals in a health promotion and well-being perspective
- reflect experience at cantonal level from which the federal level could benefit.

Three versions of the tool were developed: (a) for conducting independent HIA, (b) for conducting HIA complementary to sustainability assessment, and (c) for conducting HIA completely integrated in the sustainability assessment. The three versions were tested in studies of agriculture policy and transportation policy, and it was concluded that HIA complementary to or integrated with sustainability appraisal was better than independent HIA. Due to lack of support from other departments this conclusion was not followed up and the FOPH decided to follow the example of Geneva and focus on the introduction of HIA through legislation.

The Swiss HIA platform

The Conference of Sanitary Directors (CDS), in which the cantonal Ministers of Health meet, tried unsuccessfully to introduce HIA at cantonal level at the same time for all cantons but had to content itself with simply encouraging HIA in those cantons already inclined to do it without putting any pressure on the other cantons. Instead an exchange platform with the cantons of Geneva, Ticino, and Jura with equiterre (an NGO concerned with sustainable development) and Health Promotion Switzerland was created in 2005 to facilitate the use of HIAs in the country. This platform aims to pool and enhance knowledge by sharing experience among Swiss partners using the HIA approach. A website was created in order to facilitate these exchanges and to disseminate the relevant information about HIAs. The first national conference of the platform was held in Lugano in 2006 and the platform will shortly become an association.

The main objectives of the platform are:

- to promote HIA at different institutional levels and to advocate its intro-duction within the local authorities' political agenda
- to build, share, and spread knowledge and skills, in particular through training professionals
- to develop and shape the HIA concept and methodologies by carrying out case studies in various fields, helping to define best practices
- to make the HIA tool consistent with other decision aid tools.

In order to achieve those objectives, the Platform communicates knowledge about HIA to Swiss professionals and to anyone who would like to learn more through the production of the 'Introduction Guide on HIA in Switzerland' (in French and German), through the maintenance of the website[8] (which gives information about tools and methods for doing HIA, HIA developments in Switzerland, case studies carried out in Switzerland, and HIA-related links), and through newsletters. It also runs HIA training courses, advocates for HIA in the political arena (produces fact sheets for use by administrative and political decision makers, holds meetings with Parliament members, etc.), and promotes pilot studies of HIA.

Legal status of HIA in Switzerland

At the cantonal level only Geneva has legislated for HIA. When in 2004 the cantonal Minister of Health proposed an Article (4) in the Public Health Act requiring consideration of health impacts there was heated debate. Some members of the cantonal parliament were strongly opposed to the article because they regarded EIA as a requirement that delayed or blocked decision making and feared that HIA might become a new administrative obstacle to economic activity. Eventually a compromise version of the article that stated 'if a legislative project is likely to cause negative consequences to health then the government of Geneva can decide to require an assessment of its potential impact on health' was agreed and the Act came into force in 2006, providing a legal basis for HIA in Geneva.

At the federal level a legal basis for HIA has not yet been adopted. The legisla-tive process seems to be following the same pattern as in Geneva. The FOPH initiative led to inclusion of Article 9, which is very similar to Article 4 of Geneva's Health Act in the health promotion and prevention federal law project (LPrév), the first draft of which was presented in 2008. After a broad consultation process (232 written answers), as is usual for any federal law, the government presented the final draft to the National Parliament in 2009.

It was supported by a huge majority of cantons and all the public health institutions, but was strongly opposed by the economy lobbies. During spring 2011, the Lower Chamber voted for the LPrév, including Article 9 about HIA. In November 2011, the commission of social and health affairs of the Upper Chamber voted by 7 votes to 6 against the adoption of Article 9 while adopting the rest of LPrév. In December 2011, the plenary of the Senate voted against the LPrév by 20 votes to 19. In March 2012, the Lower Chamber confirmed its decision of spring 2011. In April 2012, the commission of social and health affairs of the Upper Chamber proposed again the adoption of LPrév, but this time, by 7 votes to 5, voted in favour of the Article 9. In June 2012, the plenary of the Upper Chamber adopted, by 20 votes to 16, a "light" version of the law project, without the Article 9. LPrév now has to go back to the National Council and if the discrepancy between the two Chambers is confirmed, then a consensus conference will be set up.

Conclusion and next steps

The weaknesses and opportunities of HIA in Switzerland can be summarized as follows.

Weaknesses:

- Few administrations encourage the use of HIA. Assessment is generally perceived as obstructive and not a constructive factor for improving policies, programmes, and projects. Nevertheless, an increasing number of decision makers acknowledge the need to introduce systematic assessment in order to foster good governance.

- The broad definition of health is not fully accepted or understood by professionals outside the public health sector. There is a need for training in the understanding of health and its determinants.

- HIA has to overcome the negative perception of EIA in the minds of many politicians.

- With the proliferation and competition of various assessment tools for public policies (EIA, SEA, sustainability assessment), HIA has still to define its place and demonstrate its added value.

- The lack of staff trained in HIA is crucial to addressing the other weaknesses.

- Last but not least, the lack of political will creates a major obstacle to making HIA compulsory and persuading institutions to undertake HIA.

Opportunities:

- The existence of a legal basis, even if only permissive, helps to build the legitimacy of HIA for non-health professionals.

- The possibility of a legal basis at the federal level could encourage cantons to develop cantonal level legal or strategic frameworks.

- HIA often serves as catalyst for an intersectoral approach between administrations, which allows better focus on the relevant determinants of health.

- Timely production of HIA results often influences the political/administrative decision-making process, stimulating increased attention to health promotion and fostering a positive image of HIA.

- The organizational framework of HIA is locally developed to match locally available resources and local political–administrative understanding. As a result the process suits the particular arrangements of each canton, conforming to the federalist system of Switzerland. This could encourage cantons not yet involved to adopt HIA.

- The strengthening of the HIA process at the international level (WHO, EU) and the integration of HiAP approaches contribute to consolidation of HIA in Switzerland.

- The work of the Swiss HIA Platform supports, encourages, and develops the practice of HIA in Switzerland and advocates its use to administrative and political decision makers.

References

1. OECD Reviews of Health Systems—Switzerland. An update of the Review of the Swiss Health System. *Paris: OECD and WHO, 2006; OECD Editions, 2011.*

2. Government of Geneva. Décision sur la politique de la santé et l'adhésion au réseau européen Villes-Santé de l'OMS. Extrait du PV du Conseil d'Etat du 6 février 1991. Republic and Canton of Geneva, Geneva, 1991.

3. WHO Regional Office for Europe. Phase IV (2003–2008) WHO European Healthy Cities Network: goals and requirements. Available at http://www.euro.who.int/en/what-we-do/health-topics/environment-and-health/urban-health/publications/2003/phase-iv-20032008-who-european-healthy-cities-network-goals-and-requirements. Accessed 30 December 2011.

4. Simos J, Cantoreggi N. Environnements urbains et santé—Des liens anciens qui méritent une actualisation. Public Health Schweiz 2008; 1: 15.

5. Simos J, Arrizabalaga Ph. Utiliser les synergies entre évaluation environnementale stratégique (EES) et évaluation d'impact sur la santé (EIS) pour promouvoir la prise en compte de l'environnement et de la santé dans les processus décisionnels publics. Soz Praventiv Med. *Social and Preventive Medicine*, 2006; 51: 133–36.

6. Cantoreggi N *et al. HIA in Switzerland: considerations concerning the experience of the Cantons of Geneva, Jura and Ticino. Italian Journal of Public Health 2007; 4: 169–75.*

7. Swiss Society of Public Health. Targets for Health in Switzerland. Health for All in 21st Century (WHO Europe). Bern: SSSP.

8. EIS plateforme. Available at http://www.impactsante.ch/spip/. Accessed 28 February 2012.

Chapter 20

Health impact assessment in France

Jean Simos and Nicolas Prisse

Introduction

While the development of HIA in France may appear delayed compared with similar countries, it is now undeniably present at the national, regional, and local levels. HIA was introduced in France through two separate routes, each influenced by different rationales and requirements:

- the state or national level (in particular, the central government)
- the local community level (including towns and cities).

Evaluation and assessment of public policies at national level

The introduction of HIA at the national level stems from the combination of three circumstances:

- the need to improve policy making by government institutions
- the need to tackle health inequality
- the opportunity to take part in an international movement.

Increasing attention has been paid to evaluation of public policies in France since 1980. Evaluation was seen as necessary in order to address a situation that was characterized by:

- a high level of uncertainty about the effectiveness of policy choices made in a complex environment
- a call from citizens and their representatives for greater transparency and a clearer understanding of the expected and achieved outcomes of policies
- a requirement to justify choices made and the use of resources
- a challenge to the view that 'expertise' was an adequate measure of effectiveness a priori or a posteriori.

In particular, the finance law of August 2001 required assessment of performance against the annual budget with indicators and comparison of intended and actual achievements for each of government's major areas of work, broken down by programme and activity. Any difference between goals and actual achievements had to be justified in a document presented to parliament and published annually.

In the field of health policy, the Public Health Act of 2004 took a new step by establishing 100 national objectives, defining five strategic plans and requiring the High Council for Public Health to:

- contribute to the definition of multiyear public health targets and monitoring of progress against objectives
- provide the public authorities with the expertise required to manage public health risks, and in conjunction with health agencies to design and evaluate policies and strategies for prevention and safety.

Currently, the High Council for Public Health evaluates the majority of national health plans. In March 2011, it added an HIA expert to its membership and is promoting HIA in France.

Participation of citizens in debates on health issues

Over the past decade the idea of 'health democracy' has grown in France alongside efforts to improve the planning and evaluation of health policy. New laws and regulations allow organizations representing users and citizens to participate in the discussion of health issues. The law concerning 'hospitals, patients, health and territories' of August 2009 created regional health agencies (RHAs) and gave an important role to the Regional Conferences for Health and Autonomy (RCHAs). These regional conferences bring together all stakeholders and user representatives in a given region and have an important role in the development of the regional strategic plans that define a region's health priorities for a period of five years. Some RHAs have gone further and organized debates and other forms of public consultation on health issues in their regions. Consequently, health democracy, or the participation of service users or citizens, can be seen as an integral component in the process of developing public policies on health.

The use of impact assessments in support of national legislation

Health policy evaluation and health democracy have helped to pave the way for the adoption of HIA. Nevertheless, the extension of systematic impact assessments from government decisions on health issues to those on other policy areas (as is also the case for the European Commission) was the decisive factor for the development of HIA in France.

The need to develop a system to assess the impacts of public policies and to strengthen the role of parliament was evidenced during the last constitutional reform of 2008 and by the law of 15 April 2009, which modified the role of Parliament so that it would not only 'vote on laws and control government activity' but also 'evaluate public policies'. In order to make 'a tool for evaluation and decision support'[1] available to Parliament, this constitutional reform required that new legislation sent to the State Council and Parliament should be supported with impact assessments. These impact studies had to conform to specific requirements set by the legislature. The ministry proposing a piece of legislation must present a precise 'assessment of the economic, financial, social and environmental consequences, as well as the anticipated financial costs and benefits, of the proposed measures for each category of public administration and for any natural or legal individuals who may be interested, also indicating the method of calculation employed'.

The General Secretariat of the Government (GSG), with the help of a network of correspondents led by central government, is at the heart of this system. The GSG, in conjunction with the prime minister, monitors that each assessment produced is adequate. The State Council and the presidents of each Assembly have the ability to block any proposal if the impact assessment is deemed non-compliant. To assist ministries in preparing impact assessments the GSG has developed an information sheet, an internal website, a guidance note, rules for the presentation of impact studies, and a handbook on how to do impact studies.

The handbook suggests five questions relating to public health in the wider framework of social impacts:

♦ Does the proposal have an impact on the health or safety of individuals or groups of citizens?

♦ Is the proposal likely to reduce the prevalence of diseases or premature deaths?

♦ Is the proposal likely to reduce the health risks associated with pollution, waste treatment, and noise pollution?

♦ Is the proposal likely to change harmful behaviours (smoking, alcohol consumption, etc.)?

♦ Does the proposal impact on particular groups? If so which?

Other questions examine the social, economic, or environmental impacts of proposals which may indirectly affect health. For example:

◆ Does the proposal promote the development or reduction of social or income inequality?

◆ Is the proposal likely to affect the labour market (e.g. in terms of access or return to work)?

◆ Does the proposal affect drinking water resources?

It therefore appears that the system of impact studies ensures *a priori* assessment of the effects of legislation. A detailed conclusion on the working of this system cannot be drawn until more time has elapsed. However, in a recent report, the French Inspector General for Social Affairs wrote that although the ownership of the new impact study system seemed satisfactory by different actors they had not had the expertise to consider health and the descriptions of direct and indirect (social, economic, and environmental) impacts on health in the assessments could have been improved.

Health and urban planning at the local level

The introduction of HIA at the local community level was initiated and supported by the WHO Healthy Cities project, to which approximately 60 French cities are linked. Significantly, phase IV of the WHO European Healthy Cities Network, which ran from 2003 to 2008, included HIA in the member cities and other national networks. In the absence of a legal basis the introduction of HIA at the local level has been less systematic than at the national level, but more rapid. The WHO European Healthy Cities Network spread knowledge of HIA and organized several training days (Paris in 2005, Turku in 2006, Geneva in 2008). Training was also organized through the French network of Healthy Cities and the Association Internationale pour la Promotion de la Santé et le Developpement Durable (S2D), who organized a two-day event for elected officials and policymakers from the area of Rennes in 2011. More extensive HIA training was also provided at the Public Health Summer School in Besançon, in June 2009.

These activities led to the first three local-level HIAs in France:

◆ the creation of a new crèche in Rennes (2009)[2]

◆ the restoration of Pontchaillou train station in Rennes (2011)

◆ the redevelopment of the area around the Saint-Quentin-en-Yvelines train station (Ecopôle project) in the Paris region (2012).

Several other projects are currently in the preparatory phase (in Toulouse, Brest, and Nanterre). The Healthy Cities of the Rhone-Alpes region

(Lyon, Grenoble, and Villeurbanne) with the National Centre for the Management of Territorial Service will be providing a comprehensive HIA training for their technical managers in 2012 and 2013.

Health inequalities

In recent years, health inequalities have become one of the central issues of national health policy. Life expectancy at birth in France is among the highest in Europe (78.1 years and 84.8 years for men and women respectively in 2010), but social inequalities in health remain wide.

The Ministry of Health has made increasing efforts to reduce health inequalities and the first objective of the 2011–2015 National Health Strategy is 'to prevent and reduce health inequalities from the early stages of life.' At the regional level, the RHAs are also required to include objectives to reduce health inequalities in their regional strategies.[3]

Most determinants of health such as working conditions, social relationships, and education, and therefore the public policy responses to health inequalities, lie outside the remit of the health sector. Certainly, government agencies, health professionals, and healthcare facilities must work to ensure equitable access to prevention and healthcare services, but they also have a major role to play in training and raising awareness of other agencies and professionals, who are in a position to improve the social determinants of health.

The National Committee of Public Health, an interministerial body that serves to share and exchange information several times addressed the issue of social determinants of health during 2010–2011, thereby supporting the idea of HiAP. Similarly, at the regional level, committees for the coordination of public policy take the lead on intersectoral actions favourable to health. However, according to many stakeholders, the tools needed to work on the social determinants of health are lacking, particularly in the local municipalities. HIA has shown that it can be a tool to reduce social inequalities as they relate to health, for two reasons:

- It considers social determinants of health within policies (particularly at the regional and local levels).
- It considers the distribution of potential health consequences among social groups.

The definition and values of HIA, incorporated into the Gothenburg consensus,[4] and the emphasis on involving stakeholders in HIA further attest to the use of HIA in reducing health inequality.

Opportunities arising from an international movement

The relative delay in the development of HIA in France is reflected among local and regional projects, in particular by a lack of experience and a strong demand for training. Deficiencies in this area are especially obvious as French academic experts in public health have until recently ignored the evolution of HIA in Anglo-Saxon countries, confining themselves to evaluations of health policies or health risks. In this respect, the confusion that remains among certain professionals concerning the impact assessment of health as introduced by the 1996 Air Quality Law (which concerned quantitative assessment of health risk) is indicative of the researchers' lack of understanding of HIA.

However, in France, as in many developed countries, EIAs have had much influence on the development of HIA. EIA aims in particular to estimate risks to the environment posed by public policies or projects, as well as potential indirect risks to human health. It has been used for over 30 years as a tool to support decision making, particularly with regard to territorial development or public works projects. In the light of the promotion of health equity, experience of EIA has been complemented by experience gathered abroad and by the international movement, including the European project on Joint Action on Health Inequalities, which focuses on the sharing of HIA concepts and tools.

Conclusion and next steps

At both the national and local levels in France the process of developing and implementing public policies (particularly in the health field) has been marked in recent decades by:

- the development of assessments
- involvement of citizens and/or their representatives
- the need to predict the consequences of public decisions and to keep the public informed regarding policy choices
- concern to reduce health inequalities and take into consideration the broad social determinants of health.

Accordingly, HIA can be considered as an approach that appears to address all these concerns.

As with the impact assessments conducted by the European Commission, HIA in France at the national level finds a place in the overall system of impact assessments that support legislation, but this mechanism will undoubtedly require adjustments in order to improve the health component. At the regional level some RHAs are already considering HIA as a promising tool to support and raise the awareness of local policy makers of the social determinants of health. Moreover, HIAs are seen as an approach that is supportive of 'health democracy' that could facilitate an HiAP approach and reduce health inequalities. The current international momentum with these issues should help France further develop its engagement with HIA.

References

1. Circular from the Prime Minister on 15 April 2009 on the implementation of the constitutional reform (legislative procedure); NOR: PRMX0908734 Paris, The French Government, Bureau of the Prime Minister.
2. Moulin E, Jourdren A. L'exemple des crèches rennaises durables. Available at http://legifrance.gouv.fr/affichTexte.do?cidTexte=JORFTEXT000022235390&categorieLien=idn. Accessed 23 March 2012.
3. Article R. 1434-2 of the Public Health Code. Brussels WHO European Centre for Health Policy.
4. WHO European Centre for Health Policy. Health impact assessment: main concepts and suggested approach—Gothenburg consensus paper 1999. WHO European Centre for Health Policy, Brussels.

Chapter 21

Health impact assessment in Italy

Fabrizio Bianchi and Liliana Cori

HIA in Italy at national and regional level

In Italy HIA is not obligatory at national or regional level, except in limited situations that are described here. The Italian National Health Service has responsibility for public health as well as cure and rehabilitation. In this domain, there is potential interest in adopting HIA as a formalized process for evaluating programmes and policies.

The organization and management of the prevention, cure, and rehabilitation services is assigned to regional health systems administered by regional governments. Although HIA could represent a useful tool to assess programmes, policies, and projects of regional and local interest, so far only a few regions have used it.

Budgets are allocated by national government to regions according to population size, age structure, and other criteria, but responsibility for management and decision making is devolved to regions. Consequently, prevention and healthcare services differ widely between regions depending on cultural, economical, and political factors,[1] and so it is to be expected that development of HIA also differs between regions.

Progress on legislation on HIA is slow and faces cultural barriers. Researchers have to surmount the difficulties of working with the many disciplines that are relevant to HIA of policy. Nonetheless more HIAs are being performed in Italy and HIA is being applied to more complex settings. The Italian experience confirms that HIA is a useful tool for informing the debates at the interface of research and policy, and the difficult questions around uncertainty and the precautionary principle.

Education and training for HIA

In Italy, education in epidemiology, prevention, and public health is covered in post-graduate courses (PhDs and Masters) of faculties of medicine. Specific training on HIA is included in a few of these courses. In addition to formal university education, the Italian National Research Council, the National Institute of Health, some regional administrations, and local health units have organized numerous training courses on HIA. The Ministry of Health and the Ministry for the Environment have supported these activities, actively participating in national seminars and working groups. In 2010, the Italian Centre for Diseases Control (CCM) financed a training and intervention project for local health operators, based on rapid HIA.

The presence in Rome of a WHO Environment and Health Office, with consolidated HIA expertise, has also represented an important source of reference for researchers, on both methodological and operational activities. The Italian Epidemiology Association (AIE) has given increasing prominence to HIA in the past decade and its journal *Epidemiologia & Prevenzione* has published several articles on HIA, creating a favourable atmosphere for the introduction of HIA into public health practice.[2] More recently, the Italian Society of Hygiene, Public Health and Preventive Medicine has also given consideration to HIA.

Research objectives

Italian researchers involved in HIA are working to pursue four main objectives:

1. To improve the involvement of stakeholders in the HIA process in local level projects (HIA-NMAC EU project—see Chapter 22).

2. To strengthen quantitative approaches to the appraisal of impacts (e.g. RAPID EU project on Risk assessment).[3]

3. To improve checklists and evaluation tools for public health staff involved in decision-making conferences. In Italy such conferences have to be convened to examine projects and programmes (MONITER and VisPA projects).

4. To make recommendations for policy makers derived from evidence-based assessment of impacts. Such recommendations are crucial when the assessment indicates a need for preventive interventions (mitigation) or precautionary actions.

Researchers are also concerned with health inequalities. A study of the health impacts of socioeconomical status involving a large group of epidemiologists, coordinated by the University of Turin working in the framework of the European Union joint action on inequalities in health, is presently in progress.[4]

HIA of waste management undertaken in Italy

EIA and SEA require an assessment of health impacts, but coverage of health has been weak or absent in most EIA and SEA reports even when there was a probability of major health impacts and strong community concern. Many initiatives have been taken in some Italian regions to enhance the health component in EIA or to undertake separate HIA.

Waste management is a topic that causes concern to both public administrations and citizens' associations. The difficulty of applying EU regulations for waste management and the heated opposition to building new disposal facilities, especially waste incineration plants, are well known. Public protests are often simplistically dismissed as symptoms of the NIMBY (Not in My Backyard) syndrome, thereby failing to recognize the specific content of the objections to the construction of waste management facilities. Several requests to perform HIA to evaluate waste management plans have been made by both public officials and citizens' associations in Italy.

Epidemiologists and public health officials operating in research bodies (National Research Council), universities (hygiene and public health departments), the National Health Service (public health and prevention services), and environmental protection agencies were the first in Italy to gain experience of doing HIA. In 2002, the province of Florence commissioned the Tuscany Health Agency and the Institute of Clinical Physiology of the National Research Council (IFC-CNR) to undertake an HIA to evaluate the potential impacts of building a new waste incineration plant at three possible locations in an industrial/commercial area.[5] Characterization of the environment, emissions modelling, and assessment of health conditions were carried out. An increase in respiratory diseases in adults and children was predicted in the area defined as exposed by diffusion models. As a consequence, the final report recommended as the best option location of the plant in an area where fewer people would be affected and made suggestions for a programme of environmental reinstatement. The plant location has not yet been decided, but several actions have been taken, such as reducing traffic flows, installing a neighbourhood heating system, and improving the local environment with a 20-hectare wooded area (specifically planned to absorb air pollution).

Other HIA in Italy

In 2008, the regional government of the Abruzzo region (central Italy) promoted a law that required the use of HIA to assess projects planned for the region. This is the only such law in Italy. There has been a rapid growth of interest in proposals for oil-prospecting activity in the region and it was proposed to use HIA to monitor these. Although in 2009 new regulations replaced the previous ones and cancelled the requirement for HIA, a training course was carried out for the administrative staff in the Abruzzo region and HIA guidelines were drafted.[6]

While the regional law allowing HIA was in force a study to address the major environmental risks in the area was carried out by the environment and health departments of the regional government, in collaboration with the research institution Consorzio Mario Negri Sud (CMNS). Now a chapter in the regional budget provides finance to maintain this activity, and to implement communication and participation activities in the region, related to high-risk areas. Meanwhile, CMNS together with IFC-CNR successfully applied to EU DG Environment funds for a project 'Participative assessment of the health, environment and socio-economic impacts deriving from the handling of urban waste, HIA21'[7], which explores how HIA could enhance participation in Local Agenda 21 processes. This project will identify critical issues along the waste chain management by a retrospective HIA of the experience of two waste-treatment plants in Italy (a large landfill and an incinerator), in the context of Local Agenda 21.

In the Tuscany region, Title II of the urban bylaw on planning and evaluation procedures for territorial changes (LR.N. 01—03 January 2005)[8] requires that all plans and programmes that could impact on the environment or resident population be evaluated from an environmental and health point of view in order to consider their sustainability and safety.

The Moniter Project

In 2007, the Emilia-Romagna Regional Government promoted the Moniter Project, which established an environment and health surveillance and assessment system in the areas where eight municipal waste incinerators are located. The project included a literature review, a consultation with experts about priorities and effective communication, a rapid appraisal of one of the existing plants (the Bologna province incinerator), and a Delphi consultation on tools, stakeholders, and HIA models in the context of incinerators.[9] Guidelines for the HIA of new plants were published in 2010.[10] The Moniter project has created new competences, strengthened a culture of precautionary practice, encouraged consideration of impacts on human health, and promoted the use of HIA to support public planning.

HIA in public administration

The VisPA project funded by the Centre for Diseases Control of the Ministry of Health aims to explore the uses of HIA in public administration. As part of this project a rapid HIA process involving production of official binding decisions by sector experts meeting in a technical decision-making conference was tested. Forty public officials belonging to the administrative bodies of four Italian regions are being trained to participate in these conferences.

A project for 'testing a model to evaluate environmental and health impacts useful for identifying risk areas' was launched in Piedmont region (northern Italy), coordinated by the Regional Environment Protection Agency (Piedmont ARPA). It involves the Piedmont health services in producing official binding opinions in technical decision-making conferences, using an HIA methodology. One of the goals is to train service staff to include consideration of health in EIA and SEA procedures. In the past EIA of projects such as a waste-incineration plant in the town of Turin, the Turin–Lyon fast railway, and a thermoelectric plant had failed to take account of health impacts. The impact assessment (EIA and HIA) for a new electric power line between Domodossola and Borgomanero used a better process of screening, scoping, and involvement of concerned citizens. Based on a systematic examination of studies of the effects of exposure to electromagnetic fields a stricter limit of 1 volt/metre was imposed for the electromagnetic field under the line. Piedmont ARPA has also been asked to assist HIA in other regions. Valle d'Aosta Region asked for their advice on an HIA comparing the effect of closing the tunnel and highway under Mont Blanc. In this case the analysis focused mainly on pulmonary diseases in the municipalities along the whole highway, and this showed appreciable impact, especially on children and older people.

The Environment Protection Agency (ARPA) of the Apulia region (southern Italy) have paid particular attention to HIA as part of EIA and SEA procedures and the use of epidemiological data. They recently carried out a risk assessment study on benzo(a)pyrene, emitted by the industrial plants in the Taranto area, as a result of which they recommended a reduction in the permitted threshold below that currently allowed by national law (1 ng/m^3) and suggested modification and re-engineering of plants found to be exceeding the limits.[11] The regional and local authorities used the HIA report to justify a remediation plan, which required the companies responsible for the pollution to modify their plants.

A further example is one of the several HIAs carried out in Lazio region by the Epidemiology Department of the regional health service in which the impact on air quality and public health of policies to reduce traffic pollution, implemented in Rome between 2001 and 2005, was assessed. The analysis, developed in the framework of the Intarese EU project, evaluated the benefits of the policy in different socioeconomic groups of the urban population.[12] The effects of the intervention were evaluated by applying the full-chain model, analysing pressure (number and age distribution of cars), emissions (PM$_{10}$ and NO$_2$ concentrations), population exposure, and years of life gained, broken down by a small-area indicator of socioeconomic position. The conclusion was that the traffic policy in Rome was effective in reducing air pollution, but that most of the health gains were found in well-off residents.[13] This type of study represents an important improvement of the appraisal phase of HIA, providing relevant information on impact on health inequalities to decision makers.

In a completely different setting, the Department of Hygiene of the University of Turin carried out an HIA on the impact of an unauthorized settlement of approximately 500 Roma people in order to address the concerns of residents living close to the camps. Since no public institutions supported the study, it was funded by the university in collaboration with an NGO, Terra del Fuoco, which was already working in the area. The HIA described the living conditions, health status, access to public services, employment, and education in the settlement, thereby increasing understanding of the present situation and helping the planning of interventions.

Conclusion

Knowledge and use of HIA in Italy is developing and it is increasingly linked with the international research groups that will strengthen methods and make HIA more effective. Stakeholders need to be more involved in the HIA process and there is a need to make progress with the legislative framework for HIA.

References

1. Costa G, Paci E, Ricciardi W. (eds). United Italy, 150 years later: has equity in health and health care improved? Epidemiologia e Prevenzione 2011; 35(5–6) suppl 2: 1–136).

2. Bianchi F, Lauriola P. HIA, health impact assessment: a multidisciplinary procedure to support decision making in public health. Epidemiologia e Prevenzione 2011; 35: 73–76.

3. University of Southern Denmark RAPID . Available at http://www.sdu.dk/om_sdu/institutter_centre/ist_sundhedstjenesteforsk/forskning/forskningsenheder/sundhedsfremme/forskningsprojekter/rapid?sc_lang=en. Accessed 29 February 2012.

4. EuroHealth Net Joint Action on health inequalities. Available at http://eurohealthnet.eu/research/joint-action-health-inequalities, Accessed 29 February 2012.

5. Bianchi F, Buiatti E, Bartolacci S *et al*. Esperienza di utilizzo della VIS per la localizzazione di un inceneritore nell'area fiorentina [Experience of HIA use for the placement of an incinerator in the Florence area.] Epidemiologia e Prevenzione 2006; 30: 46–54.

6. Pagliani T, Desiderio M. Linee guida per la valutazione di impatto sanitario (VIS). Documento redatto per l'Agenzia Regionale Sanitaria ASR Abruzzo. [Guidelines for Health Impact Assessment (HIA). Document drafted on behalf of the Abruzzo Regional Health Agency RHA.] Available at http://www.negrisud.it/ambiente/lineeguidaVIS.pdf. Accessed 29 February 2012.

7. Coordinamento Agende 21 Locali Italiane. Available at http://www.a21italy.it/IT/index.xhtml. Accessed 29 February 2012.

8. Marangoni F, Stevanin M, Cori L, La tutela dell'ambiente e della salute umana nelle normative dei piani territoriali. [Environment and human health protection in territorial planning.] Wigwam News 2008; July: 11–13.

9. Tintori A. VIS di impianti di incenerimento di rifiuti solidi urbani: indagine policy Delphi. [HIA of waste incineration plants: a policy Delphi investigation.] IRPPS Working Paper n. 32, 2010. Available at http://www.irpps.cnr.it/en/pubblicazioni/working-paper-on-line. Accessed 29 February 2012.

10. Moniter Project, Emilia-Romagna Region, Italy. Available at http://www.arpa.emr.it/moniter/. Accessed 29 February 2012.

11. Bisceglia L, Valutazione dell'impatto sanitario dell'inquinamento da idrocarburi policiclici aromatici nell'area di Taranto, communication in 'La VIS in Italia Esperienze e Prospettive', CNR and ISS, Roma,2010. Available at: http://media.src.cnr.it/evento/workshop-la-valutazione-di-impatto-sulla-salute-vis-italia-esperienze-e-prospettive. Accessed 29 February 2012.

12. INTARESE Intefrated Assessment of Health Risks Environmental Stressors in Europe. Available at http://www.intarese.org. Accessed 29 February 2012.

13. Cesaroni G, Boogaard H, Jonkers S, Porta D, Badaloni C, Cattani G, Forastiere F, Hoek G. Health benefits of traffic-related air pollution reduction in different socioeconomic groups: the effect of low-emission zoning in Rome. Occupational and Environmental Medicine 2012; 19: 133–39.

Chapter 22

Health impact assessment in new member states and pre-accession countries of the EU

Gabriel Gulis

Introduction

Twelve new countries joined the EU in 2004 and 2007. Ten of them were former communist countries and the other two were Malta and Cyprus. Negotiations have also been launched with other countries, including Turkey, Croatia, and Serbia. With the exception of Malta, Cyprus, and Turkey all these countries share a common past, having been part of the communist block for decades. As such, they operate very similar health systems oriented toward extensive hospital development, polyclinics, and traditional state-based systems of health protection covering hygiene and sanitation control.[1] Changing political and societal conditions naturally lead to changes in health systems. Health protection became more influenced by modern public health ideas of disease prevention and health promotion. The search for new ways of working furnished a reason for interest in HIA.

In most new member states and pre-accession countries the existing emphasis on health protection and environmental health provided a second reason for introduction of HIA, either as part of the mandated EIA or as part of the health protection work. The participation of many institutions from these countries in different health promotion-oriented programmes of the WHO, such as the Healthy Cities movement, Health Promoting Schools or the Regions for Health programme, provided a third reason for interest in HIA. In addition HIA has been promoted by HIA workshops organized by WHO in many of the new member states during the last decade.

The European Commission supported the development of HIA through many projects. Some new member states were included in the effectiveness of HIA project.[2] Recently the European Commission funded a project entitled 'HIA in New member states, accession and pre-accession countries' (HIA-NMAC).[3] This chapter reviews the findings of HIA-NMAC and presents other developments on HIA in new member states. Because of the shortage of published scientific information on public health themes from new member states and accession countries[4] most of the information presented in this chapter is either from HIA-NMAC work or personal observations and informal interviews conducted by author.

Review of HIA in new member states and accession countries

Within HIA-NMAC a series of workshops provided an excellent opportunity to gather information on the background, knowledge, and experience of HIA of participants. The mean age of participants from different countries varied between 36 and 44 years and one third were male. Their work positions varied from public health students to prime ministerial advisors but most attendees were heads of departments in a ministry or municipality, nurses, chief medical officers for regions, health coordinators, project developers, university professors, health inspectors, or project coordinators. An important issue was language; translation was always necessary and usually handouts in the national language were provided. A clear lesson from the workshops is that countries should be encouraged to develop teaching materials in their own language. For most participants the workshop was their first introduction to HIA. Table 22.1 shows the percentages of those who had heard of or used HIA before attending the workshop.

Various factors explain the wide differences between countries in awareness of HIA. The high percentage of participants from Bulgaria, who had heard of HIA, is because most participants worked in public health and because Bulgaria

Table 22.1 Percentages of workshop participants from different countries who had heard of or used HIA

Country	Percentage of participants who had heard of HIA before NMAC workshop	Percentage of participants who had used HIA before NMAC workshop
Turkey	37	0
Lithuania	80	57
Poland	14	0
Bulgaria	82	58
Slovak Republic	37	10
Hungary	63	25

has included HIA in its public health legislation. However, although legislation had raised awareness, people did not feel confident to do HIA as there had been no training or capacity building. Similarly, the high percentage of participants from Lithuania is accounted for by a legal obligation in that country to conduct HIA within EIA or a separate HIA for planned development projects (economic). Furthermore, Lithuania was twinned with the Netherlands in 2002–2003 in a project to encourage HIA supported by the Programme of Community Aid to Countries of Central and Eastern Europe (PHARE) and also participated in the effectiveness of HIA project (funded by DG SANCO). However, discussions in the workshops made clear that in both Lithuania and Bulgaria understanding of HIA is still very limited in health and other sectors.

Hungary has a strong tradition of using different impact assessment techniques and of public health training, which accounts for its relatively high-level awareness of HIA. An awareness-raising workshop 'Health, economy and society' had been organized by the Hungarian Ministry of Health, Social and Family Affairs and the EC (DG SANCO) in 2003, and a policy paper on HIA was produced.[5] Recently a special volume of a national journal of the Ministry of Health 'Nepegeszsegugy (Public health)' devoted a full issue to HIA and the Hungarian government is preparing to establish an HIA support unit within one of the public health institutions.

The Slovak Republic had also been introduced to HIA at least on a local level through training workshops within the PHASE project of WHO during 2003–2005. The Public Health Act no 355/2007 passed in 2007 included HIA as a responsibility of public health institutes. Although implementation of this section of the act was delayed and its content amended after January 2011, it gave public health authorities powers to request inclusion of HIA reports in any project documentation. During the time period 2007–2010 two additional capacity-building workshops (one on HIA methodology and equity and one on the development of a screening tool for use in the Slovak Republic) supported by WHO offices in Rome and Venice were organized to train a group of eight national HIA experts. These eight experts now lead work on HIA in the Republic.

The WHO office in Rome has also supported capacity-building workshops in Estonia, Romania, and Latvia. Moreover, the capacity-building workshop in Latvia in 2011 led the Latvian Ministry of Health to call for the development of a guidance document on HIA. The development of HIA in Latvia is linked to the introduction of a new public health strategy highlighting the HiAP approach. The Czech Republic is also building HIA capacity. The National Institute of Public Health published a guidance document on the use of HIA in SEA in 2006 and the region of Liberec uses HIA not only at project level but also at policy level.[6] Poland continues to participate in project work related to HIA. Rising interest at the national political level in Poland is shown by the inclusion of 'HIA and Health in All Policies' as a theme at the conference of Ministers of Health of EU member states during the Polish presidency in November 2011.

Slovenia was one of the first new EU member states to use HIA at policy level even before entering the EU[7] and is continuing to work on HIA (mostly in the National Institute of Public Health in Ljubljana). Malta and Turkey were actively involved in the HIA-NMAC project and have developed case studies, teaching modules (Turkey), and built capacity by training.

This overview demonstrates the importance of capacity-building events. More training, competence development, and a systematic forum for exchange of experience headed the list of needs to support practice of HIA in all the participating countries. Lectures on HIA are now included in undergraduate and graduate public health training programmes and within continuing professional development programmes in Lithuania, Turkey, the Slovak Republic, Hungary, and Poland.

Enablers and barriers for HIA

Any administration considering the use of HIA has to think of the enablers and barriers to implementation. Table 22.2 presents the enablers and barriers to the use of HIA most often mentioned in the capacity-building events

Table 22.2 Enablers and barriers for the use of screening and/or full HIA

Enablers	Barriers
Well-trained experts	Lack of financial, human, and technical resources
Accurate information and data	Lack of information
Demand from population/awareness	Frequent political changes
Financial resources	Time-consuming, existing rules for administration
Good, accessible literature	Uncertainties
Political demand/awareness	Hard to plan
International experience	Lack of interest
Legal requirement for HIA	Cannot answer all questions
Voluntary status of HIA	Lack of legal requirement
Reinforces civic society	Lack of knowledge

Reproduced with permission from Gulis G. Health impact assessment in new member states, accession and pre-accession countries HIA-NMAC. Final Technical Report. Esjberg: University of Southern Denmark, 2008. Available at http://ec.europa.eu/health/ph_projects/2004/action1/docs/action1_2004_frep_20_en.pdf.

for new member states (HIA-NMAC project and WHO capacity-building workshops).

The suggested enablers and barriers are heterogeneous and in some cases contradictory, reflecting different cultural, legal, and working traditions. For example, a legal requirement and the voluntary status of HIA are both listed as enablers. The availability of well-trained people together with data, tools, adequate time, and public and political support were all thought to increase the probability that HIA would be done. Lack of these factors had the opposite effect. Participants identified the following needs to support future practice of HIA in their respective countries:

- further education and training
- legal basis for HIA
- technical support, including software
- methodological support and guidelines
- financial support.

In particular all participants emphasized the need for public health education reflecting the principles of the determinants of health.

Capacity building

The key elements for capacity building are:

- workforce development
- organizational development
- resource allocation
- partnerships
- leadership.[8]

Workforce development was viewed as the most important element. The achievements of the training workshops could be enhanced by development of training modules and HIA websites in national languages. Workforce development must be sustained. The Slovak Republic provides a good example of this, where eight experts, after being trained, went on to run workshops for others within the country and to have key roles in examining and licensing potential practitioners to undertake HIA.

Organizational development through project work or specific workshops is very challenging. One possible approach is demonstrated by Hungary, which has established an HIA support unit and strengthened an HIA sub-group at the School of Public Health in Debrecen.

Resource allocation as part of capacity building for HIA must consider more than financial resources. Human resources, which are essential, can be built through training, participation, and collaborative research activities. Attendance by nationals of new member states at international HIA conferences continues to increase. Formal and informal discussion with workshop participants highlighted the need for information resources and data availability. Training modules in national languages can address that need for information resources. Participants also mentioned technical and methodological support as being important for successful implementation of HIA. Because of the nature of HIA, country-specific HIA guidelines are likely to be more useful than a single European guideline. However, as shown from our experience, participants successfully learned to develop and use their own screening tools. Again, the best way to support the development of country- and language-specific technical and methodological tools is by establishing a forum within the EU for systematic exchange of HIA experience.

In both formal evaluations and informal discussions during workshops, participants stressed the value of 'meeting people from other departments and ministries'. Bulgaria was the only country where the participants came exclusively from the public health sector and after the second workshop participants expressed their intention to work with staff from other ministries and departments when organizing further HIA training. Intersectoral partnership working on HIA has been contrasted to the regulatory-based approach. In many countries licensing procedures have a legal time framework that means that a proposal must be approved or rejected within a certain number of days. Often, this time limitation makes the consultation with partners and conduct of a full HIA impossible and leads to no HIA being done. It is easier to complete an HIA quickly where there is an established culture of partnership working.

HIA training

Personal and organizational leadership requires trained people. Isolated HIA training courses are available in various countries but these are infrequent, often too expensive for staff from new member states, and not available in all languages. Distance learning packages and discussion forums might offer a satisfactory solution to these problems in the fairly near future. A bid has been submitted to the Visegrad group (the Czech Republic, the Slovak Republic, Hungary, and Poland) to establish a Central European HIA support centre at Trnava University, and this could also organize regular training courses. However training is organized it will need to be funded.

Any project team is likely to include people expert in many different disciplines but also to lack people expert in other disciplines relevant to HIA and

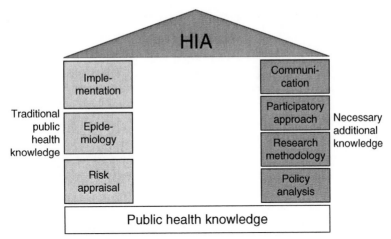

Fig. 22.1 The knowledge needed for HIA.

Adapted with permission from Gulis G. Health impact assessment in new member states, accession and pre-accession countries HIA-NMAC: Final Technical Report. Esjberg: University of Southern Denmark, 2008. Available at http://ec.europa.eu/health/ph_projects/2004/action1/docs/action1_2004_frep_20_en.pdf.

therefore to need expertise from outside the team. However, the content of general public health training also needs to be addressed. Workshop participants from all countries had strong knowledge of basic public health, medicine, epidemiology, and other, mostly medical, disciplines. However, they realized that they needed stronger understanding of the broad determinants of health and additional generic topics such as communication skills, participatory approaches, research methodology, information gathering, policy analysis, and policy theory. Schools of public health need to ensure that their courses cover not only traditional public health topics but also teach the additional topics needed to 'glue' this knowledge together as their graduates are likely to become the leaders of HIA in their countries (Figure 22.1).

Making HIA a legal requirement

The issue of whether HIA should be legally required deserves careful consideration. In some new member states (the Slovak Republic, Lithuania, Bulgaria, and Hungary) HIA is already legally required through different laws (public health law, health protection law, or within EIA) while in other new member states there is no legal requirement for HIA. There is no evidence as to which model works better. Taking account of the value base of HIA, the variety of methodological approaches, and the range of stakeholders involved in HIA one obvious question is 'What should be legally required and from whom?'.

Should authorities be obliged by law to screen each proposal for likely health impacts? If so who should do it? Among workshop participants as among the HIA community in general (see Chapter 11, page 110) there was no consensus on these points.

Many participants looked for technical and methodological support and guidelines for HIA. It is unlikely that any guideline could be suited to the needs of all European countries and indeed each country may need several different guidelines. Experience from the HIA-NMAC project shows that the best way to develop country- and language-specific materials, including screening tools, was for them to be written by nationals of those countries supported by HIA practitioners from other countries.

Examples of HIA from new member states

HIAs conducted in new member states reflect the themes that are most relevant to them and include HIA of policies relating to agriculture, public health, Roma population, and tourism. The first published case study from Slovenia addressed the impact of EU accession on Slovenian agriculture.[8] HIAs in Slovenia, Hungary,[9] the Slovak Republic, and Poland have concerned policies on wine production and foods rich in dietary fibre (unfortunately most of these are still unpublished). Turkey has led (supported by Malta and the Slovak Republic) work on HIA of tourism policies, focusing on both general summer and winter tourism and special regulations (diving policies in Malta). Hungary has lead work on policies on the Roma population,[10,11] an issue that is of great importance in new member states. In 1999 the Slovak Republic conducted an HIA of its public health policy and it is about to conduct an HIA of changes to its health system.

Conclusions

Interest in and understanding of HIA has steadily grown among the new member states of the EU and pre-accession countries during last decade. Most of that development is related to research rather than routine use. More individuals are learning to undertake HIA, and HIA is gaining importance in the public health agenda as well as in general political and social discourse. This progress is being fostered by exchange of experience and methods.

References

1. Gulis G. Health impact assessment in CEE region: case of the former Czechoslovakia. Environmental Impact Assessment Review 2004; 24: 169–95.
2. Wismar M, Blau J, Ernst K, Figueras J: The effectiveness of health impact assessment. Brussels: European Observatory on Health Systems and Policies, 2007.

3. Gulis G. Health impact assessment in new member states, accession and pre-accession countries HIA-NMAC. Final Technical Report. Esjberg: University of Southern Denmark, 2008. Available at http://ec.europa.eu/health/ph_projects/2004/action1/docs/action1_2004_frep_20_en.pdf. Accessed 29 February 2012.

4. McCarthy M, Clarke A. European Public Health Research Literatures—measuring progress. European Journal of Public Health 2007; 17(Suppl 1): 2–5.

5. Ohr M. Getting Health Impact Assessment into the Policy Process in Hungary, Budapest; Central European University and Open Society Institute, 2003. Available at http://pdc.ceu.hu/archive/00001835/01/Ohr.pdf. Accessed 29 February 2012.

6. Valenta V, Kucerova J. Integration of health impact assessment into strategic documents. Hygiena 2007; 2: 59–61.

7. Lock K, Gabrijelcic-Blenkus M, Martuzzi M, Otorepec P, Wallace P, Dora C, Robertson A, Maucec Zakotnik J. Health impact assessment of agriculture and food policies: lessons learnt from the Republic of Slovenia. Bulletin of the World Health Organization 2003; 81: 391–98.

8. New South Wales Health. A Framework for building capacity to improve health. Sydney: New South Wales Health Department, 2001. Available at http://www.health.nsw.gov.au/pubs/2001/pdf/framework_improve.pdf. Accessed 29 February 2012.

9. Adam B, Molnar A, Bardos H, Adany R. Health impact assessment of quality wine production in Hungary. Health Promotion International 2009; 24: 383–93.

10. Kosa K, Molnar A, McKee M, Adany R. Rapid health impact appraisal of eviction versus a housing policy in a colony dwelling Roma community. Journal of Epidemiology and Community Health 2007; 61: 960–65.

11. Molnar A, Adam B, Antova T, Bosak L, Dimitrov P, Mileva H, Pekarcikova J, Zurlyte I, Gulis G, Adany R, Kosa K. Health impact assessment of Roma housing policies in Central and Eastern Europe: A comparative analysis. Environmental Impact Assessment Review 2012; 33; 7–14.

Chapter 23

Health impact assessment in the USA

Andrew Dannenberg and
Aaron Wernham

Background of HIA in the USA

The use of HIA in the USA began in approximately 1999. Early HIAs by the San Francisco Department of Public Health and the University of California, Los Angeles (UCLA) examined the impacts on health of proposed living wage ordinances.[1,2] Subsequently, a number of efforts led to increasing interest in HIA as a tool to inform decision making related to the built environment, such as urban planning, redevelopment proposals, and transportation projects,[3,4] and related to policies outside the health sector that affect health.[5]

In 2002, the US Centers for Disease Control and Prevention (CDC) hosted an interdisciplinary workshop to create a research agenda for the emerging area that examines the impacts on health of the design of the built environment.[6] Out of several dozen ideas on this research agenda, HIA rose to the top as one of the most important tools for promoting healthy community design. Subsequently, in 2004, the Robert Wood Johnson Foundation and CDC hosted a second interdisciplinary workshop that identified the next steps needed to move the field of HIA forward in the USA, such as pilot tests, a database of completed HIAs, capacity building to train professionals to conduct HIAs, an evaluation of the impact of HIAs, and identification of more resources for conducting HIAs.[7]

To date, most HIAs in the USA have been carried out without a specific legislative mandate or regulatory requirement. They have been led by public health officials in local, state, or tribal health departments, by academic public health professionals, by community-based organizations seeking to promote the consideration of health, and by professionals in allied disciplines such as urban planning.[8,9] Although some local and state health departments have undertaken HIA without external sources of funding, private foundations and CDC have funded a considerable portion of HIA efforts in the USA to date.

Interest in and use of HIA appears to have increased more rapidly in recent years. Recent funding announcements by the Health Impact Project and CDC attracted hundreds of applications for HIA funding from local and state health departments, planning departments, universities, and non-governmental organizations in most states in the USA. In the last few years several universities have added HIA to their public health course offerings. Recent initiatives such as the National Prevention Strategy and Healthy People 2020 (discussed below) have underscored an emerging USA interest in cross-sector approaches to population health, a transition which both helps to explain the recent USA interest in HIA and explicitly supports it.

Major groups involved in HIA in the USA

Numerous government, foundation, academic, non-profit, and private sector organizations work with and/or provide support for HIAs in the USA (Table 23.1). On the federal level, the environmental health and chronic disease centres at the CDC conduct training and research on HIA and provide funding for HIAs. State, tribal, and local health departments have conducted

Table 23.1 Examples of organizations involved in HIA in the USA

◆ Federal government

  • US Centers for Disease Control and Prevention

    ▪ National Center for Environmental Health

    ▪ National Center for Chronic Disease Prevention and Health Promotion

  • US Department of Agriculture, Bureau of Land Management

  • US Department of the Interior, Minerals Management Service

  • US Environmental Protection Agency

◆ Tribal health departments—Alaska

◆ State government

  • Health departments, including Alaska, Arizona, California, Kentucky, Massachusetts, Minnesota, Oregon, South Carolina, Wisconsin

  • Transportation departments, including Massachusetts, Oregon, Washington

◆ Local government

  • Health departments, including San Francisco, Los Angeles, Portland, Seattle, Baltimore, North Slope Borough AK, Davidson County NC, Billings MT, Douglas County NE

  • Metropolitan planning agencies, including Nashville TN

(continued)

Table 23.1 (Continued) Examples of organizations involved in HIA in the USA

- ◆ Foundations
  - Blue Cross/Blue Shield of Minnesota
  - Kellogg Foundation
  - Kresge Foundation
  - Northwest Health Foundation
  - Robert Wood Johnson Foundation
  - The California Endowment
  - The Pew Charitable Trusts
- ◆ Universities
  - Indiana University, Indianapolis
  - Johns Hopkins University, Baltimore
  - Portland State University, Portland OR
  - University of California, Berkeley
  - University of California, Los Angeles
  - University of Minnesota, Minneapolis
  - University of Pennsylvania, Philadelphia
  - University of Washington, Seattle
- ◆ Non-profit organizations
  - Georgia Health Policy Center
  - Human Impact Partners, Oakland CA
  - Illinois Public Health Institute
  - Kansas Health Institute
  - Oregon Public Health Institute
  - Upstream Public Health, Portland OR
- ◆ Non-governmental organizations
  - American Planning Association
  - American Public Health Association
  - Association of State and Territorial Health Officials
  - National Association of County and City Health Officials
  - National Conference of State Legislators
  - National Network of Public Health Institutes

or assisted with the conduct of HIAs in many parts of the country. HIAs in health departments usually depend on external funding, but some HIAs have been done using internal resources. In a growing number of state and local jurisdictions, land use and transportation planning agencies are using HIAs or assisting in the conduct of HIAs on local projects and plans.

The Robert Wood Johnson Foundation, The Pew Charitable Trusts, The California Endowment, and other private foundations have played a major role in providing funding to advance work on HIA in the USA. Their support has been essential for the development of HIA training, workshops, conferences, and reports, as well as the conduct of numerous individual HIAs.

A number of universities have been actively engaged in advancing the field of HIA. Faculty and staff have conducted HIAs, taught courses and workshops, and contributed to the science base of the field. HIA work at UCLA[10] and the University of California, Berkeley[11] has been especially extensive.

Non-profit organizations, such as Human Impact Partners in California and Upstream Public Health in Oregon, have played an important role in advancing HIA practice through conducting HIAs and providing training and technical assistance to other groups. The availability of such assistance is critical as new organizations begin to use HIA but lack staff with prior experience in the field. Non-governmental organizations representing public health agencies and organizations and planners—such as the National Association of County and City Health Officials, the Association of State and Territorial Health Officials, the National Network of Public Health Institutes and the American Planning Association—have participated in HIA-related efforts, providing information, training, and technical assistance. Several private consulting firms based in the USA have conducted HIAs for private clients, primarily in the natural resource development sector; most of this work is proprietary and few details are publicly available.

Overview of HIAs completed in the USA

The CDC and the Health Impact Project have attempted to track the use of HIA in the USA through professional networks and through an online 'intake form'.[12] As of May 2012, the authors are aware of 103 completed HIAs and 89 additional HIAs currently in progress. These HIAs have been or are being conducted in 34 states, suggesting a wide distribution of interest in the topic.

Figure 23.1 summarizes the HIAs completed in the USA according to the sector addressed and year of completion. The built environment and transportation are the sectors most commonly addressed in HIAs. Other sectors addressed include natural resources and energy, labour and employment, and

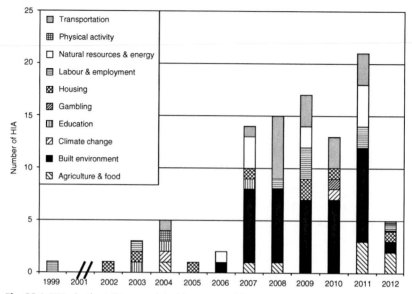

Fig. 23.1 HIAs in the USA completed by year and by sector, January 1999–June 2012 (excludes HIAs with unknown completion date).

Data from Health Impact Project map database at www.healthimpactproject.org.

food and agriculture. Website links to the completed reports are available on the Health Impact Project website for most HIAs.[13]

HIAs have been conducted in the USA by non-governmental organizations, local, state, tribal, and federal health departments, non-health agencies such as departments of planning or environmental management, and universities. Despite the varied organizations—both public and private—that have conducted or participated in HIAs, the practice is still sporadic rather than routine in most regions of the country.

Legal status of HIA

During the past decade, several legislative bills have been introduced but not enacted on the federal and state levels that would have promoted or required the use of HIAs. The Healthy Places Act (S-110-1067) was introduced into the US Senate by then Senator Barack Obama in 2007.[14] On the state level, bills to promote HIA have been introduced in Maryland and California.[15]

The first legislatively required HIA in the USA was for the State Route 520 bridge replacement project in Seattle. In 2007, the Washington state legislature adopted a bill requiring the project to 'incorporate the recommendations of a HIA to calculate the project's impact on air quality, carbon emissions, and other public health issues, conducted by the Puget Sound clean air agency and

King County public health'.[16] In 2009, the Massachusetts legislature adopted the Healthy Transportation Compact, which requires state agencies to 'implement HIA for use by planners, transportation administrators, public health administrators and developers'.[17] The Department of Transportation and the Department of Health are collaborating to work out how this requirement will be implemented.

As in the example of EIA discussed in the next section, some laws that require the analysis of health impacts may support the use of HIA to meet those requirements even when they do not specifically call for HIA. A recent research report reviewed laws in several sectors for a sample of local, tribal, and state jurisdictions, and found that many existing laws actually contain requirements for health analysis that may be met by conducting an HIA.[18]

Links between EIA and HIA

The National Environmental Policy Act of 1970 (NEPA)[19] can be interpreted to require an assessment of health impacts as part of the EIA process[8] (see Chapter 9, page 90). As required by NEPA, the federal government conducts over 500 environmental impact statements a year, and thousands of briefer environmental assessments. Collectively, these laws apply to a wide range of activity with potential importance to health, such as housing and land-use decisions, natural resource extraction, and motor vehicle fuel economy standards. Congress's purpose in adopting NEPA included 'to…stimulate the health and welfare of man' (Sec. 101[42 USC § 4331]). A number of states have adopted similar state-level requirements for EIA. The regulations that established the federal environmental impact statement (EIS) process as the mechanism for implementing NEPA defined health as one of the effects that must be considered (40 CFR § 1508.8). However, available evidence suggests that health is often considered narrowly in NEPA compliance, often with a focus on pollution-related effects, or indirectly,[8,20,21] or not at all. For example, the discussion of air pollution (such as a predicted change in ozone levels) in an EIS seldom describes the health consequences of such air pollution (such as the associated predicted change in the number of asthma cases).

Recently, HIAs have been used to accomplish a more systematic consideration of health in the EIA process. In this context HIAs have been used to inform a number of EIA-based decisions, such as housing redevelopment and land-use decisions in San Francisco,[3] oil and gas leasing in Alaska,[22] and planning a transit corridor in Oregon.[23]

The degree to which the HIA and EIA analyses are integrated varies depending on the relationship of the team conducting the HIA and the agency responsible for leading the EIA. HIAs have been conducted independently and submitted as a comment letter on a draft EIA (for example the I-5 Columbia River Crossing HIA[24]). The agency conducting an EIA is generally required to respond to comments that raise substantive new issues or data sources that were not included in the draft analysis. On the other hand, more formal collaborations between health experts and agencies leading EIAs have led to HIAs being integrated into an EIA[9] or conducted in parallel with the EIA and included as an appendix or referenced in discussions of health in the EIA (Lake Oswego to Portland Transit Project,[23] Point Thomson Oil Extraction[25]). In Alaska, the state health department has recently begun an HIA programme and now routinely participates as a formal part of the team conducting all project-level EIAs in the state.[26]

The National Research Council (NRC) recently reviewed HIA practice in the USA and concluded that the consideration of health in NEPA compliance is required by law, and that HIA provides an effective way to meet that requirement. The NRC recommended federal guidance to assist agencies to better integrate health considerations.[8] With hundreds of EIAs done each year, capacity will be an important question if agencies begin requesting HIAs more frequently. While health departments and non-governmental organizations such as public health institutes may be able to meet some of this demand, the budget strain and cuts facing many public health agencies will compound the challenge. In Alaska, the HIA programme is funded in part by permit fees, which may be one avenue through which health departments could defray the costs of participating in an EIA. The US Department of Health and Human Services has delegated the CDC authority to provide comments related to health in EIAs[27] but with no dedicated resources for this role, the involvement of CDC in the EIA process has been minimal in recent years.

Political environment for HIA in the USA

In the past decade, and particularly in the past three years, there has been a surge of interest in multisectoral approaches to health promotion. The concept of HiAP appears to be achieving more traction.[28] The governor of California, for example, issued an executive order mandating that California agencies adopt an HiAP approach (California Executive Order S-04-10,[29]). In other cases the term HiAP may not be used explicitly, but the need for interdisciplinary collaboration between public health and other sectors has become a prominent theme. This focus on cross-sectoral approaches to health promotion has sparked growing interest in HIA as a practical means to implement the principle. The NRC found that 'substantial improvements in public health will occur only by ensuring that health considerations are factored into projects, programs, plans, and policies in non-health-related sectors' and that 'HIA is a particularly promising approach for integrating health implications into decision-making'.[8]

Similarly, the National Prevention Strategy issued by the National Prevention Council (comprising the Surgeon General and 17 primarily non-health agencies) states that 'opportunities for prevention increase when those working in housing, transportation, education, and other sectors incorporate health and wellness into their decision making' and that HIA 'can be used to help decision makers evaluate project or policy choices to increase positive health outcomes and minimize adverse health outcomes and health inequities'.[30]

The White House Task Force on Childhood Obesity encourages the use of HIA, stating that 'communities should be encouraged to consider the impacts of built environment policies and regulations on human health. Local communities should consider integrating HIAs into local decision-making processes, and the Federal government should continue to support the development of an HIA approach, tools, and supporting resources that promote best practices.'[31] Other recent national documents that encourage the use of HIA include the Department of Health and Human Services Healthy People 2020 report[32] and the CDC's Transportation and Health Policy statement.[33]

The major opposition to expanded use of HIA is an antiregulatory political environment in the USA. While opposition to environmental regulations is not a new phenomenon, the recession and high unemployment rates have intensified concerns about bureaucratic requirements. The EIA process is often perceived as slow and cumbersome. The conduct of an HIA requires time and resources, and some project proponents fear that use of HIA could compound the already lengthy process of securing approval for a proposed project. In addition, high priority is often given to short-term costs and benefits, yet in many cases any health benefits that could be realized by implementing HIA may not be manifest for many years. In this climate, even when HIA is conducted independent of an EIA or on an entirely voluntary basis, these concerns are still common among some stakeholder groups.

Building capacity to conduct HIAs

As interest in HIA increases in the USA there is a need to train professionals in public health and other disciplines such as urban planning and environmental management in the skills required to conduct and interpret HIAs. Various short courses on HIA, typically lasting one to three days, have been and are being taught in the USA. These courses vary in depth and breadth; some are intended primarily to raise awareness of HIA while others aim to provide enough information to enable participants with sufficient experience in public health to conduct an HIA with minimal guidance. One detailed short course in HIA is offered annually by the San Francisco Health Department.[34]

With support from CDC, the American Planning Association offers a free six-hour online course about HIA intended to convey the basics of the topic.[35] This course has attracted thousands of users, including many planners, who receive free continuing education credits for taking the course.

At least eight universities in the USA now teach graduate level courses focused on HIA, typically lasting 10 to 14 weeks. These schools include Indiana University, Johns Hopkins University, University of Portland, University of California Berkeley, University of Pennsylvania, University of Virginia, University of Washington, and University of Wisconsin. Many of these courses attract students from multiple disciplines, including public health, urban planning, public policy, and other areas.

Various guides for the conduct of HIA, ranging in length from 8 to 76 pages, have been developed by the USA. HIA practitioners and working groups.[36–41] Numerous websites have been developed for those who need more information about HIA, including websites developed by UCLA,[10] the San Francisco health department,[42] the Health Impact Project,[43] Human Impact Partners,[44] the Minnesota Design for Health team,[45] and CDC.[46]

Research and scholarship on HIA

The first review of HIAs completed in the USA covered the period 1999–2007 and identified 27 HIAs, of which 15 (56%) had been conducted in California.[4] Of the approximately 80 HIAs completed in the USA over the past decade, a few have been published in peer-reviewed journals. These include HIAs about the San Francisco living wage ordinance,[1] the Los Angeles living wage ordinance,[2] the San Francisco Trinity Plaza housing redevelopment,[3] the Alaska North Slope oil development,[21] the Humboldt County Comprehensive Plan,[47] menu labelling,[48] local food procurement policy,[49] the Page Avenue, Missouri redevelopment project[50] the Atlanta Beltline transit, trails, and parks project,[51] and California climate change policy.[52]

Some work has been done on tools that can be useful for conducting HIAs, such as models of injuries[53] and of traffic noise[54] associated with built environment projects, and a process evaluation of specific HIA tools has been undertaken.[55] Other work has analysed existing datasets to provide quantitative estimates that could be used in HIAs, such as the amount of walking associated with the use of public transit.[56] HIA has also spurred development of other health-based tools such as the Healthy Development Measurement Tool,[57] a comprehensive evaluation metric to consider health needs in urban development plans and projects. This tool, which grew out of an HIA of a San Francisco land-use plan, includes over 100 indicators of social, environmental, and economic conditions, a checklist of development targets associated with each indicator, and a menu of policies and design strategies to advance community health objectives.

Evaluation of the impact of HIAs—on decisions, on the health of affected populations, on improving public participation in decision-making, and on promoting improved intersectoral collaboration—is an important need of the field. Two examples of HIAs that are known to have made an impact on decisions are described in Box 23.1. Funded by the Robert Wood Johnson Foundation, an extensive evaluation of HIAs in the USA is now underway, led by the Group Health Research Institute Center for Community Health and Evaluation in Seattle.[58]

Box 23.1 Examples of HIA success stories

Atlanta BeltLine HIA

The Atlanta BeltLine is a multibillion dollar project encompassing transit, bicycle, and pedestrian trails, parks, and redevelopment that is revitalizing many areas of the city of Atlanta, Georgia (www.beltline.org). With colleagues from CDC and the local health department, Professor Catherine Ross at the Georgia Institute of Technology conducted an HIA of the BeltLine project in 2005–2007. The HIA provided new information on how the BeltLine proposal might affect neighbouring communities and provided practical recommendations for enhancements that would maximize the health benefits of the project. Used as a reference by community members and decision makers, the HIA report determined that the project would have a largely favourable impact on community health through improving the availability of greenspace, creating opportunities for physical activity, reconnecting people and places previously separated by the rail corridor, and increasing transportation options. The HIA revealed how developers could strategically place parks, residential areas, civic buildings, transit routes, and grocery stores to increase residents' health and decrease potential health problems. As a result of the HIA's findings, local donors gave $5 million for new trail construction, the BeltLine's board of directors and citizen advisory committee now include health experts, construction of greenspace is a top priority, and project and funding decisions are taking health into account.

Adapted from Making Healthy Places, by Andrew L. Dannenberg, Howard Frumkin, and Richard J. Jackson. Copyright © 2011 Andrew L. Dannenberg, Howard Frumkin, and Richard J. Jackson.[59]

Box 23.1 Examples of HIA success stories *(continued)*

Massachusetts Low Income Home Energy Assistance Program (LIHEAP) HIA

The Boston University Child HIA Working Group conducted an HIA of LIHEAP to examine the health risks for low-income children associated with unaffordable energy costs. Some of the pathways and health issues explored included the trade-offs that families face between paying energy bills and buying food—sometimes referred to as 'heat or eat'—and the resulting nutritional risks to children. They also studied the health risks—such as burns and carbon monoxide poisoning—that can result when families use unsafe heating sources when energy bills become too high. Finally, they identified the unhealthy living conditions faced by families who were no longer able to afford adequate housing because of high energy costs (e.g. exposure to pests, water leaks and mould, peeling lead paint, and the resulting health hazards, such as asthma, injuries, and lead poisoning). Recommendations from the report included: (1) fully funding LIHEAP, (2) increasing LIHEAP benefit levels to vulnerable families, (3) extending outreach services to clinicians in healthcare settings, (4) creating an initiative that addresses the needs of families on LIHEAP waiting lists, (5) enforcing required data collection on arrearages and disconnections from utility companies, and (6) exploring the rise of the home energy insecurity scale. The HIA ultimately contributed to a decision to increase the level of funding to the programme. Groups in Rhode Island used the report to advocate for increased levels of funding.

Reproduced by permission of Island Press, Washington, D.C. Adapted with permission from Health Impact Project Massachusetts Low Energy Assistance Programme available from http://www.healthimpactproject.org/hia/us/massachusetts-low-income-energy-assistance-program.[60]

Opportunities for growth of HIA in the USA

This appears to be a period of growing interest in and use of HIA in the USA, fuelled in part by the emerging focus on intersectoral approaches to health promotion. The number of people trained to conduct HIAs in short courses, graduate school courses, and online continues to grow. In 2011 a new professional organization, the Society of Practitioners of Health Impact Assessment (SOPHIA)[61] was created, primarily for HIA practitioners in North America but open to all interested personnel. The third HIA in the Americas conference was held in Oakland, California, in October 2011 for experienced HIA practitioners, and an inaugural National HIA Conference was held in Washington, DC, in April 2012, designed for a broader audience, including public health professionals and those from other disciplines, and policy makers. For at least the last five years, HIA practitioners from the USA have participated in and presented talks at the international HIA conferences held in Europe, gaining valuable insights from the experiences of their HIA colleagues in other countries.

The recent NRC report[8] provides helpful guidance on what is needed to move the field forward in the USA. This report suggests ensuring the quality and credibility of HIA, including peer review of HIA reports, incorporating HIA into the EIA process, providing quantitative information in HIAs where it is possible and likely to improve the HIA's effectiveness, ensuring robust engagement of stakeholders in the HIA process, evaluating the impacts of HIA, promoting cross-disciplinary training, and managing expectations regarding the role that HIA can play in decision making relative to all other considerations that influence policy decisions.

Funding for public health in the USA remains relatively low, and many states and municipalities have experienced severe budget cuts during the recession. This presents a challenge for developing a more widespread and stable practice of HIA. As the practice expands and more people are aware of it, more questions regarding its validity and effectiveness are likely to be asked, and evaluation to document the value of HIA will be important. Furthermore, if HIA is perceived as adding to the bureaucratic delays that impose an undue burden on projects moving forward, there will be opposition to making HIA more standard practice.

Among the most encouraging developments in the field—and a model that shows promise as a means to achieve a more stable and enduring practice of HIA—are the regional collaboratives that have developed. In Alaska, efforts by tribes and tribal health organizations led to the formation of a joint state-tribal-federal working group on HIA, and now a formal HIA programme at the state health department. In San Francisco, the health department has practiced HIA for over 10 years with minimal outside funding, and this has helped build a robust regional practice of HIA, with non-governmental organizations, community advocacy groups, the University of California, and several health departments collaborating to undertake HIAs, to conduct HIA training, and to develop tools that improve the quality of HIAs. The prospects for increasing use of HIAs in the USA appears more promising now than at any time in the past.

References

1. Bhatia R, Katz M. Estimation of health benefits from a local living wage ordinance. American Journal of Public Health 2001; 91: 1398–1402.

2. Cole BL, Shimkhada R, Morgenstern H, Kominski G, Fielding JE, Wu S. Projected health impact of the Los Angeles City living wage ordinance. Journal of Epidemiology and Community Health 2005; 59(8): 645–50.

3. Bhatia R. Protecting health using an environmental impact assessment: a case study of San Francisco land use decisionmaking. American Journal of Public Health 2007; 97: 406–13.

4. Dannenberg AL, Bhatia R, Cole BL, Heaton SK, Feldman JD, Rutt CD. Use of health impact assessment in the U.S.: 27 case studies, 1999–2007. American Journal of Preventive Medicine 2008; 34: 241–56.

5. Cole BL, Fielding JE. Health impact assessment: a tool to help policy makers understand health beyond health care. Annual Review of Public Health 2007; 28: 393–412. Available at http://international.uiowa.edu/centers/global-health/documents/ Healthimpactassessment.pdf.

6. Dannenberg AL, Jackson RJ, Frumkin H, Schieber RA, Pratt M, Kochtitzky C, Tilson HH. The impact of community design and land-use choices on public health: a scientific research agenda. American Journal of Public Health 2003; 93: 1500–1508.

7. Dannenberg AL, Bhatia R, Cole BL, Dora C, Fielding JE, Kraft K, McClymont-Peace D, Mindell J, Onyekere C, Roberts JA, Ross CL, Rutt CD, Scott-Samuel A, Tilson HH. Growing the field of health impact assessment in the United States: an agenda for research and practice. American Journal of Public Health 2006; 96: 262–70.

8. National Research Council, Committee on Health Impact Assessment. Improving Health in the United States: The Role of Health Impact Assessment. Washington, DC: National Academies Press, 2011. Available at http://www.nap.edu/catalog.php?record_ id=13229. Accessed 1 March 2012.

9. Wernham A. Health impact assessments are needed in decision making about environmental and land-use policy. Health Affairs (Millwood) 2011; 30: 947–56.

10. UCLA Health Impact Assessment Clearing House Learning and Information Centre. Available at http://www.hiaguide.org/. Accessed 1 March 2012.

11. UC Berkeley Health Impact. Available at http://sites.google.com/site/ucbhia/. Accessed 1 March 2012.

12. Health Impact Project. Tell us about your Health Impact Assessment. Available at www.healthimpactproject.org/tell. Accessed 1 March 2012.

13. Health Impact Project—HIA in United States. Available at http://www. healthimpactproject.org/hia/us. Accessed 1 March 2012.

14. S1067 Healthy Places Act 2007. Available at http://www.govtrack.us/congress/bill. xpd?bill=s110-1067. Accessed 1 March 2012.

15. Farquhar D, Health Impact Assessments: A tool to Assess and Mitigate the Effects of Policy Decisions on Public Health. Available at http://www.ncsl.org/documents/ environ/HIA.pdf. Accessed 1 March 2012.

16. Seattle and King County Public Health SR 520. Health Impact Assessment: A bridge to a healthier community 2008. Available at http://www.kingcounty.gov/healthservices/ health/ehs/hia.aspx. Accessed 1 March 2012.

17. Massachusets Department of Transportation. Healthy Transportation Compact. Available at http://www.massdot.state.ma.us/GreenDOT/ HealthyTransportationCompact.aspx. Accessed 1 March 2012.

18. Health Impact Project and Sandra Day O'Connor School of Law, Arizona State University. Legal Review Concerning the Use of Health Impact Assessments in Non-Health Sectors 2012. The Pew Charitable Trusts. Washington, D.C., USA. Available at http://www.healthimpactproject.org/resources/legal-review-concerning-the-use-of-health-impact-assessments-in-non-health-sectors. Accessed June 2012.

19. US Environmental Protection Agency. National Environmental Policy Act 1970. Available at http://www.epa.gov/compliance/basics/nepa.html. Accessed 1 March 2012.

20. Steinemann A. Rethinking human health impact assessment. Environmental Impact Assessment Review 2000; 20: 627–45.

21. Bhatia R, Wernham A. Integrating human health into environmental impact assessment: an unrealized opportunity for environmental health and justice. Environmental Health Perspectives 2008; 116: 991–1000.

22. Wernham A. Inupiat health and proposed Alaskan oil development: Results of the first Integrated Health Impact Assessment/Environmental Impact Statement of proposed oil development on Alaska's North Slope. EcoHealth 2007; 4: 500–13.

23. Oregon Public Health Institute. Lake Oswego to Portland Transit Project: Health Impact Assessment. Available at http://www.healthimpactproject.org/resources/ document/portland-to-lake-oswego-transit-project.pdf. Accessed 1 March 2012.

24. Portland Health Impact Assessment Working Group. Columbia River Crossing Health Impact Assessment 2008. Available at http://www.healthimpactproject.org/hia/us/hia-report/HIA-Report-1-5-Columbia-River-Crossing.pdf. Accessed 1 March 2012.

25. Point Thomson Project EIS. Available at http://www.pointthomsonprojecteis.com/ documents.htm. Accessed 1 March 2012.

26. McLaughlin J, Castrodale L. Alaska's Health Impact Assessment Program. State of Alaska Epidemiology Bulletin. No. 19. 2011. Available at http://www.epi.alaska.gov/ bulletins/docs/b2011_19.pdf. Accessed 1 March 2012.

27. National Center for Environmental Health. Public Health Impact Assessment in the National Environmental Policy Act (NEPA) of 1969: CDC's Review and Commenting Program. Available at http://www.cdc.gov/healthyplaces/factsheets/Public_Health_ Impact_Assessment_factsheet_Final.pdf. Accessed 1 March 2012.

28. Collins J, Koplan JP. Health impact assessment: a step toward health in all policies. Journal of the American Medical Association 2009; 302(3): 315–17.

29. State of California Executive Order S-04-10 2010. Available at http://sgc.ca.gov/hiap/ docs/about/Executive_Order_S-04-10.pdf. Accessed 1 March 2012.

30. National Prevention Council, National Prevention Strategy, Washington, DC: US Department of Health and Human Services, Office of the Surgeon General, 2011. Available at http://www.healthcare.gov/prevention/nphpphc/strategy/report.pdf. Accessed 1 March 2012.

31. White House Task Force on Childhood Obesity. Report to the President. Solving the problem of childhood obesity within a generation. May 2010. Available at http://www. letsmove.gov/white-house-task-force-childhood-obesity-report-president. Accessed 1 March 2012.

32. US Department of Human Services. Healthy People 2020. Available at http://www.healthypeople.gov/2020/TopicsObjectives2020/pdfs/HP2020_brochure_with_LHI_508.pdf. Accessed 1 March 2012.

33. Centers for Disease Control and Prevention. CDC Transportation Recommendations 2011. Available at www.cdc.gov/transportation. Accessed 1 March 2012.

34. San Francisco Department of Public Health. HIA Practitioners Summer Training Course. Available at http://www.sfphes.org/HIA_Training.htm. Accessed 1 March 2012.

35. American Planning Association. Planning for Healthy Places with Health Impact Assessments. Available at http://professional.captus.com/Planning/catalog.aspx. Accessed 1 March 2012.

36. Agyekum G *et al.* UCLA HIA training manual. UCLA-CLIC. 2008. Available at http://www.ph.ucla.edu/hs/hiaclic/methods/training_resources.htm#uclatraining. Accessed 1 March 2012.

37. Bhatia R. A guide for health impact assessment. California Department of Public Health. 2010. Available at http://www.apho.org.uk/resource/item.aspx?RID=104502. Accessed 1 March 2012.

38. Bhatia R. Health Impact Assessment: a guide for practice. Oakland, CA: Human Impact Partners. 2011. Available at http://www.sfphes.org/publications/HIA_Guide_for_Practice.pdf. Accessed 1 March 2012.

39. Forsyth A (ed). Rapid health impact assessment toolkit. University of Minnesota, Design for Health. 2008. Available at http://www.designforhealth.net/pdfs/HIA/BCBS_Rapidassessment_011608.pdf. Accessed 1 March 2012.

40. National Association County & City Health Officials. Health impact assessment: quick guide. 2008. Available at http:www.apho.org.uk/resource/item.aspx?RID=82413. Accessed 1 March 2012.

41. North American HIA Practice Standards Working Group. Minimum elements and practice standards for health impact assessment: version 2. 2010. Available at http://www.humanimpact.org/doc-lib/finish/11/9. Accessed 1 March 2012.

42. San Francisco Department of Public Health. Environmental Health Program on health, equity and sustainability. Available at http://www.sfphes.org/default.htm. Accessed 1 March 2012.

43. Health Impact Project—Home. Available at http://www.healthimpactproject.org./ Accessed 1 March 2012.

44. Human Impact Partners. Available at http://www.humanimpact.org/. Accessed 1 March 2012.

45. Design for Health. Health Impact Assessment. Available at http://www.designforhealth.net/resources/healthimpact.html. Accessed 1 March 2012.

46. Center for Disease Control and Prevention. Healthy Places Health Impact Assessment. Available at http://www.cdc.gov/healthyplaces/hia.htm. Accessed 1 March 2012.

47. Harris EC, Lindsay A, Heller JC, Gilhuly K, Williams M, Cox B, Rice J. Humboldt County General Plan Update Health Impact Assessment: A Case Study. Environmental Justice 2009; 2(3): 127–134.

48. Kuo T, Jarosz CJ, Simon P, Fielding JE. Menu labeling as a potential strategy for combating the obesity epidemic: a health impact assessment. American Journal of Public Health 2009; 99: 1680–86.

49. Gase LN, Kuo T, Dunet D, Schmidt SM, Simon PA, Fielding JE. Estimating the potential health impact and costs of implementing a local policy for food procurement to reduce the consumption of sodium in the county of Los Angeles. American Journal of Public Health 2011; 101: 1501–1507.

50. Hoehner CM, Rios J, Garmendia C, Baldwin S, Kelly CM, Knights DM, Lesorogol C, McClendon GG, Tranel M. Page Avenue health impact assessment: building on diverse partnerships and evidence to promote a healthy community. Health and Place 2012; 18: 85–95.

51. Ross CL, Leone de Nie K, Dannenberg AL, Beck LF, Marcus MJ, Barringer J. Health Impact Assessment of the Atlanta BeltLine. American Journal of Preventive Medicine 2012; 42: 203–213.

52. Richardson M, English P, Rudolph Ll. A health impact assessment of California's proposed cap-and-trade regulations. American Journal of Public Health. Published online ahead of print July 19, 2012; e1–e7. doi:10.2105/AJPH.2011.300527.

53. Wier M, Weintraub J, Humphreys EH, Seto E, Bhatia R. An area-level model of vehicle-pedestrian injury collisions with implications for land use and transportation planning. Accident Analysis and Prevention 2009; 41(1): 137–45.

54. Seto EY, Holt A, Rivard T, Bhatia R. Spatial distribution of traffic induced noise exposures in a US city: an analytic tool for assessing the health impacts of urban planning decisions. International Journal of Health Geographics 2007; 6: 24.

55. Slotterback CS, Forsyth A, Krizek KJ, Johnson A, Pennucci A. Testing three health impact assessment tools in planning: A process evaluation. Environmental Impact Assessment Review 2011; 31: 144–53.

56. Besser LM, Dannenberg AL. Walking to public transit: steps to help meet physical activity recommendations. American Journal of Preventive Medicine 2005; 29: 273–80.

57. Health Development Measurement Tool. Available at http://www.thehdmt.org/. Accessed 1 March 2012.

58. Robert Woods Johnson Foundation. Identifying the critical elements of successful health impact assessments. Available at http://www.rwjf.org/grants/grant.jsp?id=69004. Accessed 1 March 2012.

59. Dannenberg AL, Frumkin H, Jackson RJ. Making Healthy Places: Designing and Building for Health, Well-being and Sustainability. Washington, DC: Island Press, 2011. Available at www.makinghealthyplaces.org. Accessed 1 March 2012.

60. Health Impact Project Massachusetts Low Energy Assistance Programme. Available at http://www.healthimpactproject.org/hia/us/massachusetts-low-income-energy-assistance-program. Accessed 1 March 2012.

61. Society of Practitioners of Health Impact Assessment. Available at http://habitatcorp. com/sophia/Welcome.html. Accessed 1 March 2012.

Chapter 24

Health impact assessment in Canada

Louise St-Pierre and Anika Mendell

Introduction

The practice and institutionalization of HIA in Canada has been characterized by highs and lows. Indeed, at both the federal and provincial levels, significant gains have been made but have not necessarily been sustained. At the local level, HIAs are carried out on selected projects across the country but are not systematically used. Consequently, it can be said that unlike EIA, HIA is not yet an established process in Canada. Rather, implementation of HIA continues to be a work in progress.

However, over the last two decades in Canada there has been HIA-related activity at all levels of government and in various sectors. Indeed, the federal government has produced an internationally recognized guide,[1] two provinces (Quebec and British Columbia) have legislated HIA within the context of renewed Public Health Acts, and various public health units are exploring the implementation of HIA in their regions. Some public health organizations use what is called the 'expert-driven model' of HIA, while the Quebec provincial government has structured HIA practice built on the 'decision-support' model.[2] In Nova Scotia, the People Assessing Their Health (PATH) Network has developed a community-led HIA process. Furthermore, EIA occasionally covers more holistic dimensions of health as defined in HIA. As a result, there is no doubt that Canada continues to be an interesting case study of how HIA emerges as a practice, and the factors that foster and hinder its sustainability.

The Canadian health system at a glance

In Canada health is publicly funded and the Canadian constitution specifies that health is the responsibility of the ten provinces and three territories. The provinces and territories administer and deliver health services, although the federal government shares responsibility for the health of certain populations, such as 'registered' Aboriginal peoples.[3] Public health is also a shared responsibility: while services are structured and delivered at the provincial/territorial level, the Public Health Agency of Canada (PHAC) at the federal level aims to facilitate the coordination of public health efforts across the country and supports knowledge development and transfer.

Historically, the federal level has played an important role in the development and promotion of ideas surrounding healthy public policy. For example, the leadership of the Canadian Health Department during the first International Conference on Health Promotion in 1986, in Ottawa, is widely recognized.[4] More recently, the PHAC has been actively involved in work supporting the WHO Commission on the Social Determinants of Health and this agency also promotes the use of equity-focused health impact assessment (EFHIA).[5] Other national organizations contribute to the development of knowledge on healthy public policy.

However, provinces differ widely with respect to the structure of health systems and their capacity to work on policies developed outside the health sector and, thus, to implement HIA. The size of the population, resources available, public health competencies, and views regarding the role of the public health sector explain this variation. Although the vast majority of the provinces/territories have comprehensive health policies and recognize the social determinants of health, public health resources are primarily focused on functions such as surveillance, infectious diseases, and disease prevention, and less on health promotion and healthy public policy.[6,7]

HIA within environmental impact assessment

In the 1990s, Canada was in the avant-garde of the integration of social determinants of health, within EIA. A group of environmental health professionals (under the leadership of Health Canada) noted the lack of integration of human health issues into project assessments in EIA. Consequently in 1992, the Federal/Provincial/Territorial Committee on Environmental and Occupational Health established a task force with the objective of facilitating the integration of broadly defined health concerns into the EIA process.[8] This involved developing various documents and tools, including the three-volume *Canadian Handbook on HIA*,[1] which received international recognition and was probably better appreciated and used outside Canada than within.[9]

At the provincial level health is generally taken into account in the context of EIA, albeit in a highly variable manner from one region to another. The tendency is to restrain the concept of health to its physical dimension.[10] Exceptions can be found in situations where formal mechanisms for public participation in EIA process exist, such as in British Columbia (Environmental Assessment

Office, www.eao.gov.bc.ca/) and Quebec (Bureau d'audience publique sur l'environnement, www.bape.gouv.qc.ca).

HIA as a means to promote healthy public policy

Moving from environmental health to health promotion, the idea of healthy public policy has been explored at both federal and provincial levels. In 2005, the Government of Canada established the National Collaborating Centres for Public Health Programs, including one centre devoted to Healthy Public Policy (NCCHPP). This centre, funded by the federal government and based in the province of Quebec, emphasized the importance of healthy public policy within the Canadian public health sector (at least at the federal level) and the readiness to share the Quebec experience in this area with the rest of the country. The centre documents Canadian HIA practice and also provides training and support to local and regional public health units across Canada. In a few cases, the concept of healthy public policy has been applied at the provincial level. Indeed, over the course of two decades, HIA has been mandatory in two provinces: British Columbia and Quebec.

British Columbia—a first attempt at HIA institutionalization

In the wake of the first International Conference on Health Promotion,[11] the Ministry of Health of British Columbia created an Office of Health Promotion, which began to promote HIA as a tool for healthy public policy. This cause gained momentum in 1991, when the British Columbia Royal Commission on Health Care and Costs recommended evaluating the potential health effects of all provincial programmes or legislation 'to include studies of potential health effects in all environmental impact assessments'. In 1993, HIA was integrated into the policy analysis process at the cabinet level. By 1995 HIA had come to the forefront of the policy agenda and 'a series of 86 workshops and 26 presentations were held across the province to increase awareness of the determinants of health and to familiarize potential users of the HIA with a guidelines document'.

However, a year later the situation in British Columbia changed dramatically. Following the election in 1996, the provincial government shifted its orientation and set about making major political changes. The Office of Health Promotion, which had become the Population Health Resource Branch, was dismantled, projects were transferred to various government departments, and various champions of HIA left the health sector. Consequently, there was no follow-up to the training sessions and a section in the guidelines was changed so that analysis of health impact was no longer interpreted as mandatory. After reviewing uptake of the HIA training sessions and guidelines, in 1998 the Ministry of Health concluded that the practice had not shown any effect on 'creating policy or program changes consistent with the determinants of health perspective'. Following this report, practice of HIA ceased at the provincial level in British Columbia for over a decade.

Although short lived, this first HIA experience in British Columbia inspired initiatives both internationally and in Canada. Moreover, HIA recently resurfaced through the renewal of the Public Health Act.[12] Section 61 of this Act mandates the Minister of Health 'to evaluate, and advise the government on, those actions of government that may impact public health'. This has translated into general reflection of how to include HIA in the governmental context, but no concrete implementation of HIA. The story of HIA in British Columbia has been well described and analysed by Banken.[13]

Quebec—building on British Columbia's experience

During the same period (the 1990s), various government reports recommended the use of intersectoral initiatives to improve the health of the population in Quebec. In 2000, the Commission d'étude sur les services de santé et les services sociaux (Clair Commission) recommended assessment of the impacts of public policies on health.[14] In 2001 these reports, coupled with an out-of-date Public Health Act (over 30 years old) led to a new public health law, which included provision for HIA.

A working group was created with the mandate to propose guidelines for the amended Act. The mandate of this group was to ensure that the four core public health functions, including health promotion, would be strengthened by the new Act. For this, the group turned to various fundamental texts in the area of health promotion, including the Gothenburg consensus on HIA[15] and descriptions of HIA initiatives around the world. In addition, the temporary disappearance of HIA in British Columbia was used as an argument to convince legislators to integrate HIA into the new Public Health Act. These efforts bore fruit and Section 54 of the Public Health Act obliges government ministries to ensure that proposed legislative provisions do not have potentially negative effects on health. It also mandates the Ministry of Health and Social Services (MSSS) to support other ministries in achieving this obligation. The implementation of Section 54 has led to a form of institutionalization of HIA in Quebec at the central level of the government. The implementation of this section is supported by professionals at the MSSS responsible for Section 54, a new mechanism for integrating HIA into the decision-making process, an HIA guide, a network of professionals from all other ministries (who participate in biannual meetings and receive bulletins), and a research programme to develop new knowledge related to healthy public policy.[14] A recent evaluation of Section 54 of the Public Health Act has shown that, between 2003 and 2008, 183 legislative proposals were submitted to the MSSS under this section from a variety of ministries, including the Ministries of Sustainable Development, Environment and Parks (34%), of Agriculture, Fisheries and Food (14%), and of Employment and Social Solidarity (12%).[16]

Growing interest in HIA

Currently, pockets of HIA activity can be identified across the country. In the province of Alberta, where a cross-ministry team has developed tools, a number of pilot projects have been completed and HIA is in the early stages of implementation. In Ontario, both the Ministry of Health and Long-Term Care and Public Health Ontario have launched health equity impact assessment frameworks and tools, as well as pilot projects. In the province of Manitoba, the cross-departmental initiative Healthy Child Manitoba paired up with the University of Manitoba in 2010–2011 to conduct an equity-focused HIA on a public health programme aimed at adolescents.

Activity is also taking place at the regional and local levels. In Ontario, different regional health authorities with community and municipal partners are exploring both training and implementation of HIA with a particular focus on equity within their institutions. For example, Sudbury and District Health Region (located in north-eastern Ontario) identified equity-focused HIA as one of their ten promising practices to reduce social inequities in health.[17] They have since engaged in HIA training in partnership with the National Collaborating Centre for Healthy Public Policy and are planning HIA pilot projects. Toronto Public Health has also engaged in HIA.[18]

In eastern Canada, the People Assessing Their Health (PATH) network has practiced community HIA in a range of settings in the province of Nova Scotia and abroad, and two regional health authorities have embarked on HIA training sessions with community partners and specific groups of the population (Acadian and Aboriginal).

HIA development and the triple I model

Despite all of these encouraging developments, in Canada very few HIAs have been done which correspond with 'classically defined' criteria (prospective assessment, complete procedure, appropriate type of policy, programme or project assessed, right timing etc.), and there is no consistent community of practice in HIA. It is reasonable to affirm that HIA practice is still young in this country.

In order to go beyond these initial observations to better understand what we call the 'tentative emergence of HIA' in Canada, it may be useful to turn to theories of public policy development. The triple-I model,[19] which considers the importance of Ideas (beliefs and values), Institutions (norms, rules, and government structures), and Interests (who bears benefits and costs) in the emergence of policies, has been particularly helpful in our attempts to explain the Canadian situation with regards to HIA.

The 'idea' of HIA

From the Lalonde report[20] in 1974 to the creation of the National Collaborating Centres for Public Health ideas have proliferated about the determinants of health and the need for action outside the healthcare sector. HIA featured in prominent reports such as the Senate Sub-Committee report on Population Health[21] and the Canadian Health Council report[22] on the same subject. Growing concern for health equity can be observed in various provinces at various levels, and interest in the HiAP approach has also gained momentum in Canada. However, governments in Canada do not have the same stimulus as European countries, where the EU has committed to HIA and HiAP.

Some provinces are models for the others, and inspire action. British Columbia inspired Quebec, which in turn attracted the interest of other provinces in the establishment of mechanisms that allow for the integration of HiAP, therefore the idea of HIA being necessary, because all governmental sectors are involved (directly or indirectly) in shaping the health status of the population, is recognized and accepted. However, this idea alone is not sufficient to take action. Considering how ideas do or do not translate into institutional support can provide further insight into HIA practice in Canada.

Institutions that shape norms and structure support for HIA

The EIA processes in which the impact on human health can be taken into consideration have been a lever for HIA practice. Generally speaking, Canada is well equipped in terms of public health organizations, including research capacities, academics, and networks in public health, to further HIA. While certain parts of the country do not have the resources to implement HIA that other, more populous regions do, this factor does not seem to be directly connected to the emergence of HIA practice. It seems, rather, that the norms and governmental orientations regarding the roles and mandates of public health may influence the capacity and the legitimacy for public health actors to work outside the traditional frontiers of the health sector. Indeed, where we find inclusive governmental public health plans, as in Quebec, specific units on Healthy Public Policy, as in Alberta, or official standards of practices that invite the public health sector to work with communities on social determinants of health, as in Ontario, HIA finds its way into practice more easily.

Interest for HIA: who wins, who loses

The last aspect is interest for HIA, which we believe is lacking in Canada. There is, of course, interest for HIA within the public health sector, as the idea of the determinants of health becomes increasingly accepted in various areas of public health, not just in the field of health promotion. However, real interest has to be transformed into resource allocation, as it has been in Quebec, but not in many other provinces.

Besides the direct cost assumed by the public health sector there is also a political cost of HIA. The engagement of other sectors outside of health is inherent to HIA but a convincing case has not yet been made to present HIA as a truly 'win-win' procedure for all sectors. In fact, other sectors already grappling with EIA consider it to be an arduous inconvenience. Furthermore, it is not necessarily politically profitable for decision makers outside the health sector to dig into their proposals and seek new problems unrelated to the main policy objective. As such, it is not necessarily in the best interest of decision makers to be involved in HIA unless it is valued by the population they serve. Even those decision makers within the health sector who are already uncomfortable with the proportion of the government's budget consumed by health may not want to be in the delicate position of opposing a decision from within their government.

Conclusion

Based on this very brief analysis, we can say that HIA as a tool to develop healthy public policy is relatively well recognized across Canada and that various levers (for example, the ideas of HiAP and health equity, and the institutionalization of holistic EIAs) have promoted the use of HIA. The federal government, as well as the more populous provinces, might have the resources to support work beyond the traditional frontiers of the health sector to address the social determinants of health. These factors have brought more than one province to consider and even adopt HIA legislation. However, concrete implementation seems to need additional willingness, as well as champions to overcome the resistance inherent to activities that require power sharing both outside and from within the health sector.

References

1. Health Canada. The Canadian Handbook on Health Impact Assessment. Volumes 1-4, CD Health Canada 2004. Available at http://publications.gc.ca/collections/Collection/H46-2-99-235E-1.pdf. Accessed 2 March 2012.

2. Harris-Roxas B, Harris E. Differing forms, differing purposes: a typology of health impact assessment. Environmental Impact Assessment Review 2010; 30: 396–403.

3. Health Canada First Nations, Inuit & Aboriginal Health. Health Canada 2011. Available at http://www.hc-sc.gc.ca/fniah-spnia/index-eng.php. Accessed 2 March 2012.

4. Raeburn J. Ottawa Charter: reflections from down under. Promotion & Education 2007; 10(Suppl. 2): 41–42.

5. PHAC Consultation Workshop on Equity-Focused Health Impact Assessment. Briefing Note for Participants. International Workshop at Ottawa (Canada), 23–24 October, WHO, 2009.

6. Bernier N. Canadian Approaches to Public Health: A Comparative Overview of Policy Content and Organization, Article presented to the 17th reunion of the Society for the Advancement of Socio-Economics, Budapest, Hungry, 30 Juin to 2 July 2005. Available at http://www.cacis.umontreal.ca/Bernier_NF.SASE.pdf. Accessed 2 March 2012.

7. Paradis G. 'F' for public policy. Canadian Journal of Public Health 2011; 102: 163.

8. Shademani R, Von Schirnding Y. Health Impact Assessment in Development Policy and Planning. Report of an Informal WHO Consulting Meeting, Cartagena, Colombia, 28 May 2001. Geneva: WHO. Available at http://www.who.int/mediacentre/events/HSD_Plaq_02.4_def1.pdf.

9. NCCHPP Report on the Canadian Roundtable on Health Impact Assessment (HIA) 2007. Available at http://www.ncchpp.ca/133/Publications.ccnpps?id_article=175. Accessed 2 March 2012.

10. Noble B; Bronson J. Practitioner survey of the state of health integration in environmental assessment: The case of northern Canada. Environmental Impact Assessment Review 2005; 26: 410–24.

11. WHO. The Ottawa Charter for Health Promotion. Geneva: World Health Organization, 1986.

12. British Columbia. Bill 23-2008 Public Health Act 2008. Legislative Session: 4th session, 38th Parliament. Available at http://qp.gov.bc.ca/38th4th/1st_read/gov23-1.htm. Accessed 2 March 2012.

13. Banken R. Strategies for institutionalizing HIA. Health Impact Assessment Discussion papers, Number 1. Brussels: WHO European Center for Health Policy, 2001. Available at http://www.euro.who.int/document/e75552.pdf. Accessed 2 March 2012.

14. NCCHPP. The Quebec Public Health Act's Section 54. Briefing Note. National Collaborating Centre for Healthy Public Policy, Institut national de santé publique du Québec, 2008. Available at http://www.ncchpp.ca/docs/Section54English042008.pdf. Accessed 2 March 2012.

15. WHO. European Centre for Health Policy Health Impact Assessment: main concepts and suggested approach. Brussels: WHO Regional Office for Europe, 1999. Available at http://www.apho.org.uk/resources/item.aspx?RID=44163. Accessed 2 March 2012.

16. Héroux de Sève J. À la frontière des responsabilités des ministères et des organismes publics: l'application de l'article 54. Bilan et Perspectives. Québec: Ministère de la Santé

et des Services sociaux du Québec, 2008. Available at http://publications.msss.gouv. qc.ca/acrobat/f/documentation/2008/08-245-02.pdf. Accessed 2 March 2012.

17. Sutcliffe P, Snelling S, Laclé S. Implementing local public health practices to reduce social inequities in health. EXTRA/FORCES intervention project. Sudbury: Sudbury and District Health Unit, 2010.

18. Toronto Public Health. Mixed Waste Processing Study Health Impact Assessment. Staff report/Action required, document from Medical Officer of health to the Board of Health. City of Toronto. Available at http://www.toronto.ca/garbage/mwp/pdf/mwps_ hia_report_and_attachments.pdf. Accessed 2 March 2012.

19. Heclo H. Ideas, Interest and Institutions, in Lawrence C, Dodd IC, Jillson C (eds), The Dynamics of American Politics: Approaches and Interpretations. Boulder CO: Westview Press, 1993.

20. Lalonde M. A New Perspective on the Health of Canadians. A working document. Ottawa: Ministry of National Health and Welfare, 1974. Available at http://www. phac-aspc.gc.ca/ph-sp/pdf/perspect-eng.pdf. Accessed 2 March 2012.

21. Keon W J, Pépin L. Population health policy: Issues and Options. Fourth report of the Subcommittee on Population Health of the Standing Senate Committee on Social Affairs. Ottawa: Canadian Senate, 2008.

22. Health Council of Canada. Stepping it Up: Moving the Focus from Health Care in Canada to a Healthier Canada. Toronto: Health Council of Canada, 2010. Available at http://publications.gc.ca/collections/collection_2011/ccs-hcc/H174-22-2010-2-eng.pdf. Accessed 2 March 2012.

Chapter 25

Health impact assessment in Australia

Ben Harris-Roxas, Patrick Harris, Marilyn Wise, Fiona Haigh, Harrison Ng Chok, and Elizabeth Harris

Introduction

For almost 20 years public health leaders and organizations in Australia have supported the development of HIA. Some of the world's first HIA guidance was developed in Australia. Despite this it has been difficult to locate a 'home' for HIA in Australian policy and planning processes. While EIA has long been mandated in legislation at state and federal levels for major projects, there is no equivalent mandate for HIAs, of either major projects or policy proposals. Despite recognition that health is an important issue to consider across a range of government and private sector planning there is strong opposition from most jurisdictions within Australia to making HIAs a discrete legally compulsory process. One path that has been explored to address this problem within the Australian context has been to legislate that health should be one of the factors considered within EIAs. Another path has been to include HIA in social impact processes and so in triple bottom line sustainability assessments, especially at local government level where findings can be fed in to social and municipal health plans. There are also some limited examples of community-led and advocacy HIAs carried out independently from policy and planning processes.[1]

A brief history of the development of HIA in Australia

Australia is a federation comprised of six states, two territories, and a federal government. There is legislation in all of these jurisdictions requiring EIA of major developments but no equivalent nationally consistent legislation requiring HIA, and no systematic framework or triggers for undertaking HIA. Despite this, each of the jurisdictions in Australia has had some level of HIA activity over a number of years.[2] A comprehensive description of the development of HIA in Australia has recently been published by Harris and Spickett,[3] and gives detailed information on the development and current practice of HIA in Australia.

The purpose of and process for undertaking HIA in Australia have been contested since the National Health and Medical Research Council released the first National Framework for Environmental and Health Impact Assessment in 1994.[4] The preamble to that report outlined the issues clearly. Some saw inclusion of a wider understanding of health in EIA as a radical agenda for restructuring society and some consumer advocates stated that a process centred around social and political aspects of the decision making would be more useful than one based on risk assessment techniques. The debate had already begun on whether environmental health impact assessment (EHIA) needed a strong legislative base with unambiguous guidelines on sources and use of evidence. Concern was expressed that without these safeguards EHIA was an invitation to unwieldy, unpredictable, unscientific, and unaffordable processes with no proven benefits. These arguments reflected both a traditional 'health risk' approach that viewed scientific evidence as the objective and only credible source of evidence, and an emerging new public health approach that incorporated evidence from a range of sources using a variety of methods and viewed HIA as a tool for positively promoting health by influencing the social determinants of health.[1,5,6]

In 1994 there was also concern over the unequal power and access to resources of different stakeholders involved in the EHIA process and over the role of proponents (those putting forward the proposal) in determining how issues were described and scoped. In some ways these concerns were the origins of what we now refer to as community-led or advocacy HIA. There was also pressure to widen the range of projects subject to EHIA to include strategic regional planning, cumulative regional planning, monitoring, licensing, and control procedures. To date except in huge coastal mining developments there has been little call in Australia for the development of cumulative, integrated, or strategic impact assessments.

Since the 1994 report, and in line with the founding values of HIA of democracy, equity, sustainable development, and ethical use of evidence emphasized in the Gothenburg consensus paper,[7] increased attention has been paid to the distribution of impacts. This has led to the emergence of EFHIA, discussed later in this chapter (page 239), in which Australia has been a world leader,[8–10]

Environmental health impact assessment

In 2001 national guidelines for HIA were produced by the National Environmental Health Council[11] and these are currently being updated. A review of legislative and administrative frameworks for HIA in 2005 reiterated earlier calls for health considerations to be included within EIA processes,[12] although it was recognized that this was difficult to achieve. The authors' work in New South Wales reveals the limited consideration given to health concerns, apart from risk assessments of air quality, soil contamination, and the safety of the water supply. A recent study investigating coverage of health in a random sample of EIAs of major state developments in Australia[13] found that although environmental impacts directly related to health, such as air quality, soil contamination, occupational safety, and traffic, were included, health was not considered as a stand-alone concept. Social and economic impacts were included, although the brief for the EIAs did not specify them. Overall, across all types of impacts assessed there was no use of health data to inform assessments, no consideration of health or well-being, no characterization of the causal pathway between an assessed impact (e.g. air quality, access to facilities such as schools or hospitals) and eventual health outcomes, and no mention of the distribution of impacts on different population groups.[13]

The increased political emphasis in Australia on smaller government, reducing regulation, and decreasing cost burdens on developers means that there is little political support for the introduction of additional, potentially expensive, assessment processes. The current challenge is to find ways of building health considerations within EIA while promoting the systematic considerations of health in policy and programme development.

The use of HIA on polices, projects, and programmes

While much of the initial impact assessment focus was on projects, Mahoney and Durham urged that HIA should also be applied to policy and programme development.[2] Their argument was later supported by the New South Wales (NSW) Health and Equity Statement.[14] The Victorian and the NSW governments each funded HIA capacity-building projects with a focus on local government.[15–17] An evaluation of the NSW project showed that it had had considerable influence.[18] Although there are no longer any funded HIA capacity-building projects in Australia, activity continues around the country.[19–22] The author's centre at the University of New South Wales has to date supported more than 39 HIAs of a range of proposals, including land use and population planning, urban regeneration, health sector policies and plans, sustainability, and education.

A significant challenge to mandating the use of HIA has been the reorienting of the health sector and embedding of HIA in public health (including health promotion and environmental health). This requires the larger and more powerful health system to recognize the legitimacy of HIA as a mechanism for improving both internal 'health policy' and external 'public policy'. At the same time cross-government support is required for incorporating health and well-being as a policy concern, as has been done with the development of HiAP in South Australia.[23,24]

In retrospect, while progress in formally adopting HIA has been slow and largely opportunistic, consistent progress has been made in building capacity to undertake and provide technical support for HIA. This has been assisted by increased international legitimacy of HIA, evidence of the effectiveness of HIA, recognition that humans are part of the environment, a growing evidence base for identifying and assessing impacts, and growing diversity in how HIA is understood, undertaken, and adapted to local conditions.

People being understood as part of the environment

At the present time the most feasible way of promoting use of HIA in Australia appears to be through strengthening the way health is considered within EIA. This will not only increase the number of HIAs undertaken but over time improve their quality through routine peer review processes being undertaken on EIA by consultants.

In NSW incorporating human health as part of 'the environment' is seen by EIA practitioners as problematic. Human health and well-being were not clearly articulated as part of the environment within the NSW Environmental Planning and Assessment Act (1979). Nonetheless, growing interest in the relationship between the man-made urban environment and health has resulted in the development of guidance for Australian town planners and other stakeholders on better design of cities and suburbs.[25,26] More recently a high-level report on the sustainability of the Murray/Darling river system commissioned by government caused outrage because it failed to consider the impacts of proposed changes on local people as well as on the natural environment.[27] The interconnectedness between the health of the river and the health of local people and communities has now been widely debated.

The potential health impacts of developments are often significant concerns when the broader community and stakeholders provide input into planning, project assessment, and determination. For example, current challenges to coal seam gas exploration from community stakeholders, who feel they have limited opportunity to engage with decision makers, rest largely on health concerns. Increased recognition of humans as part of the environment provides opportunities to contribute to EIAs in a more integrated way. Proponents are increasingly being asked to consider health in their assessments and consultants undertaking EIAs are now more likely to include an HIA.

Increased evidence of the effectiveness of HIA

The effectiveness of HIA was considered in Chapter 7. Review of three HIAs of policies[28] and case studies of various HIA[8,29,30] in New Zealand and Australia have consistently found that HIAs lead to changes in the planning and implementation of proposals, improved stakeholder relationships, and introduced relevant information into decision-making processes. The extent to which this occurs seems to vary depending on context, and it is often difficult to attribute changes solely to the HIA. Preliminary findings from research into HIA's effectiveness in the Australian context[31] and the factors that influence it[32] indicate that most HIAs have some degree of direct effectiveness (resulting in changes to decisions) and that even those that did not directly influence the intended decision result in outcomes such as influencing and informing other decisions and future planning, providing an evidence base for planning and decision making, technical, conceptual, and social learning, developing, strengthening, and providing a framework for stakeholder relationships, and informing future HIAs. This review of effectiveness is proving useful in engaging policy makers and enlisting their support to undertake HIAs on their policies and plans. Over time a pool of people who have had positive experiences in undertaking HIAs and who support its ongoing use despite the lack of government funding has been built.

Developing HIA for real world use

Many Australian policy makers have called for an HIA process that can be undertaken in an afternoon. They say this reflects the reality of the time frames available for comment on the policies of other sectors. On the other hand academics and those wishing to professionalize HIA are interested in developing a more structured and standardized approach. The reality in Australia is that there is a wide diversity of approaches that have been developed to reflect local needs and opportunities. Box 25.1 outlines some of the various approaches currently being used to institutionalize consideration of health and labelled as HIA. They range from legally mandated HIAs, HIA permitted when necessary under state public health acts, health lenses to assess potential health impacts, and HIA called for by local civil society groups and community groups. In the Australian context blurred understanding of the boundaries and roles in the policy development of HIA, HiAP, and healthy public policy may distract from practical action and create unnecessary competition.[20]

At this point, rather than focusing on the standardization of an approach that ensures that health and public policy contribute to promoting health and

---

Box 25.1 Approaches to institutionalizing consideration of health impacts in Australia

- Require health to be considered as part of EIAs or broader impact assessment (EIA legislation in most jurisdictions).

- Require stand-alone HIAs on specified types/categories of proposal (e.g. Tasmania requires that a stand-alone HIA be conducted on projects beyond a certain scale).

- Give health officials the right to conduct HIAs where they deem it necessary or appropriate (Victoria's Public Health Act empowers the Minister for Health to require HIAs on proposals that the Minister identifies).

- Regulations or policies that support HIA's discretionary use but do not require it (many local governments and authorities in New South Wales, Victoria and Western Australia, the New South Wales Population Health Plan).

Approaches that are not exactly requirements for HIA but are related, or may lead to HIA use:

- Require a health review or screening of government policies (New South Wales Aboriginal Health Impact Statement).

- Discretionary use of non-HIA processes to look at health issues intersectorally (South Australia's Health Lens and their HiAP initiative).

---

health equity, it may be more useful to focus on identifying the essential components of HIA and ensuring its quality.

Essential components should include:

- a documented and transparent process that the assessment follows
- a clear statement of the HIA's goals and purpose
- a rigorous, documented approach to gathering and assessing evidence
- clear predictions of impacts
- recommendations for enhancement and mitigation
- self-identified indicators of how the HIA's effectiveness will be judged (these will vary markedly depending on context).

An evidence base to support HIAs

Some organizations in Australia are collecting systematic reviews, review papers, and materials from other HIAs[33,34] in order to help those undertaking

HIA to find relevant evidence and identify potential impacts. The University of New South Wales Healthy Built Environment programme has undertaken a review of the role of the built environment in supporting human health.[35] There are also resources on regeneration, urban density, and working in disadvantaged communities. At present there is no central collection of these reviews but this seems an obvious next step. There is also increasing recognition of the need to draw on a wider range of evidence than risk assessments to identify potential impacts.[6,21]

Equity considerations and equity-focused HIA

The Australian Collaboration for Health Equity Impact Assessment developed a framework for EFHIA[10,36] and a focus on the distribution of impacts across the population. By international standards Australians have excellent and improving health but health gains are not shared equally.[37] The most glaring example of health inequity is between indigenous and non-indigenous Australians, where there is a 17-year gap in life expectancy. There are consistent inequities related to rurality, place of residence, level of education, income, and country of birth across health service use, behavioural risk factors, and quality of life.[38,39]

Although many argue that these issues should be routinely addressed in all HIAs without an explicit requirement to look at distributional impacts, they are often overlooked.[8,20,40,41] This reflects the complex process for assessing impacts often in the absence of data on distributional impacts. The focus on equity is seen by some partners within and outside the health system as a 'value add' to their planning processes, and helps to reduce the anxiety of stakeholders that participation in an HIA implies that their planning is poor.[42–44]

Conclusion

In our quest to encourage the use of HIA there may be a chance that the HIA community has forgotten why it is promoting its use. If we fixate on the number of HIAs being conducted alone we may be disappointed as HIAs use ebbs and flows with levels of government funding and support. However, if we think about HIA as part of a broader healthy public policy agenda, in which HIA is an important tool that can be used selectively and strategically not only to inform and guide decision making but to change ways of working and understanding of health, we will see more signs for hope and encouragement.

Australian experience has been that HIA is useful in building effective cross-sectoral partnerships that focus on real issues and make transparent and evidence-informed decisions about planning and implementation. This does not mean that HIAs should be conducted on all proposals, but it does mean that our partners have a much better and more practical understanding of health, its determinants, and how their actions influence them.

Acknowledgement

We acknowledge Associate Professors Lynn Kemp and Pat Bazeley from the University of New South Wales with thanks for their ongoing support of our HIA work and their contribution to our thinking.

References

1. Harris-Roxas B, Harris E. Differing Forms, Differing Purposes: A Typology of Health Impact Assessment. Environmental Impact Assessment Review 2011; 31: 396–403.
2. Mahoney M, Durham G. Health impact assessment: A tool for policy development in Australia. Melbourne: Health Impact Assessment Unit, Deakin University, 2002.
3. Harris P, Spickett J. Health impact assessment in Australia: A review and directions for progress. Environmental Impact Assessment Review 2011; 31: 425–32.
4. NHMRC National Framework for Environmental and Health Impact Assessment, Canberra. National Health and Medical Research Council, 1994. Available at http://www.nhmrc.gov.au/publications/synopses/eh10syn.htm. Accessed 2 March 2012.
5. Harris E. Contemporary Debates in Health Impact Assessment: What? Why? When? New South Wales Public Health Bulletin 2005; 16: 107–108.
6. Vohra S, Cave B, Viliani F, Harris-Roxas B, Bhatia R New international consensus on health impact assessment. Lancet 2010; 376: 1464–65.
7. WHO European Centre for Health Policy Health Impact Assessment: Main concepts and suggested approach—Gothenburg consensus paper. European Centre for Health Policy, Brussels. WHO Regional Office for Europe. 1999. Available at www.apho.org.uk/resource/view.aspx?RID=44163. Accessed 2 March 12.
8. Harris-Roxas B, Harris P, Harris E, Kemp L. A Rapid Equity Focused Health Impact Assessment of a Policy Implementation Plan: An Australian case study and impact evaluation. International Journal for Equity in Health 2011; 10: 6. Available at http://www.equityhealthj.com/content/10/1/6. Accessed 2 March 2012.
9. Harris-Roxas B, Simpson S, Harris E. Equity Focused Health Impact Assessment: A literature review. Newcastle, NSW: CHETRE on behalf of the Australasian Collaboration for Health Equity Impact Assessment, 2004. http://www.hiaconnect.edu.au/files/Harris-Roxas_B_(2004)_Equity_Focused_HIA.pdf. Accessed 2 March 2012.
10. Mahoney M, Simpson S, Harris E, Aldrich R, Stewart Williams J. Equity Focused Health Impact Assessment Framework. Newcastle, NSW: Australasian Collaboration for Health Equity Impact Assessment, 2004. Available at http://www.hiaconnect.edu.au/files/EFHIA_Framework.pdf. Accessed 2 March 2012.
11. enHealth Health Impact Assessment Guidelines, National Public Health Partnership, Commonwealth Department of Health and Aged Care Australian Commonwealth Department of Health and Aged Care, Canberra. Available at http://www.health.gov.au/internet/main/publishing.nsf/content/health-pubhlth-publicat-document-metadata-env_impact.htm. Accessed 2 March 2012.

12. NPHP Health Impact Assessment: Legislative and administrative frameworks, Canberra. National Public Health Partnership, 2005. Available at http://www.nphp. gov.au/workprog/lrn/hia_legframe.htm. Accessed 2 March 2012.

13. Harris P, Harris E, Thompson S, Harris-Roxas B, Kemp L. Human Health and Wellbeing in Environmental Impact Assessment in New South Wales, Australia: Auditing health impacts within environmental assessments of major projects. Environmental Impact Assessment Review 2009; 29: 310–18.

14. NSW Health. NSW Health and Equity Statement: In All Fairness, Sydney. New South Wales Department of Health, 2004. Available at http://www.health.nsw.gov.au/ pubs/2004/pdf/fairness.pdf. Accessed 2 March 2012.

15. Harris E, Simpson S. New South Wales Health Impact Assessment Project: Phase 1 report. Sydney: Centre for Health Equity Training, Research and Evaluation (CHETRE), University of New South Wales, 2003. Available at http://www.hiaconnect. edu.au/files/Simpson_S_(2003)_NSW_HIA_Project_Phase_1_Report.pdf. Accessed 2 March 2012.

16. Harris-Roxas B, Simpson S. The New South Wales Health Impact Assessment Project. NSW Public Health Bulletin 2005; 16: 120–23.

17. Harris E. NSW Health Impact Assessment Capacity Building Program: Mid-term review. Sydney: Centre for Health Equity Training, Research and Evaluation, University of New South Wales, 2006. Available at http://www.hiaconnect.edu.au/files/ HIA_Mid-Term_Review.pdf. Accessed 2 March 2012.

18. R Quigley, C Watts. Evaluation of Phase Three of the New South Wales Health Impact Assessment Project, Sydney. Final report. Quigley and Watts Ltd, 2008. Available at http://www.hiaconnect.edu.au/files/NSW_HIA_Project_Evaluation_Report.pdf. Accessed 2 March 2012.

19. Harris P, Spickett J. Health impact assessment in Australia: A review and directions for progress. Environmental Impact Assessment Review 2011; 31: 425–32.

20. Harris E, Harris-Roxas B. Health in All Policies: A pathway for thinking about our broader societal goals. Public Health Bulletin of South Australia 2010; 7: 43–46.

21. Spickett JT, Brown HL, Katscherian D. Adaptation strategies for health impacts of climate change in Western Australia: Application of a Health Impact Assessment framework. Environmental Impact Assessment Review 2011; 31: 297–300.

22. Harris P, Harris-Roxas B, Wise M, Harris L. Health Impact Assessment for Urban and Land-use Planning and Policy Development: Lessons from Practice. Planning Practice and Research 2010; 25: 531–41.

23. Government of South Australia. South Australia's Strategic Plan: through a health lens. Adelaide: South Australian Department of Health, 2008. Available at http://www. health.gov.au/internet/nhhrc/publishing.nsf/Content/458/$FILE/458%20-%20O% 20-%20SA%20Health%20-%20SASP%20...through%20a%20health%20lens.pdf. Accessed 2 March 2012.

24. WHO and Government of South Australia. Adelaide Statement on Health in All Policies: Moving towards a shared governance for health and wellbeing. Adelaide: World Health Organization and South Australian Government, 2010. Available at http://www.who.int/social_determinants/hiap_statement_who_sa_final.pdf. Accessed 2 March 2012.

25. Sutherland E, Carlisle R. Healthy by Design: An innovative planning tool for the development of safe, accessible and attractive environments. NSW Public Health Bulletin 2007; 18: 228–31.

26. Harris P, Harris-Roxas B, Harris E. An Overview of the Regulatory Planning System in New South Wales: Identifying points of intervention for health impact assessment and consideration of health impacts. NSW Public Health Bulletin 2007; 18: 188–191.

27. Murray Darling Basin Authority. Murray-Darling Draft Basin Plan, Sydney. Murray Darling Basin Authority, 2011. Available at http://www.mdba.gov.au/draft-basin-plan. Accessed 2 March 2012.

28. Ward M. Health Impact Assessment in New Zealand: Experience at a policy level, Wellington. Public Health Advisory Committee, 2006. Available at http://www. hiaconnect.edu.au/files/HIA_in_New_Zealand_Experience_Policy_Level.pdf. Accessed 2 March 2012.

29. Mathias K, Harris-Roxas B. Process and Impact Evaluation of the Greater Christchurch Urban Development Strategy Health Impact Assessment. BMC Public Health 2009; 9: 97.

30. Harris-Roxas B, Harris P. Learning by doing: The value of case studies of health impact assessment. New South Wales Public Health Bulletin 2007; 18: 161–63.

31. Harris E, Baum F, Harris-Roxas B, Kemp L, Spickett J, Keleher H, et al. The effectiveness of health impact assessments conducted in Australia and New Zealand, $190,000. Canberra: Australian Research Council, 2010.

32. Harris-Roxas B, Harris E. Conceptual Framework for Evaluating the Impact and Effectiveness of Health Impact Assessment in Health Impact Assessment, in O'Mullane M (ed), Integrating Health Impact Assessment into the Policy Process. Oxford: Oxford University Press (forthcoming), 2012.

33. PCAL. Evidence Papers. Sydney: Premier's Council for Active Living, 2011. Available at http://www.pcal.nsw.gov.au/resources/evidence_papers. Accessed 2 March 2012.

34. NSW Health. Healthy Urban Development Checklist: A guide for health services when commenting on development policies, plans and proposals. Sydney: New South Wales Department of Health, 2009. Available at http://www.health.nsw.gov.au/pubs/2010/ pdf/hud_checklist.pdf. Accessed 2 March 2012.

35. Kent J, Thompson S, Jalaludin B. Healthy Built Environments: A review of the literature. Healthy Built Environments Program. Sydney: City Futures Research Centre, University of New South Wales, 2011. Available at http://www.be.unsw.edu. au/healthy-built-environments-program/publications. Accessed 2 March 2012.

36. Simpson S, Mahoney M, Harris E, Aldrich R, Stewart-Williams J. Equity-Focused Health Impact Assessment: A tool to assist policy makers in addressing health inequalities. Environmental Impact Assessment Review 2005; 25: 772–82.

37. Turrell G, Stanley L, de Looper M, B O Health Inequalities in Australia: Morbidity, health behaviours, risk factors and health service use. Health Inequalities Monitoring Series No. 2. Canberra: Queensland University, 2006.

38. Paradies Y, Harris R, Anderson I. The Impact of Racism on Indigenous Health in Australia and Aotearoa: Towards a research agenda, Melbourne. Cooperative Research Centre for Aboriginal Health, 2008. Available at http://www.lowitja.org.au/files/crcah_ docs/Racism-Report.pdf. Accessed 2 March 2012.

39. Australia Fair. A Fair Go for All Australians: International Comparisons 2007—10 Essentials, Canberra. Australian Council of Social Services, 2007. Available at http://www.chpcp.org/resources/3517__Australia%20fair%20numbers%20and%20stories.pdf. Accessed 2 March 2012.

40. Harris E, Harris P, Kemp L. Rapid Equity Focused Health Impact Assessment of the Australia Better Health Initiative: Assessing the NSW components of priorities 1 and 3. Syndey: Centre for Primary Health Care and Equity, University of New South Wales, 2006.

41. Harris P, Harris-Roxas B, Harris E, Kemp L. Health Impact Assessment and Urbanisation: Lessons from the NSW HIA Project. NSW Public Health Bulletin 2007; 18: 198–201.

42. Gunning C, Harris P, Mallett J. Assessing the health equity impacts of regional land-use plan making: An equity focussed health impact assessment of alternative patterns of development of the Whitsunday Hinterland and Mackay Regional Plan, Australia. Environmental Impact Assessment Review 2011; 31: 415–19.

43. Wells VL, Gillham KE, Licata M, Kempton AM. An Equity Focused Social Impact Assessment of the Lower Hunter Regional Strategy. NSW Public Health Bulletin 2007; 18: 166–68.

44. Tugwell A, Johnson P. The Coffs Harbour 'Our Living City Settlement Strategy' Health Impact Assessment. Environmental Impact Assessment Review 2011; 31: 441–44.

Chapter 26

Health impact assessment in Thailand

Siriwan Chandanachulaka

HIA was first introduced to Thailand during the national health system reform process begun in 2000.[1] Initially, it aimed to be a social learning process for healthy public policy formulation. Earlier reports of HIA in Thailand have been published.[2]

Legal status of HIA in Thailand

There are three pieces of legislation governing HIA in Thailand. The National Health Act (NHA) 2007[3] and the Thai Constitution 2007[4] clarify the nature and purpose of HIA while the Enhancement and Conservation of National Environmental Quality Act (NEQ)[5] 1992 specifies how EIA should be undertaken.

The 'Community Right' part of the Constitution (section 67 paragraph 2) states that:

> Any project or activity which may seriously affect the community with respect to the quality of the environment, natural resources and health shall not be permitted, unless, prior to the operation thereof, its impacts on the quality of the environment and on public health have been studied and assessed and a public hearing process has been conducted for consulting the public as well as interested persons and there have been obtained opinions of an independent organization, consisting of representatives from private organizations in the field of the environment and health and from higher education institutions providing studies in the field of the environment, natural resources or health.

Section 11 of the NHA states that an individual or group of people has the right to request an evaluation of the health impacts resulting from public policy and to participate in that evaluation. It further states that they have a right to receive information, explanations, and underlying reasons before approval is granted for a policy or activity that may affect their health or the health of the community, and that they have the right to express their opinions on such matters. Section 25 (5) gives the National Health Committee powers to specify how impact assessment should be performed: 'To prescribe rules and procedure for monitoring and evaluation in respect of national health system and the impact on health resulting from public policies, both in the level of policy making and implementation.'

The NEQ states that for projects or activities that may impact on the environment an EIA must be conducted and approved by an expert committee. The permitting authority must make the measures proposed in the EIA report a condition for permission. Currently there are 34 (increased from the previous 22) types of project/activity for which an EIA should be conducted. Four aspects have to be covered in an EIA: physical and biological natural resources, environment, benefit to humans, and quality of life, in which health is included. However, health in EIA reports tends to concentrate on occupational health besides giving a brief description of morbidity and mortality from important diseases at the provincial level, and numbers of health personnel and facilities in the province.

In 2010, 11 types of project/activity were specified in Section 67 of the Constitution as requiring an EHIA.[6] The definition of EHIA in the Thai context is slightly different to that of Fehr,[7] who defined it as 'a component of EIA dealing specifically with impact on human health'.

Map Ta Phut and the development of legislation on EHIA

In June 2009, people living in the Map Ta Phut area became concerned about the health impacts of developments proposed for the nearby industrial estate and sued government organizations for granting permission for 76 projects in breach of Section 67, paragraph 2 of the Constitution. They demanded suspension of these projects. The court ordered temporary suspension of 65 projects in December 2009. This legal challenge prompted the development of rules and regulations filling the gap between the provisions of the Constitution and the existing laws and regulations, which provided for EIA but had no legal basis for resolving any problems identified.

In response to events in Map Ta Phut, the government designated a Committee for Solving Problems of Implementation of Section 67 Paragraph 2 of the Constitution (a panel comprising academics, government, private sector and public representatives) headed by a former prime minister, Anand Panyarachun. This committee proposed five documents to the government:[8]

1. Draft rules and regulations for preparation and consideration of EHIA (December 2009).

2. Draft notification by the Prime Minister establishing a temporary independent organization (January 2010).

3. List of projects/activities specified as seriously harmful (August 2010).

4. Proposals for town planning and buffer areas around industrial zones.

5. Important issues to be resolved for the Map Ta Phut industrial area.

The first two documents apply to the whole country, while the other three are specific to the Map Ta Phut area.

Finally, in 2010, the Central Administrative Court ruled that only two of the temporarily suspended projects needed an EHIA before being permitted.[9] However, about 30 of the projects had meanwhile undertaken EHIA on a voluntary basis. Guidelines for conducting EHIAs are based on Ministry of Natural Resources and Environment (MONRE) guidelines (December 2009), which describe the process for conducting EHIA, including a time-consuming public hearing and method for announcing results of the hearing. The opinion of Japanese companies affected by the Court Ruling is described in Chapter 27 (page 253).

The National Health Committee also responded to events in Map Ta Phut by issuing guidelines that apply to all areas for HIA[10] in four contexts (in 2009):

1. projects specified in section 67 of the Constitution

2. public policies where an HIA may be appropriate

3. any projects or policies for which an HIA is requested in accordance with the public right stated in section 11 of the constitution

4. projects or policies for which HIA can be conducted as a community learning process.

Comparison of EIA and EHIA processes

The four main ways in which EHIA differs from EIA are as follows:

1. EHIA applies to various sizes and types of project/activity (notified in August 2010), for example large-scale petrochemical plants, large-scale power-generation plants, all scales of production, disposal, and treatment of radioactive materials, nuclear power generation plants, and all industrial estates that include petrochemical industries or steel production.

2. For EHIA there is a time-consuming public hearing process and a role for stakeholders and others involved.

3. In EHIA impacts are identified and assessed in terms of health. This covers changes in condition and use of natural resources, production, transportation, and storage of hazardous substances, exposure to pollution and health-threatening substances, change and effect on occupation, employment, and local working conditions, change and effect on relationship of

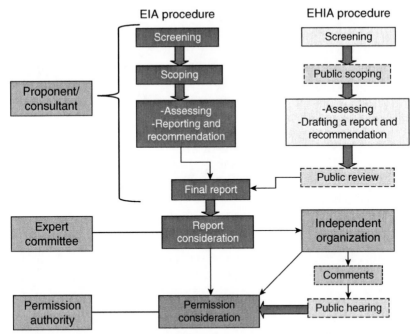

Fig. 26.1 Comparison of EIA and EHIA processes.

Data from Chandanachulaka S. HIA Legislation and Practice in Thailand Presented in the Workshop for HIA of Air Pollution in Southeast and East Asia. South Korea.

people and communities, change in areas that are important for cultural heritage, specific impact on particular groups of people, and resources and capacity of public health services.

4. EHIA gives a role to concerned organizations, e.g. independent organizations, permitting authority, and the Office of Natural Resources and Environmental Policy and Planning (ONEP).

The EHIA and EIA processes are compared in Figure 26.1.

Relation of HIA and EIA

Legislation makes two separate organizations responsible for EIA and HIA: an expert committee of MONRE with a secretariat provided by ONEP is responsible for considering and reviewing EIA reports, and an HIA commission designated by the National Health Committee is responsible for establishing systems and procedures as specified in the NHA for HIA. The constitution gives responsibility for providing an opinion on any project or activity that may cause serious harm to natural resources, environment, or human health to a third organization, which will be established soon.

The NHA allows individuals or groups to request that an HIA be conducted separately from the EIA. HIA can also be combined with EIA to form an EHIA, in which case it must be conducted according to the regulations issued by MONRE. Many more EIAs now explicitly include health and for some projects or policies a separate HIA is conducted.

Case studies of HIA done in Thailand

A review of four different EIA/EHIAs was undertaken. These were a compulsory EHIA in Map Ta Phut, a voluntary EHIA in Map Ta Phut, an EHIA of a steel production plant, and an EIA of an oil and gas exploration project. This review revealed the following:

- A separate chapter on health impacts was included in all reports.
- Health baseline data more relevant to projects was included. Sub-district or district level data were given rather than more general provincial level data, and morbidity and mortality data were for diseases or symptoms relevant to the project.
- Vulnerable subgroups such as children, the elderly, and pregnant women were not included in the population baseline data.
- The reports were organized around the five stages of the HIA process: screening, scoping, appraising, reporting and recommendation, and monitoring and evaluation.
- Recommendations included protective and mitigation measures as well as monitoring measures.
- One project described the process without explicitly presenting an assessment of impact on human health.
- HIAs were conducted for construction and operational phases and in one case for the decommissioning phase.
- Two projects included assessment of the impacts of chemicals on human health, including toxic and carcinogenic effects.
- The impact on the community was assessed as well as impact on workers. Two reports analysed impacts for different risk groups and areas.
- Impacts on health facilities and service capacity were assessed where there was a possibility of the project causing serious health impacts.

Section 11 of the NHA allows people to request an HIA separate from EIA and this was the case for biomass power generation plants in Chiangrai and Ubonratchatani Provinces, iron mining in Lumpang Province and a coal power plant in Chachoengsao Province. HIA of policy has been conducted on the ASEAN Free Trade and Medicine Patent Treaty.

Obstacles and challenges for HIA in Thailand

Expanding coverage of health in EIA statements has proved relatively easy. However, guidelines for HIA are too broad and its practice is under-developed. The first obstacle is that there has previously been little experience of considering health. The second obstacle is a lack of experts with experience of conducting HIA and the third obstacle is that project proponents tend to concentrate on the process of HIA rather than assessing real health impacts. Moreover, all relevant organizations and people involved need to reach a common understanding of the definition, process, and limitations of HIA. Health data sets, health indicators, and health criteria for HIA need to be improved. Guidelines for HIA of specific projects and activities are required and local people need better understanding of EIA and HIA.

Conclusion

Inclusion of HIA in three major pieces of legislation, the Enhancement and Conservation of Environmental Quality Act (1992), the Constitution (2007), and the National Health Act (2007), suggests that it is well developed. As a result of the legal challenge from local people in the Map Ta Phut area and the ruling of the Administrative Court that government organizations had breached Section 67, paragraph 2 of the Constitution, development of HIA was driven forward. Regulations based on the Constitution and related legislation have been established and have been effective since December 2009. HIA in Thailand is now in an early stage of development and further development is required.

References

1. National Health Commission Office. HIA for HPP Towards Healthy Nation: Thailand's Recent Experiences, 2nd edn. Nonthaburi, Thailand: National Health Commission Office, 2007.
2. Phoolcharoen W, Sukkumnoes D, Kessomboon P. Development of health impact assessment in Thailand: recent experiences and challenges. Bulletin of the World Health Organization 2003; 81: 465–67.
3. National Health Act B.E. 2550. Available at http://whothailand.healthrepository.org/bitstream/123456789/590/1/National%20Health%20Act_2007.pdf. Accessed 2 January 12.
4. Constitution of the Kingdom of Thailand B.E. 2550. Available at http://www.asianlii.org/th/legis/const/2007/1.html. Accessed 2 January 2012.
5. The Enhancement and Conservation of the Environmental Quality Act B.E. 2535. Available at http://www.wipo.int/clea/docs_new/pdf/en/th/th031en.pdf. Accessed 2 January 2012.

6. Ministry of Natural Resources and Environment. Thailand Notification of Rule, Procedure, Method and Guideline for Preparation of the Environmental Impact Assessment Report for Project or Activity which may Seriously Affect Community with respect to Quality of Environment, Natural Resources and Health. Bangkok, Office of Natural Resources and Environmental Policy and planning, 2010.

7. Fehr R. Environmental Health Impact Assessment, Evaluation of a Ten-Step Model. Epidemiology 1999; 10: 618–25.

8. Office of the Prime Minister. Result of Committee for Solving Problems of Implementation of Section 67 Paragraph 2 of the Constitution (Bangkok, Office of the Prime Minister: 2011. Thai version).

9. MCOT. Court allows 74 Map Ta Phut industrial projects to resume operation. Available at http://www.mcot.net/cfcustom/cache_page/97952.html. Accessed 15 December 2011.

10. National Health Commission Office. Rules and Procedure for Assessing Health Impact from Public Policy (Nonthaburi, Thailand; National Health Commission: 2009. Thai version).

11. Chandanachulaka S. HIA Legislation and Practice in Thailand Presented in the Workshop for HIA of Air Pollution in Southeast and East Asia. Seoul, South Korea. 27 July 2011 (unpublished).

Chapter 27

Health impact assessment in Japan

Yoshihisa Fujino

Although few HIAs have been performed in Japan, interest in HIA among public health professionals has increased rapidly. No HIA has been formally commissioned by national or local government, and the term 'HIA' has not appeared in any governmental statement, including statements on EIA. Experience of HIA to date has been limited to a few academic studies done on a voluntary basis.[1–3]

Japan is now at the stage of spreading interest in and awareness of HIA. In 2008 an English language book on HIA[4] was translated into Japanese and published. After publication, the translators, under the auspices of the Japanese Society of Public Health, called together an HIA discussion group, in which about 50 public health professionals took part and started to learn about HIA. In 2009 and 2010, this group invited two HIA consultants from the UK to conferences at Tokyo, Nagoya, and Fukuoka. These consultants also made presentations to the Ministry of Land, Infrastructure, Transport and Tourism, and the Ministry of Health, Labour and Welfare. These activities raised interest in HIA, particularly among public health professionals.

The major factor driving interest in HIA in Japan is the increased attention given to issues of health inequity. As in other countries, inequality has become a major social problem in Japan, although only since 2000, i.e. a decade after other countries. The final report of the WHO Commission on the Social Determinants of Health[5] has played a particularly important role. One of its three major recommendations concerns the implementation of HIA at the national level, and this has successfully raised the profile of HIA and given it credibility at a time when very few people knew about it. The most interest in and understanding of HIA is currently found in the field of social epidemiology, where the ideas of the social determinants of health and the socioenvironmental model of health[6,7] have become major research fields. Although EIA has been suggested to be one of the three origins of HIA, alongside social determinants of health, and health inequality,[8] HIA has received little attention from environmental experts.

HIA guidelines from the Japanese Society of Public Health

The most obvious progress in HIA in Japan is the publication of HIA guidelines by the Japanese Society of Public Health in November 2011. The Japanese Society of Public Health has more than 8000 health professional members, including public health practitioners, researchers, academicians, and local and national government officials. By publishing HIA guidelines the society aims to spread knowledge of HIA among its members, particularly local government staff.

The guidelines were informed by guidelines previously published in other countries.[9–14] They describe the basic concepts of HIA and explain links between policy and health based on the socioenvironmental model of health. The largest section of the guidelines suggests how to conduct screening. They also emphasizes the importance of HIA in non-health sector policy, and provides the context of Japanese policy formulation.

The guidelines describe three cases of HIA screening as examples. The first case is an HIA for transition to a core city.[3] Transition to a core city is a decentralizing process, which has been promoted nationally with the aim of transferring as much authority and financial resource as possible to regional government. The second case is an HIA of the Japanese Government's proposal to introduce a so-called 'white-collar exemption' into the Japanese labour market[1] by revising the Labour Standards Law to exempt white-collar workers from work-hour regulations so that they would not be entitled to receive overtime pay. The third case is an HIA for the Government's proposal to combine the current system of separate 'nursery schools' and 'kindergartens'. In Japan, there are two types of child-care facility. Nursery schools are overseen by the Ministry of Health, Labour and Welfare, and provide basic care services for children while their parents are at work. Kindergartens are overseen by the Ministry of Education, Culture, Sports, Science and Technology, and provide early childhood education. This proposal aims to provide sufficient volume of service and a high standard of education for children in order to address a persistent lack of capacity in nursery schools.

Barriers to HIA

There are several barriers to the development of HIA in Japan. First, little information about HIA is available in the Japanese language, and some technical terms that are commonly used in the HIA world do not have appropriate equivalents in Japanese. For example, the terms 'scoping', 'terms of reference', and 'strategic' cannot be directly translated into commonly used Japanese, and these concepts are difficult for Japanese people to understand. The term 'health impact assessment' itself implies a prediction of the future based on precise quantitative risk assessment.

Second, the legitimacy of HIA has been questioned. While practitioners in local government acknowledge the usefulness of HIA, they suggest that it requires to be legitimized by a law or instruction from the national government. Third, as often pointed out in other countries, the intersectorial approach is difficult in local government settings. For example, it is difficult for the health department of a local government to address the policies of other departments, a problem which would be eased if HIA was required by law or explicit instruction.

Fourth, the wide variety of methods by which HIAs are conducted is also an obstacle. Although basic processes such as screening, scoping, appraisal, reporting, and monitoring, which are common to other impact assessment processes, have been agreed, no standard HIA method has yet been established. Previously published HIA case reports have not always complied with the agreed basic processes. Moreover, the flexible use of both quantitative and qualitative methods in HIA has advantages and disadvantages. This flexibility and variety of HIA methods can cause confusion among those starting to learn HIA, particularly in other languages. The training of health professionals, including public health practitioners, has generally been based on quantitative methods, such as epidemiology and risk assessment approaches.

Finally, the ideas of the social determinants of health and the socioenvironmental model of health, although spreading, are still unfamiliar to many people.

The Map Ta Phut experience

While HIA remains virtually unknown in Japanese society, it has unfortunately been perceived as a 'global risk' by Japanese companies involved in development outside Japan. A number of Japanese were involved in industrial developments at Map Ta Phut in Thailand where the Supreme Administrative Court of Thailand ordered a temporary suspension of operations following demands from local residents for assessment of health impacts (see Chapter 26, page 245). Although this was initially reported in Japan as due to a lack of adequate 'environmental impact assessment', the companies eventually became aware that the issue was one of HIA rather than EIA.

As information about HIA in Japan was very limited, the author was asked to explain to several Japanese companies the background and requirements of HIA. This experience led him to understand that the companies had little understanding of HIA or how to implement it. The issue was primarily dealt with by corporate risk management departments, where staff were trained in risk assessment and quantitative methods. The public health terms and concepts, such as social determinants of health, participatory approach, and health concern, including physical, mental, and social well-being, were totally unfamiliar to them. Without clear legal guidance, they preferred to stop projects even with the huge costs of cancellation rather than to undertake an HIA with uncertain requirements. Staff in one company said, 'We would be happy to do an HIA if we knew what was required. Without guidelines or explicit specifications, preferably by the Thai Government itself, we cannot accept the risk of repeated reattempts of assessment'. It seems that the impact assessment needed for Map Ta Phut was seen as a special form of EIA and the companies tended to approach the issue within the framework of an EIA, so that important features of HIA, such as 'public participation', 'public review', and 'social determinants of health', were overlooked, although these were the very issues on which the people of Map Ta Phut wanted to focus.

As a result of Map Ta Phut HIA has unfortunately come to be considered as a 'global risk' by business firms before Japanese society has had the opportunity to learn of its essential merits and importance. This experience may in turn impact on future discussion on the use of HIA in various fields, including environment, business, and health. Even SEA is perceived to some degree to be a burden for business and has not been legislated for in Japan. Moreover official guidance for SEA announced by the national government excludes electric power plants because of arguments from stakeholders, such as electric companies.

HIA in occupational health

Although HIA has not been used by national or local governments in Japan, it has already been adopted for use in occupational settings. The basic idea of HIA in occupational settings derives from the fact that the company, regardless of its size, is a community in which people share the same purpose, culture, and behaviours. Many corporate activities have a significant impact on the health of employees, their families, and the surrounding community. These activities are generally guided by business objectives, with little consideration for health and well-being, and occupational health professionals have very few opportunities to play a role in decision making for business-related issues. Pilot studies of HIA conducted in various occupational settings have been concerned with the following issues:

- closure and relocation of an office
- opening of a new factory abroad
- introduction of a shift-work schedule for women in a factory

- extension of retirement age
- business consolidation
- ban on smoking in a workplace
- closure of a clinic in a workplace
- closure of bachelor apartments.

Several rationales may be identified for the conduct of HIAs in occupational settings. Many corporate activities have a significant impact on the health of employees, their families, and local residents through changes in the social determinants of health. There are particular factors in occupational settings that may affect how groups are impacted by corporate activities, for example:

- employment status (regular employment/part-time/temporarily employed/ retired worker)
- age (junior/middle-age/veteran)
- sex (men/women/pregnant women)
- job position (administrative/rank and file)
- functional class (engineering work/officer)
- family structure (married/bachelor/husband transferred without family/ worker caring for child or aged relative).

Consideration of the health impact of corporate activities is necessary for corporate social responsibility. Conducting and documenting HIA is a good tool for corporations to use to clearly demonstrate their company's concern for health and to manage corporate risk arising from unintended future adverse health effects.

A series of pilot studies have recognized the health impacts which result from corporate activities, and occupational physicians claim that HIA represents a promising approach to expanding the scope of occupational health. In general, the consideration of health associated with business has had low priority, even when a significant negative health impact could be anticipated by health staff within the company, and opportunities for positive health impacts have not been taken. HIA could also facilitate negotiations with stakeholders, such as labour organization and local residents.

The University of Occupational and Environmental Health introduced a training course for HIA in occupational settings in 2009. This is the first and still the only such training course in Japan. Up to 2011 about 50 occupational physicians have participated in the course.

Challenges for HIA in Japan

There are many challenges for HIA in Japan. First, real HIA experience, meaning involvement in and advising the decision-making process, is necessary.

This is a dilemma because policy makers often want to have evidence of the practical usefulness of HIA before they commission an HIA report. Second, awareness of HIA among health professionals must be raised since many public health staff in Japan are still unfamiliar with HIA. Although HIA emphasizes the importance for health of non-health sector policy, health administration managers need to understand HIA if they are to take leadership in approaching and working with the non-health sector. Third, capacity building for HIA is important. Very few people are currently engaged in HIA work, and most HIA projects are characterized as voluntary or academic. A training course designed primarily for local government staff is required, particularly given the increasing demand for HIAs by health departments in local government. Fourth, as has been discussed in other countries, institutionalization for HIA is a major issue (see Chapter 11, page 110). Legislation that mandates HIA may not be a good solution, given concerns over the problems of EIA legislation. Rather, a systematic scheme that requires HIA for any policy proposal is required at both the local and national government levels. Fifth, although the environmental field has paid no attention to HIA, the time has now come to talk with environmental experts about health and it will probably be acceptable to discuss HIA as an element of SEA (see Chapter 9, page 92). However, the different understanding of 'impact assessment' stemming from the different disciplines may engender tension between health and environmental professionals.

It is hoped that the guidance of the Japanese Society of Public Health will increase awareness of HIA and encourage people in local government who are willing to use their discretionary power to conduct HIA. HIA conducted on an academic basis may play a health advocacy role and put health higher on the agenda.

References

1. Fujino Y, Matsuda S. Health impact assessment of 'white-collar exemption' in Japan. Journal of Occupational Health 2007; 49: 45–53.
2. Fujino Y, Nagata T, Kuroki N, Dohi S, Uehara M, Oyama I, et al. Health Impact Assessment of Occupational Health Policy Reform at a Multinational Chemical Company in Japan. Journal of Occupational Health 2009; 51: 60–70.
3. Hoshiko M, Hara K, Ishitake T. Health impact assessment of the transition to a core city in Japan. Public Health 2009; 123: 771–81.
4. Kemm J, Parry J, Palmer S. Health Impact Assessment: Concepts, Theory, Techniques, and Applications. New York: Oxford University Press, 2004.
5. WHO Commission on Social Determinants of Health. Closing the gap in a generation: health equity through action on the social determinants of health. Final report of the Commission on Social Determinants of Health. Geneva, Switzerland: World Health Organization, 2008.

6. Dahlgren G, Whitehead M. Policies and strategies to promote social equity in health. Stockholm: Institute for Future Studies, 1991.

7. Marmot M, Wilkinson R. Social Determinants of Health. New York: Oxford University Press, 1999.

8. Harris B, Harris E. Differing forms, differing purpose: A typology of health impact assessment. Environmental Impact Assessment Review 2011; 31: 396–403.

9. Abrahams D, Pennington A, Scott-Samuel A, Doyle C, Metcalfe O, Broeder L, *et al.* European Policy Health Impact Assessment (EPHIA) A Guide. Brussels: European Union, 2004.

10. enHealth Health Impact Assessment Guidelines. National Public Health Partnership, Commonwealth Department of Health and Aged Care. Available at http://www.health. gov.au/internet/main/publishing.nsf/content/health-pubhlth-publicat-document-metadata-env_impact.htm. Accessed 2 March 2012.

11. Health Promotion Division. Developing health impact assessment in Wales. Cardiff: National Assembly of Wales, 1999.

12. NHS Executive London. A Short Guide to Health Impact Assessment: Informing Healthy Decisions. London: NHS Executive, 2000.

13. Public Health Advisory Committee. A Guide to Health Impact Assessment: A Policy Tool for New Zealand, 2nd edn. Wellington: National health Committee, 2005.

14. Scott-Samuel A, Birley M, Ardern K. The Merseyside Guidelines for Health Impact Assessment, 2nd edn. Liverpool: International Health Impact Assessment Consortium, 2001.

Chapter 28

Health impact assessment in Korea

Eunjeong Kang

In Korea as in many other countries there are two streams of HIA. One stream considers health impacts in the frame of EIA and the other uses HIA as a tool to enhance population health through healthy public policy.[1]

HIA in the frame of EIA

EIA was introduced in Korea in 1977 in order to prevent environmental problems resulting from population growth and concentration of industry. The focus of EIA was on assessing the negative impacts that development projects might have on the environment. Although assessment criteria have been strengthened and some consideration of health impacts has been added, the focus of EIA on environmental pollution limited its capacity to consider health and impacts on people. Meeting national environment standards did not guarantee the absence of health impacts because cumulative and additive effects were not adequately considered. Furthermore, pollution by heavy metals such as nickel and cadmium is not currently covered by EIA. These limitations of EIA were the main impetus for the introduction of a new system of HIA within EIA.

The Ministry of Environment (MoE) in 2005 announced a 10-year comprehensive Master Plan of Environmental Health. Based on this plan, the ministry enacted the Environmental Health Act in 2009 to implement environmental policies intended to protect population health. Article 13 of this Act states that the relevant administration or the proponent who is planning a project that is subject to EIA must assess the impact of environmental risk factors on the population's health.

Examples of projects for which an EIA must be undertaken include:

- development of an industrial complex with an area larger than 150,000 m^2
- construction of a fired power plant with a capacity larger than 10,000 kW
- construction of an incinerator with a capacity larger than 100 tons/day

- construction of a landfill site with an area larger than 300,000 m^2
- construction of night soil treatment facilities with a capacity larger than 100 kl/day.

The steps of an HIA are project analysis, screening, scoping, appraisal, plan for mitigation measures, and plan for monitoring. Qualitative assessment methods are used to compile the scoping matrix and quantitative assessment methods are used to compile the risk index and assess cancer risk. The physical determinants of health (air, including odour, water, noise, and vibration) are assessed. Particular attention is paid to:

- materials known to be hazardous
- materials for which emissions can be calculated
- materials for which risk assessment is possible.

Between 1 January 2010 and 30 June 2011, HIA was carried out for 32 of the 96 projects that were subject to EIA. The types of project most frequently suject to an HIA were industrial complexes (75%) and fired power plant (16%).[2] Of the 32 projects for which an HIA was conducted, 25 used a quantitative analysis, which showed that 13 were expected to exceed environmental standards although these problems would not have been detected under the existing EIA system. Proposals for mitigation measures and a monitoring plan were further benefits of the HIA.

It may be too early to evaluate HIA in EIA in Korea since they have only been implemented for less than two years, but the experience may be helpful to other countries. Although HIA in EIA was mandated by the Environmental Health Act, the Act is a 'sunset' policy whose life is limited to three years so this regulation is temporary. It is therefore important that enough evidence should be gathered during these three years to show that the benefits to society of HIA in EIA are far greater than the costs to developers.

Because of the regulatory features of EIA, the aspects of health assessed are limited to a few physical determinants of health, while socioeconomic determinants and their health implications are unlikely to be considered. As long as EIA is considered to be an 'obstacle' to development projects, it will be difficult to expand the determinants considered to include socioeconomic ones. For this reason an alternative system of doing HIA initiated by the health sector may be needed.

Furthermore, numerous development projects such as urban construction, energy production, road construction, and river development that may affect population health are not required to have HIA in EIA. One of the biggest barriers to expansion of HIA to cover these projects may be getting acceptance from the relevant sectors, including the Korean Ministries of Land, Transport, and Maritime Affairs. Efforts to increase understanding of HIA by different ministries are crucial.

Lastly, the current HIA in EIA is applied to projects but not to programmes or policies, which occupy a higher position in the regulatory hierarchy. Korea has a pre-environmental review system (PERS) to consider environmental impacts of programmes and policies, and it has been suggested that HIA should be introduced to PERS in order to consider health impacts from the earliest stages of developments.

HIA as an environmental approach to public health

The environmental approach to public health, based on the realization that health is determined by social, economic, and environmental factors as well as individual lifestyle, has been the other motivator of HIA in Korea. Health promotion policy in Korea began with the National Health Promotion Act in 1996, but policies and programmes were primarily aimed at individual behavioural changes. In 2001, the government tried to introduce an environmental approach to public health by including 'creation of healthy environments' as one of the four core features of the long-term national health promotion plan (Health Plan 2010). 'Creation of healthy environments' was concerned with food safety, clean air, safe water, and other environmental aspects, and also with reducing health inequalities. While Korea recognized the importance for public health and health inequalities of sectors outside the health sector, it did not have a specific strategy or tool to address these sectors so HIA started to be viewed as a solution to this problem.

HIA and the Korea Institute for Health and Social Affairs

The Korea Institute for Health and Social Affairs (KIHASA,) which is a government-funded research institute under the prime minister's office, started a research programme on HIA in the health sector. The budget for this research programme comes from the Ministry of Planning and Finance. The programme started in 2008 and every year needs approval from this ministry for continued funding.

KIHASA's research activities for HIA are four-fold:

◆ conduct HIA demonstration projects
◆ develop HIA guidelines for local government
◆ accumulate evidence on use of HIA
◆ involvement in international networks.

The HIA demonstration projects are mostly located in healthy cities. A healthy city is 'one that is continually creating and improving the physical and social environment and expanding those community resources which enable people to mutually support each other in performing all the functions of life and in developing to their maximum potential'.[3] HIA can contribute to healthy public policy, which is a key feature of healthy cities, by serving as a systematic framework for decision makers to consider the health and well-being of the community when developing policies, programmes, or projects. Table 28.1 shows the programmes and projects in healthy cities in which HIAs were conducted in 2009 and 2010.

The HIA guidelines for local governments developed by KIHASA are based on internationally available guidelines and the lessons learned in HIA projects undertaken earlier.[4]

The evidence for HIA in different policy arenas accumulated by KIHASA will be used as an 'off-the-shelf' database to help local governments with limited resources to conduct an HIA.[5] In addition, an advisory committee, workshops, conferences, and other promotional activities will support HIA activity in local government.

Lastly, since 2010 KIHASA has been actively involved in the international network for HIA in the Asia region, serving as the chair institution for the HIA working group in the Regional Forum on Environment and Health in East Asia and Southeast Asia. This working group developed a three-year plan (2010–2012) with three specific objectives:

1. to share knowledge on HIA practices, guidelines, and tools, and evidence on health effects in various projects, programmes, and policies

2. to develop and promote HIA as an integral part of the decision-making process in countries in the region

3. to enhance the skills and knowledge of those involved in HIA and related topics by building capacity, disseminating information and ideas, and developing cooperative projects between countries in the region.

Other HIA initiatives

While KIHASA has been working to develop HIA through its various research activities, the Ministry of Health and Welfare and the Korea Centre for Disease Control have also been developing HIA. The Ministry of Health and Welfare published the Health Plan 2020, which is the 10-year master plan for health promotion in Korea and includes HIA as one of 31 core tasks. The plan sets three specific objectives with annual targets (Table 28.2).

Table 28.1 HIA conducted in healthy cities by KIHASA in 2009 and 2010

Year	City	Name of project/programme/ plan/policy	Sector	Assessment methods	Type of hia
2009	Gangnamgu, Seoul	Carbon mileage program	Energy	Community profiling, literature review, interest group workshop	Rapid
	Changwon, Gyoungnam	Bicycle policy	Transportation	Community profiling, literature review, community survey and focus group interview, policy analysis, consulting with experts	Intermediate
	Gwang Myeong, Gyunggido	Artificial turf in school playgrounds	Education	Literature review, product test, student/teacher survey, consulting with experts	Comprehensive
		Lighting of schools at night	Education	Literature review, case study, community survey, consulting with experts	Rapid
		Aegi-Neung water-slide park plan	Park and green space	Literature review, interest group workshop	Rapid
2010	Siheung, Gyunggido	Healthy apartment project	Housing	Community profiling, literature review, secondary data analysis, consulting with experts, case study, interest group workshop	Rapid
	Donggu, Gwangju	Dong Juck Gol walking path project	Park and green space	Community profiling, literature review, secondary data analysis, consulting with experts, interest group workshop	Rapid
	Jinju, Gyoungnam	Regeneration project for low-income residents	City planning	Community profiling, literature review, community survey, interest group workshop	Rapid
		Free vaccination programme for children	Healthcare	Community profiling, literature review, case study, community survey, consulting with experts, GIS space analysis, interest group workshop	Rapid
	Gangdonggu, Seoul	Bus rapid transit between Seoul and Hanam City	Transportation	Community profiling, literature review, secondary data analysis, pedestrian safety environment survey	Rapid

Adapted with permission from Kang E et al, Building and operating a system for health impact assessment, 2009, Korea Institute for Health and Social Affairs: Seoul, 2009 and Kim DJ et al, Health Impact Assessment and capacity building in healthy cities in Korea. Pt. 1. Korea Institute for Health and Social Affairs: Seoul, 2010.

Table 28.2 HIA objectives and annual targets in the Health Plan 2020

Objectives	Annual target numbers					
	2008	**2009**	**2010**	**2011**	**2015**	**2020**
Number of central governments conducting two or more HIAs per year	1	1	1	1	5	10
Number of local governments conducting two or more HIAs per year	–	3	5	10	30	100
Number of private institutions accredited as 'health-friendly corporations'	–	–	–	–	10	30

Reproduced with permission from Choi EJ, Detailed strategies to establish the Third National Health Promotion Master Plan 2020, Ministry of Health and Welfare, Korea Institute for Health and Social Affairs, 2011.

In order to achieve these objectives, three sets of activities are planned. First, building and operating a technical support system for HIA, which will involve developing guidelines and tools, constructing an HIA warehouse where HIA reports can be found, creating a national website for HIA, evaluating HIAs conducted, providing education and training programmes, and doing HIA demonstration projects. Second, a legal basis will be established in order to legitimate HIA activity by local and central government and the private sector. Third, financial and non-financial incentives and innovative programmes will be developed to involve local government and the private sector with HIA. One innovative programme is 'community health-keepers', in which committees of residents in a community are organized to survey local administration activities from the perspective of health. Another innovation is accreditation of corporations that have demonstrated consideration of health in their business activities as 'health-friendly corporations'.

The Korea Centre for Disease Control has also supported HIA by developing indicators for monitoring the activities of healthy cities, including their HIA practices.[6] The Ministry of Health and Welfare is preparing guidelines and evaluation criteria for HIA and these will be finished by the end of 2011.

In summary, starting from a research programme at the KIHASA, more and more local governments, especially healthy cities in Korea, are showing interest in HIA. Although Korea does not have a legal basis at the national level for HIA, one local government (Mujoo in Junnam) has included HIA in its healthy cities ordinance. This shows that HIA in Korea is gradually being recognized as a useful tool for socioecological health promotion.

HIA is emerging as a tool for health promotion and therefore has several challenges. First, since the concept and the usefulness of HIA are disputed, consistent efforts are needed to communicate about HIA and its usefulness in different sectors, including the health sector.[5] Although HIA guidelines and a monitoring tool for HIA have been developed, more time is needed to communicate these to people who are unfamiliar with HIA.

Second, unlike HIA in EIA, which has the Environmental Health Act as its legal basis, there is no legal requirement or framework for HIA in the public health field. The HIA research programme of KIHASA is funded on a yearly basis. The strongest form of regulation for HIA is the national Health Plan 2020 but it is uncertain how effectively this plan will be implemented. There are no serious sanctions for failing to implement this plan and government officers change their posts every two years or so. This is why some kind of legal foundation is necessary.

Conclusion and research agenda

Korea has two streams of HIA: one originated from EIA and the other from an environmental approach to public health. The former has a strong but temporary legal foundation but its scope is too narrow to encompass all aspects of health impact. The latter takes a broad health model but does not have a legal foundation. Both streams need further legal support. Academia has a critical role in providing the information needed to convince society of the need for HIA. Priorities for research are developing underlying theories, assessment methods and tools, and economic evaluations to show the value of HIA.

References

1. Harris JP, Harris E, Thompson S, Harris-Roxas B, Kemp L. Human health and wellbeing in environmental impact assessment in New South Wales, Australia: Auditing health impacts within environmental assessments of major projects. Environment Impact Assessment Review 2009; 29: 310–18.
2. Park YM, Joo HS, Jo GJ, Lim HS, Kang YJ, Kim YK. Operating status and improvement measures of health impact assessment II. Seoul: Ministry of Environment, Korea Environment Institute, 2011.
3. Hancock T, Duhl L. Promoting Health in the Urban Context. WHO Healthy Cities Paper No. 1. Copenhagen: FADL, 55.
4. Kang E, Park HJ, Kim JE. Building and operating a system for health impact assessment, 2009. Seoul: Korea Institute for Health and Social Affairs, 2009.
5. Kang E, Lee Y, Harris P, Koh K, Kim K. Health impact assessment in Korea. Environmental Impact Assessment Review 2011; 31: 438–40.
6. Park YH, Koh KW, Kim KY, Jhang WG, Kim JH, Kang E, Kim DJ, Lee BO, Im SM, Park KJ. Development of the operating measures of a long-term surveillance system for healthy cities using demonstration projects. Seoul Korea Center for Disease Control, Soon Chun Hyang University, 2010.
7. Ministry of Health and Welfare, Seoul Korea Institute for Health and Social Affairs, 2011.

Chapter 29

Health impact assessment in developing countries

Gary Krieger, Burton Singer,
Mirko Winkler, Mark Divall,
Marcel Tanner, and Jürg Utzinger

Introduction

Many perceive HIA as a relatively new and exciting approach that has the
potential to raise the profile of health within the policy formation and programme planning and assessment cycle of large-scale projects of diverse
types.[1,2] In developing countries, extractive industry projects in the mining,
oil/gas, water resource, and agriculture/bioenergy sectors are obvious targets
for HIA, especially since there is a 40-year long history of performing EIAs for
such large industrial projects.[3]

HIA—too Eurocentric?

The methods, procedures, and tools of performing HIA have quietly developed over the last two decades with a strong Eurocentric—or more broadly
'western'—focus on transportation, housing, and social programmes and
policies (e.g. roads, housing, living wages, etc.). The WHO has taken an essen-
tially 'western' tack with a strong emphasis on economic sectors such as transport, agriculture, and housing,[4] and many of the HIA examples on its website
are focused on various aspects of the urban built environment of relatively
wealthy countries. This 'western' focus is evident in the core values of HIA
(democracy, equity, sustainability, and ethical use of evidence) listed in the
Gothenburg consensus document (Chapter 6, page 63) and reiterated on the
WHO website.[5] More recently a fifth value of 'comprehensive approach to
health' has been emphasized, recognizing that physical, mental, and social
well-being are determined by myriad factors from various sectors, as detailed
in the social determinants of health framework.[6,7]

In sharp contrast to the largely Eurocentric values, in developing countries
'democracy' is often not respected or practiced in those settings where many

extractive industry projects are being developed, 'equity' is a relative term when projects are developed in rural settings that are impoverished and marked by different neglected population groups, extractive industry projects by their very nature are inherently unsustainable in that the target resource is exhausted over a specified time (e.g. the lifespan of a mine or gas/oil field is typically 20–30 years), objective 'evidence' is not readily available in many settings where there are little or no vital statistics or functioning health information systems,[8,9] and the social determinants of the health framework are impractical for the private sector to apply.[10]

The enthusiasm for HIA on the western stage has not been reflected in the actual practice of HIA for industrial projects in the developing world. Indeed only 6% of the published work pertaining to HIA had an explicit focus on developing world settings.[11] For the current chapter, we reviewed our over 10-year experience of performing HIA. As shown in Figure 29.1, we have performed over 75 HIAs in more than 35 countries, mainly in the developing world. Several of the major HIA projects have been published in the peer-reviewed literature and text books,[8,9,12,13] or presented at professional meetings of World Water Week and the International Association for Impact Assessment.

This experience raises several questions:

- What are the important lessons to be learned from the 6% of published HIAs which have been done in developing countries?
- Should HIA be incorporated into the existing EIA and SIA models that are already applied to developing country industrial projects?
- What is a reasonable path forward so that HIA can serve as a useful guide for potential negative impacts in advance of project implementation and for long-term monitoring and surveillance to guide adaptive tuning of plans and interventions to yield better effects on health and well-being?

Specifics of developing country HIA

In contrast to the broad HIA agenda articulated by WHO and other international organizations, a more focused and limited set of HIA processes and procedures have been developed by the private sector (particularly the mining and oil/gas industry[14,15] and the IFC (Figure 29.2). This approach has emphasized integrating health within the existing EIA and SIA processes.

The impact assessment of communities directly affected by corporate development projects has been increasingly codified by the IFC through a series of detailed performance standards that include community health as a component of performance standard 4 (community health, safety, and security).[16]

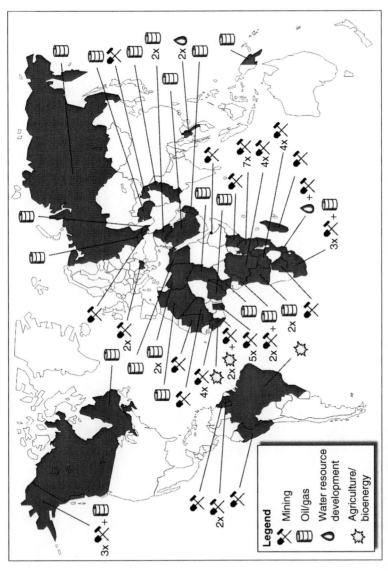

Fig. 29.1 World map showing the countries where our group has carried out HIA for different types of project.

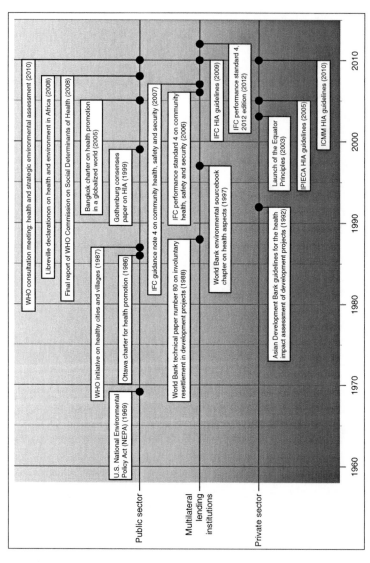

Fig. 29.2 Key developments in the public and private sectors and multilateral lending institutions that have shaped the HIA landscape over the past 50 years. ICMM, International Council on Mining and Metals; IFC, International Finance Corporation; IPIECA, International Petroleum Industry Environmental Conservation Association; WHO, World Health Organization.

Additionally, the IFC also produced a series of technical guidance notes to the standards, industry specific environmental, health, and safety guidelines, guides explaining their environmental health methodology and a dedicated HIA toolkit that further explains and presents methods for performing HIA within the existing EIA and SIA processes. The IFC methodology builds upon work in the late 1990s by the World Bank[17] demonstrating that almost half of the measurable health improvement in sub-Saharan Africa was unrelated to the health system per se, but rather due to improvements in four sectors: (i) housing, (ii) water and sanitation, (iii) transportation, and (iv) communication. The analysis further suggested that linking infrastructure to the health sector can result in improved health outcomes.

This type of environmental–health linkage strategy is appealing to private industrial corporations and major financial institutions as it capitalizes on the existing engineering and logistical skills inherent to industrial projects, while correctly avoiding placing private companies in the de facto role of ministries of health. Hence, project proponents have generally been strong supporters of the overall IFC approach, which is considered to be a highly successful set of benchmark performance standards. Importantly, the IFC performance standard framework has been operationalized and adopted by a large consortium of multilateral lending institutions known as the Equator Principles Financial Institutions (EPFI).[18] Since EPFI incorporate the IFC performance standards as part of loan covenants, this provides a clear enforcement mechanism. Major IFC (and also World Bank) supported projects have mandatory quarterly project reviews performed by independent peers. Increasingly, the major lending institutions have themselves empowered external review panels regardless of whether World Bank or IFC funding was present. EPFI specialists already receive specific IFC-sponsored training on the implementation of the entire suite of performance standards, not just those intimately involved in project finance.

For example, the Papua New Guinea liquid natural gas (PNG LNG) project, a huge US$18 billion investment lead by ExxonMobil, is subject to quarterly reviews by an independent panel of environmental, social, and health specialists employed by the lenders. The lender review panel compares specific pre-negotiated environmental, social, and health commitments made by the project against the IFC performance standards and usually publishes its reports.[19]

The corporation–government–financial institution linkages that accompany the large developing country projects described above are very different to the activities of WHO and the Eurocentric initiatives, which are much less tied to the private sector.[10] While WHO does not have an explicit regulatory role for these projects, it can be active in capacity building, particularly for host country officials, and could strengthen its normative role alongside these new

approaches of public–private partnerships for large-scale development programmes, particularly with regard to sustainability measures when projects are
ending.

The role of Chinese direct investment

Although the multilateral financial institutions are critical actors, they are far
from the only players. An important driver of the debate about the role of
impact assessments is the growing influence of Chinese direct investment in
extractive industry projects in the developing world.[11,20] For example, by 2006,
the Export-Import Bank of China (China Exim Bank) maintained relations
with 36 African countries and had 259 African projects in its portfolio, with a
financial value that has outgrown the World Bank and all other export credit
agencies in terms of investment book value.[21] In May 2007, the China Exim
Bank pledged to commit approximately US$20 billion for loans to Africa over
the next 3 years. Among other projects, the China Exim Bank portfolio includes
multibillion dollar hydroelectric projects in Ghana and Mozambique, and oil/
gas projects in Nigeria and Angola.[22] In comparison, the World Bank approved
projects worth US$4.8 billion for Africa in 2006.[21]

Chinese investments in developing country extractive industry projects have
yet to impose EIA or SIA, let alone HIA requirements. The competition for
financing infrastructure, hydroelectric, and extractive industry projects is
intense and multilaterals do not wish to be at a competitive disadvantage
because of comprehensive impact assessment requirements. However, there is
now movement from China in regard to its actions on international cooperative agreements.[22] For example, through the efforts of the IFC, the China
National Bank has joined the EPFI.

Thus, in the developing world there are two models at play. First, a 'western'
multilateral lending/development approach that ties projects to defined environmental, social, and health performance standards. Second, a more commercial strategy that is being implemented by the Chinese Exim Bank that has
been termed the 'Angola model'[23] and ties resource (commodity) development agreements with the provision of infrastructure in the contracting country. Infrastructure financed by the loan can include water, health, education,
fisheries, road/rail, and airport public works for which the contract must typically be awarded to Chinese contractors.[23]

From a net health impact perspective, the infrastructure model cannot be
discounted given the marked improvement in population level health that can
be obtained by focused infrastructure sector development.[18] Our group is unaware of any published data that compares the community health performance
of Chinese financed projects versus their EPFI competitors. The key issue is

that post-project monitoring is problematic regardless of whether the subject is environmental, social, or health. With few exceptions, the lack of long-term fully funded monitoring, evaluation, and surveillance systems is a glaring deficiency in most projects. The need for these systems accompanied by adaptive tuning of prevention and mitigation strategies cannot be sufficiently emphasized.[24,25]

Lessons learned

Developing country HIA tends to be project-focused and triggered by large infrastructure projects such as the extractive industries.[10] For developing countries, Eurocentric policy and programme HIA are luxuries that are not on the immediate horizon. Because of their size, technical complexity, and cost, extractive projects require considerable external management and professional resources, which are insufficiently present in most host countries. Complex financing arrangements are also a hallmark of these projects. While most countries have legal requirements for EIA, very few countries require formal HIA.[26] Unlike a legally mandated EIA, HIA reports may or may not be publically released.

Nevertheless, there is an increasing demand for HIA triggered by (i) multilateral financial institutions, (ii) internal corporate polices often driven by corporate social responsibility functions, and (iii) major industry trade associations. These HIAs are project focused and performed within the impact assessment methodology developed by the IFC that emphasizes the linkages between project activities and a defined set of environmental health categories, as summarized in Table 29.1.[12,27] In-migration resulting from a project often has to be included in the environmental health issues considered.

HIAs are generally performed and directed by the project proponents and their technical contractors. In this setting, the HIA is often used as an internal planning document or as a tool for developing an integrated community development support strategy, and may not be publically available. World Bank and IFC-funded HIA are typically publically available and disclosed. Project proponents will analyse and mitigate impacts that can be demonstrated to be causally project-related, and make voluntary contributions that are part of an overall strategy to maintain a 'license to operate'.[28] The HIA can serve as a road map for achieving these objectives by directing resources towards real impacts and away from one-off 'show piece' projects, such as building hospitals/clinics when no trained staff are available to operate them. These problems are not unique to HIA and similarly bedevil social outreach activities. The HIA team must work closely with the SIA team so that health is reasonably integrated in their efforts.[29]

Table 29.1 Environmental health areas framework utilized by our group in conducting HIAs of large industrial projects

Environmental health area	Description
Communicable diseases	Transmission of communicable diseases (e.g. acute respiratory infections, pneumonia, tuberculosis, meningitis, plague, leprosy) that can be linked to inadequate housing design, overcrowding, and housing inflation
Vector-related diseases	Mosquito-, fly-, tick-, and lice-related diseases (e.g. malaria, dengue, yellow fever, lymphatic filariasis, leishmaniasis, human African trypanosomiasis, onchocerciasis)
Soil-, water- and waste-related diseases	Diseases that are transmitted directly or indirectly through contaminated water, soil, or non-hazardous waste (e.g. diarrhoeal diseases, schistosomiasis, hepatitis A and E, poliomyelitis, soil-transmitted helminthiases)
Sexually-transmitted infections, including HIV/AIDS	Sexually-transmitted infections such as syphilis, gonorrhoea, *Chlamydia*, hepatitis B, and, most importantly, HIV/AIDS
Food- and nutrition-related issues	Adverse health effects such as malnutrition, anaemia, or micronutrient deficiencies due to changes in agricultural and subsistence practices, or food inflation; gastroenteritis and food-borne trematodiases
Non-communicable diseases	Cardiovascular diseases, cancer, diabetes, and obesity
Accidents/injuries	Road traffic or work-related accidents and injuries (home and project related)
Veterinary medicine and zoonotic diseases	Diseases affecting animals (e.g. bovine tuberculosis, swinepox, avian influenza) or that can be transmitted from animal to human (e.g. rabies, brucellosis, Rift Valley fever, monkey pox, Ebola, and leptospirosis)
Exposure to potentially hazardous materials, noise, and malodours	Exposure to heavy metals, pesticides, and other compounds, solvents or spills and releases from road traffic; air pollution (indoor and outdoor); noise and exposure to malodours
Social determinants of health	Including psychosocial stress (e.g. due to resettlement, overcrowding, political and economic crisis), mental health, depression, gender issues, domestic violence, ethic conflicts, security concerns, substance misuse (drug, alcohol, smoking), family planning, and help-seeking behaviour
Cultural health practices	Role of traditional medical providers, indigenous medicines, and unique cultural health practices
Health systems issues	Physical health infrastructure (e.g. capacity, equipment, staffing levels and competencies, future development plans); programme management delivery systems (e.g. malaria-, tuberculosis-, HIV/AIDS-initiatives, maternal and child health)

Adapted with permission from the IFC 2009, Introduction to Health Impact Assessment, Washington, USA and Environmental Impact Assessment Review, Volume 30, Issue 1, Mirko S. Winkler *et al.*, Assessing health impacts in complex eco-epidemiological settings in the humid tropics: Advancing tools and methods, pp. 52–61, © 2010, with permission from Elsevier.

The enthusiasm for adding HIA to the suite of impact assessment is rarely matched by a methodical long-term plan for executing a formal monitoring and evaluation (M&E) system and surveillance programme after the project enters its long-term operations phase. While efforts are directed at establishing a pre-project baseline, there is often a severe fall-off in the funding available for a practical, cost-effective monitoring and evaluation effort that will operate over the life of the project.[26,30] Follow-up monitoring and evaluation with documentation of mitigation or even enhancement is most likely to be successful when it is formally mandated either in the concession agreement between a corporation and a government or in the commitments registry associated with the project finance arrangements. For example, the PNG LNG project has developed a sophisticated, integrated health and demographic surveillance system with the PNG Institute of Medical Research as part of the forward execution plan.[19]

The ongoing monitoring, surveillance, and mitigation of health problems that have already been implemented as a consequence of upfront formally negotiated concession agreements deserves close examination as a model for future corporate projects in developing countries. This strategy would also be effective for the Angola model. Mitigation, and even health improvements, derived from the concession agreements in the frame of major hydroelectric power projects (e.g. the Nam Theun 2 Power Company and the Hongsa Power Company) in Lao People's Democratic Republic are, admittedly, targeted at project-impacted communities, but they provide an example of what might be done on a broader scale.

Finally, as part of the initial impact assessment planning process, it is beneficial to include host country ministry of health HIA training. Funding for such training could be included as part of the overall finance package. Similar strategies are utilized in the USA, where regulatory agencies 'bill-back' project proponents for specific services. The State of Alaska Department of Health Services has established a formal HIA programme that is self-funded using monies from project proponents for performing the HIA.[31] This is a sustainable model that can effectively be adapted and enhanced for developing country settings.

Impact assessment reports

According to Shakespeare, 'brevity is the soul of wit' (*Hamlet*, Act 2, Scene 2) but not for impact assessments! A generic feature of HIA, as well as EIA and SIA, has been the production of reports that can total many thousands of pages.[8] These reports are hardly read or understood by local communities. Aside from the very real problems of presenting voluminous and highly technical reports to a general audience, in many rural developing country communities there are issues related to language and literacy. Low literacy levels and local languages are the norm, not the exception. In order to address this issue, many stakeholder engagement efforts use pictorial handouts and posters. This has motivated us to develop and promote short video reports, conveying the key findings in an attractive and readily understandable manner while greater detail is provided as technical appendices.[29] Virtually any visit to a local health clinic will confirm that pictures appear to be the communication media of choice, and this is at the root of our HIA visualization strategy.[13] Commercially available software can create materials that include photos, video, graphs, and occasional tables, but very few written words. Our videos are presented using battery-powered pico projectors so they can be used in any setting, even where there is no electricity. We believe that these HIA visualization techniques will become a critical stakeholder deliverable.[13,30]

Looking ahead

The large multilateral lending institutions (e.g. the IFC, the Asian Development Bank, and the World Bank) and EPFI have moved towards placing health on an equal footing with environmental and social issues. The pace of developing country industrialization is increasing and there are opportunities that the major multilateral financial institutions, international health agencies, and the host governments can and should seize. HIA is more than a set of tools and methods; it is an effective approach that leads to a common methodological and resources platform for improving the long-term health and well-being of local communities as part of industrial development in any social-ecological or sociopolitical setting.

Effective communication of findings is as important as the critical discussion of solutions and mitigation strategies. Much of the criticism of the limited impact of even the best-conducted HIA could be alleviated by the effective use of visualization technology in the reporting, assessment, and monitoring phases of a project as described in the previous section. Integrating HIA with EIA and SIA into an overall visual ESHIA is also easily done.[30]

Practically planned and executed HIAs can make a difference in the health and well-being of host communities. In order to fulfil this goal, particularly in a developing country context, HIA must be coherently performed and validated to demonstrate to all stakeholders that it can translate aspirations into meaningful, sustainable actions and be part of socially responsible development at local, national, and global levels.

References

1. Scott-Samuel A. Health impact assessment: an idea whose time has come. British Medical Journal 1996; 313: 183–84.

2. Mindell J, Boltong A, Forde I. A review of health impact assessment frameworks. Public Health 2008; 122: 1177–87.

3. NEPA, National environmental policy act of 1969. Washington, D.C.: US Environmental Protection Agency, 1970.

4. World Health Organization Health Impact Assessment. Available at http://www.who.int/hia/en/. Accessed 19 February 2012.

5. World Health Organization Health Impact Assessment—Why use HIA? Available at http://www.who.int/hia/about/why/en/index.html. Accessed 19 February 2012.

6. Bhatia R. Health impact assessment: a guide for practice. Oakland, CA: Human Impact Partners, 2011.

7. Friel S, Marmot MG. Action on the social determinants of health and health inequities goes global. Annual Review of Public Health 2011; 32: 225–36.

8. Utzinger J, Wyss K, Moto DD, Yemadji N, Tanner M, Singer BH. Assessing health impacts of the Chad–Cameroon petroleum development and pipeline project: challenges and a way forward. Environmental Impact Assessment Review 2005; 25: 63–93.

9. Winkler MS, Divall MJ, Krieger GR, Balge MZ, Singer BH, Utzinger J. Assessing health impacts in complex eco-epidemiological settings in the humid tropics: the centrality of scoping. Environmental Impact Assessment Review 2011; 31: 310–19.

10. Krieger GR, Utzinger J, Winkler MS, Divall MJ, Phillips SD, Balge MZ, Singer BH. Barbarians at the gate: storming the Gothenburg consensus. Lancet 2010; 375: 2129–31.

11. Erlanger TE, Krieger GR, Singer BH, Utzinger J. The 6/94 gap in health impact assessment. Environmental Impact Assessment Review 2008; 28: 349–58.

12. Krieger GR, Balge MZ, Chanthaphone S, Tanner M, Singer BH, Fewtrell L, Kaul S, Sananikhom P, Odermatt P, Utzinger J. Nam Theum 2 hydroelectric project, Lao PDR, in Fewtrell L, Kay D (eds), Health Impact Assessment for Sustainable Water Management. London: IWA Publishing, 2008, pp 199–232.

13. Winkler MS, Divall MJ, Krieger GR, Singer BH, Utzinger J. Health impact assessment of industrial development projects: a spatio-temporal visualization. Geospatial Health 2012; 6: 299–301.

14. IPIECA. A guide to health impact assessment in the oil and gas industry. London: International Petroleum Industry Environmental Conservation Association, 2005.

15. ICMM. Good practice guidance on health impact assessment. London: International Council on Minerals and Metals, 2010.

16. IFC. Performance standards—2012 edition. Washington, D.C.: International Finance Corporation, 2012.

17. Listorti JA, Doumani FM. Environmental health: bridging the gaps. World Bank discussion paper No. 422. Washington, D.C.: The World Bank Group, 2001.

18. EPFI. The equator principles. London: The Equator Principles Association, 2006.

19. PNG LNG. Environmental and social reports. Available at http://pnglng.com/quarterly_reports/. Accessed 29 February 2012.

20. Bosshard P. China's environmental footprint in Africa. Johannesburg: China in Africa Project of the South African Institute of International Affairs, 2008.

21. Moss T, Rose S. China Exim Bank and Africa: new lending, new challenges. Washington, D.C.: Center for Global Development, 2006.

22. OECD. Environmental performance reviews. Paris, China: OECD Publishing, 2007.

23. Davies M. Background paper for the perspectives on Global Development 2010: shifting wealth. How China is influencing Africa's development. Paris: OECD Development Centre, 2010.

24. Scudder T. The future of large dams. London: Earthscan, 2005.

25. World Bank. Environmental governance in oil-producing developing countries. Washington, D.C.: The World Bank Group, 2010.

26. Harris-Roxas B. Health impact assessment in the Asia Pacific. Environmental Impact Assessment Review 2011; 31: 393–95.

27. Winkler MS, Divall MJ, Krieger GR, Balge MZ, Singer BH, Utzinger J. Assessing health impacts in complex eco-epidemiological settings in the humid tropics: advancing tools and methods. Environmental Impact Assessment Review 2010; 30: 52–61.

28. Harrison M. Beyond the fence line: corporate social responsibility. Clinics in Occupational and Environmental Medicine 2004; 4: 1–8.

29. Krieger GR, Bouchard MA, Marques de Sa I, Paris I., Balge Z, Williams D, Singer BH, Winkler MS, Utzinger J. Enhancing impact: visualization of an integrated impact assessment strategy. Geospatial Health 2012; 6: 303–306.

30. Winkler MS, Divall MJ, Krieger GR, Schmidlin S, Magassouba ML, Knoblauch AM, Singer BH, Utzinger J. Assessing health impacts in complex eco-epidemiological settings in the humid tropics: modular baseline health surveys. Environmental Impact Assessment Review 2012; 33: 15–22.

31. State of Alaska—Alaska HIA program. Available at http://www.epi.alaska.gov/hia/. Accessed 19 February 2012.

Chapter 30

Health impact assessment in Ghana

Kwaku Poku Asante and Seth Owusu-Agyei

About Ghana

Ghana is a developing country located on the West Coast of Africa. Until its independence from British colonial rule it was referred to as the Gold Coast because of the abundance of gold deposits in the country. Ghana is currently classified as a low-middle income country with a population of about 24 million, a gross domestic product (GDP) per capita of US$1.1290, 7% GDP growth, and poverty ratio of about 28%.[1] The stable economy, free of civil wars and unrest in the last two decades, has attracted industrial investment especially since the country returned to democratic rule after a long period of military leadership. Ghana's economy has gradually expanded as a result of a growing agriculture industry (e.g. cocoa and cotton), mining (e.g. gold, diamond, salt, bauxite, and salt), construction (e.g. roads and dams), and recently oil and gas. These industries are likely to further expand given Ghana's aim to ensure that industrialization is achieved by 'anchoring industrial development on the conversion of Ghana's natural resources into value-added products with emphasis on agro-based manufacturing, downstream oil and gas industries and value-added minerals processing and manufacturing'.[2] This expansion is likely to bring with it health challenges, thus the need for HIAs.

The most common illness in Ghana is malaria, which accounts for about 40% of all outpatient visits. Other diseases such as respiratory illnesses and diarrhoea are common. Non-communicable diseases such as diabetes mellitus and hypertension are on the increase and may be an indirect impact of the improving socioeconomic status and changing lifestyles that accompany industrialization. In communities where investment of industrial capital is proposed it is therefore important to undertake HIA to identify disease patterns and plan for prompt interventions.

Legal framework of HIA in Ghana

HIA in Ghana has traditionally been done as part of EIA before projects such as mining, road construction, and dam building but with limited aims. In the pre-colonial days there was some emphasis on the protection of human health, with local government byelaws such as the 1897 Beaches Obstruction Ordinance (Cap 240). After the 1972 Stockholm Convention, concern for environmental protection led to the establishment of the Environmental Protection Commission, which in 1994 became the Environmental Protection Agency under Act 490. However, the terms of reference of this organization paid little attention to human health compared to other environmental issues until the Environmental Assessment Regulations passed in 1999 made a clear commitment to ensuring the safety of the environment and humans as demonstrated in Part 1 section 1 (2), which states 'No person shall commence activities in respect of any under-taking which in the opinion of the Agency has or is likely to have adverse effect on the environment or public health unless, prior to the commencement, the undertaking has been registered by the Agency in respect of the undertaking'. With regards to the methods of assessing health impacts the regulations (Part II Section 14 (1)) only state that 'an environmental impact statement shall also include information on the possible health effect of the undertaking on persons within and around the vicinity of the proposed undertaking'.

The Ghana Environmental Protection Agency has tried to monitor adherence to their regulations. The Agency currently implements a project called AKOBEN, which rates adherence to environmental performance and disclosure of industrial projects, including mining.[3] The performance ratings depend on indicators such as operational performance, compliance with mandatory regulations, risk minimization from toxic/hazardous wastes, and company commitment to social responsibilities and community relations. These indicators are skewed towards minimizing environmental impacts rather than health impacts and do not address indicators of a project's performance in preventing public health impacts.

Examples of HIA in Ghana
The Volta River Project

The Volta River Project was initiated in 1962 to generate hydroelectric power for Ghana. The Akosombo Dam was constructed with a surface area of about 8500 km^2 and a live storage capacity of 148 cubic kilometres along the Volta River.[4] The first hydroelectric power was generated in 1965. In 1982, a second dam, the Kpong Dam, was built 25 km downstream of the first dam to generate further power. These two dams were intended to generate enough power to support the country's developmental needs, especially in the aluminium smelting and mining sectors. The Volta River Authority was established under the Volta River Development Act (Act 46 of 1961) primarily to manage power generation in the Volta River Project and secondarily to develop facilities and assistance for fisheries, lake transportation, and lakeside health.

During the construction of the Akosombo and Kpong Dams, a total of about 14,000 inhabitants were resettled from the banks of the Volta River. There was no HIA before construction of the Akosombo Dam despite the huge resettlement involved. After the resettlement process, various health research programmes were instituted in response to an upsurge of diseases such as shistosomiasis and diarrhoea. In some areas, the prevalence of schistosomiasis increased from 5% before the dam construction to about 90% after.[5,6] On the other hand, diseases such as onchocerciasis which require fast flowing water for their transmission were eliminated due to the slowing of the dammed river. The upsurge of diseases was a result of poorly planned social amenities such as water sources and latrines.[5] The main constraints to the project that led to these health impacts are described by Clark and colleagues as 'inadequate time span and administrative capacity', 'insufficient political will and finances', and 'absence of prior commitment and meaningful local involvement' for the project. Major lessons were learnt during the process, in particular the need for adequate assessment and mitigation plans for potential health problems prior to dam construction using a multidisciplinary approach and including community members, adequate funds for a comprehensive health impact assessments, and political will.

To address the public health challenges that were associated with the Volta River Project, several activities, which are still continuing, were instituted. These include:

1. the establishment in 1963 by the University of Ghana of the Volta Basin Research Project, which is a multidisciplinary effort that researches the potential impact of the Volta River Project on public health, agriculture, and other issues, and aims to provide evidence to plan interventions in public health and other sectors[7]

2. public health programmes to control schistosomiasis and other diseases through health education, case identification, treatment of new cases; and environmental control of disease vectors

3. provision of basic health needs through community outreach programmes using a medical boat.

The lessons learnt from the Volta River Project have been used in planning for another hydroelectric project in Ghana, the Bui Hydroelectric Power

Project (the Bui Project).[8] The Bui Project is being constructed on the Black Volta River at the Bui Gorge in north-western Ghana, about 150 km upstream of the Volta River Project. About 350 inhabitants living in seven communities will be permanently displaced. Major impacts on the burden of diseases such as schistosomiasis and HIV/AIDs are expected. Public health programmes, including a baseline health assessment, have been planned to mitigate negative health impacts. It is expected that these plans will be implemented and ensure good health for the population within the project area.

The Newmont Ahafo Project

The Ahafo Project is a gold-mining project located in Kenyasi, a mainly rural area, within the Brong Ahafo Region of Ghana. It is approximately 300 km northwest of the capital city, Accra. The mine resources are estimated to be 105 million tonnes of ore containing 6.8 million ounces of gold, and the project is expected to produce approximately 7.5 million tonnes of ore annually over a 15-year period. The project will take an area of about 2174 hectares of land for construction and mine operation facilities.[9] The Ahafo Project will have a significant economic impact on Ghana's economy, generating about 10% of Ghana's total exports, 4.5% of total foreign direct investment, and 1.3% of GDP. The project resettled about 5185 people living in 823 households within the project area and also led to economic displacement of 878 households (4390 people) who possessed farmlands within the area.[10]

Various surveys, including baseline health surveys, were conducted in 2005 prior to the start of construction by Newmont Ghana Gold Limited (NGGL) in partnership with Opportunities Industrialization Centre International. A more intensive health survey was conducted by the Kintampo Health Research Centre in 2006. Findings from this survey were important in establishing health interventions for the area. Other activities carried out for the HIA were a review of hospital records and reports of previous surveys. Major potential negative impacts on public health were identified, including an increase in the prevalence of HIV/AIDs, violence and abuses, malaria and diarrhoeal diseases, and non-communicable diseases such as diabetes mellitus and hypertension.

The potential impact of the project on health was included in the EIS and reviewed by the Environmental Protection Agency as required by law. Subsequently, measures to mitigate the negative health impacts have been managed collectively by various stakeholders in round table conferences and by various initiatives engaging stakeholders in public health within the Ghana Health Service/Ministry of Health, traditional and political leaders, and non-governmental agencies. The Community Health and Well-Being Initiative is one such initiative begun in 2006 and sponsored by NGGL with the objective of establishing a sustainable programme to ensure the well-being of the population within the Ahafo project area. The initiative refurbished health facilities and provided health equipment to meet the health demands resulting from the mine activities. The activities of this initiative were taken up by the Newmont Ahafo Development Foundation, which provides an equitable distribution of resources, including health and other social amenities, to the communities in the project area.[11]

In 2010, a Demographic Surveillance System (DSS), which identifies each person and address in the population of the project area, was established. It monitors in-migration, uptake of public health interventions, socioeconomic characteristics, and trends of medical issues such as accidents and violence. The DSS is currently being managed by the Kintampo Health Research Centre, which is a Ghana Health Service institution with extensive experience in population surveillance. As part of the HIA for this project, an evaluation survey will be conducted in 2012 using the DSS as a platform.

The Jubilee fields

The discovery of oil and gas discovery in Ghana has led to the latest extractive industry. The first oil well was commissioned in 2010, approximately 40 months after discovery of the Jubilee fields located about 60 km from the coast line in the Western Region of Ghana. In its EIA, the operators of the Jubilee fields, Tullow Ghana Limited and their partners, identified potential health impacts after a review of existing baseline data and stakeholder consultations. The impacts identified included traffic accidents, security incidents, and prostitution. As part of their mitigating actions, the operators planned to establish grievance procedures for communities likely to be affected and to implement corporate social responsibility programmes.[12]

Ghana's oil industry is likely to expand as new discoveries are made. The Ghana government and local communities are committed to ensuring that the potential health and other social impacts of the oil industry are managed adequately. Ghana has learnt lessons from the oil industry in the Niger Delta Region in Nigeria, where the oil industry has had an enormous health impact, including an increase in HIV/AIDs and inadequate health care.[13] These impacts have been attributed to lack of baseline data, poor compliance with impact statements and their mitigating programmes, lack of human resource, and poor political commitment.[14] It is hoped that the potential health risk identified before the start of Ghana's oil industry will be guided by Nigeria experience and managed appropriately.

Other industries

The cocoa industry, one of the largest agricultural industries in Ghana, is made up of small to medium sized plantations owned by rural families. The majority of cocoa plantations have been in existence for many years and it is unlikely that HIAs were conducted prior to their establishment since concerns about health impacts are relatively new. A recent survey examined child labour and found major potential health impacts in cocoa-farming activities in southern Ghana. About 90% of children were exposed to carrying heavy cocoa pods, 75% exposed to cutlass injury, and about 50% exposed to pesticide toxicity.[15]

Increasing recognition of HIA in Ghana

There is increasing awareness and recognition of the need for HIA by health professionals, non-governmental agencies, community members, and civil society groups. This awareness may be a result of growing interest in the health and environmental impact of projects by media organizations. For example, a cyanide spillage that occurred in October 2009 at the Ahafo Project was widely publicized in local and national media.

The 29th Annual Conference of the International Association for Impact Assessment, held in May 2009 in Accra, further recognized the importance of impact assessments in developing countries such as Ghana.[16]

The way forward for HIA in Ghana

HIA seems to be low on the agenda of those establishing projects and businesses probably because of the competing interests of various stakeholders, such as the government, the community, and private businesses. It is therefore difficult to obtain funds to conduct HIAs. Within the current legal framework in Ghana, HIA is embedded in EIA but the scope is unclear. Explicit law is needed to ensure HIAs are carried out and followed through during and after the implementation of industrial projects.

The obligation to conduct HIAs and act on HIA reports currently rests with project developers and the responsible government agency. Communication between these two parties may not reach other stakeholders who are responsible for health in the communities where the projects are implemented. There is a need for transparency and wide dissemination to stakeholders of HIA findings. This should include dissemination to community members in areas where projects are located, local government agencies such as health authorities, non-governmental organizations, and the local government. This will provide stakeholders with the knowledge to advocate and argue for health programmes to prevent negative impacts while promoting the positive impact of the projects. They will also be equipped with real data with which to engage the responsible government agencies and ensure that health assessments are implemented before, during, and after the projects.

There is a need for strong political will to ensure that:

1. HIAs are conducted as stand-alone assessments for all industrial developments in Ghana—this will avoid health issues being buried within the EIA
2. programmes to mitigate identified health risks are adequately implemented under a legal framework
3. adequate logistics and human capacity are developed to meet the needs of increasing industrial development.

Conclusion

Ghana is a country with large mineral deposits and natural resources. This makes it an attractive destination for large industrial projects with potential impacts on health and socioeconomic growth. HIAs are therefore needed to protect the health of the population in and around project areas. Comparison of two projects in 1960 and 2000 that led to large population resettlements suggests a marked improvement in the implementation of HIA and plans to mitigate potential impacts. There is, however, a need for HIAs to be conducted for smaller informal industries such as agricultural projects. The increasing awareness of health and HIA should be backed by clear policies and method guidelines to ensure adherence by industry.

References

1. The world bank on Ghana. Available at http://go.worldbank.org/FCHKSTVFC0.
2. The coordinated programme of economic and social development policies, 2010–2016. An Agenda for Shared Growth and Accelerated Development for a Better Ghana. Presented by H.E. Prof. John E President of the Republic of Ghana to the 5th Paliament of the 4th Republic, December 2010. Available at www.ghana.gov.gh/documents/coordinatedprogramme.pdf. Assessed 26 March 2012.
3. Ghana Environmental Protection Agency (AKOBEN). Environmental rating and disclosure programme. Available at http://www.epaghanaakoben.org/. Accessed 26 March 2012.
4. Volta River Authority. Available at http://www.vra.com/AboutUs/history.html. Accessed 26 March 2012.
5. Clarke BD, Gilad A, Bissett R, Tomlinson P. Perspective of Environmental Impact Assessment., D. Reidel: Dordrecht, Netherlands, 1984, pp 121–32.
6. Wen St, Chu KY. Preliminary schistosomiasis survey in the lower Volta River below Akosombo Dam, Ghana. Annals of Tropical Medicine and Parasitology 1984; 78: 129–33.
7. Gordon C, Amatekpor, JA. The Sustainable Integrated Development of the Volta Basin in Ghana. Volta Basin Research Project, Accra, 1999. Available at http://water-mwrwh.com/The%20sustainable%20integrated.pdf. Accessed 26 March 2012.

8. Ministry of Energy/Bui Development Committee, Ghana. Environmental and Social Impact Assessment Study of the Bui Hydroelectric Power Project, January 2007. Environmental Resources Management Reference 0042911. http://library.mampam.com/Final%20ESIA%20-%20Bui%20HEP.pdf. Assessed on 12 March 2012.

9. Newmont Ghana Gold Ltd Environmental and Social Impact Assessment Ahafo South Project, 2005 Available at http://www.newmont.com/africa/ahafo-ghana/public-disclosure-documents Accessed 26/3/12

10. Kapstein E, Kim R. The Socio-Economic Impact of Newmont Ghana Gold Limited. Stratcomm Africa, 2011 Available at http://www.newmont.com/sites/default/files/Socio_Economic_Impact_of_Newmont_Ghana_Gold_July_2011_0.pdf. Accessed 26 March 2012.

11. Newmont Ahafo Development Foundation. Available at www.nadef.org. Accessed 26 March 2012.

12. Tullow Oil PLC Ghana. Available at http://www.tullowoil.com/index.asp?pageid=50. Accessed 26 March 2012.

13. Udonwa NE, Ekpo M, Ekanem IA, Inem VA, Etokidem A. Oil doom and AIDS boom in the Niger Delta Region of Nigeria. Rural Remote Health 2004; 4(2): 273. Epub 12 May 2004.

14. Agha GU, Irrechukwu DO, Zagi MM. Environmental Impact Assessment and the Nigerian Oil Industry: A Review of Experiences and Learnings, SPE International Conference on Health, Safety and Environment in Oil and Gas Exploration and Production, 20–22 March 2002, Kuala Lumpur, Malaysia. Available at www.onepetro.org/mslib/servlet/onepetropreview?id=00074074. ISBN978-1-55563-947-1.

15. Ministry of Man Power, Youth and Employment. Labour Practices in Cocoa Production in Ghana. National Programme for the Elimination of Worst Forms of Child Labour in Cocoa. April 2007. Available at http://www.worldcocoafoundation.org/addressing-child-labor/documents/MMYEPilotchildlaborsurvey.pdf

16. IAIA2009 International Conference Proceedings. Available at http://www.iaia.org/iaia09ghana/default.aspx. Accessed 26 March 2012.

A perspective on health impact assessment, global health, and the role of the WHO

Carlos Dora

A brief history of HIA in WHO

The development of HIA in WHO headquarters was initially driven by the need to control vector-borne diseases through non-chemical means, in relation to water projects. A WHO/FAO/UNEP Panel of Experts on Environmental Management for vector control (PEEM) was created in 1981 to develop institutional frameworks for intersectoral and interagency collaboration. Methods were developed to forecast diseases in water management projects.[1] The World Commission of Dams, established in the 1990s, expressed concern over the health impacts of water projects[2] and in cooperation with WHO included HIAs as part of its deliberations.[3]

Starting in the 1980s WHO EURO has also supported training for including health in EIAs.[4,5] Other WHO regional offices, including Eastern Mediterranean Regional Office[6] and Pan American Health Organisation,[7] have also prepared HIA guidelines with a focus on addressing the environmental determinants of health. The PAHO guidelines have been widely used in the region as a reference for HIA. A training package for HIA was developed by WHO HQ in cooperation with the Danish Bilharzia Laboratory in 1999.[8] It included modules for training HIA practitioners and for institutionalizing HIA, and guidance on supporting government cross-sectoral policy making. It was subsequently used in a capacity-building programme that covered several countries, including Lao and Vietnam.

In the late 1990s WHO EURO extended the work on HIA to include:

- applications in specific sectors of the economy (transport and agriculture) as part of cross-sectoral policy making
- a contribution to the institutionalization of HIA through inclusion of health in the new protocol for SEAs
- clarification of the role of HIA as a tool for HiAP
- capacity building and community of practice for applications of HIA in cities.

The WHO EURO European Centre for Environment and Health in Rome led work on HIA of transport and later of agriculture policies. This work urged consideration of all determinants of health in policies in non-health sectors, but had a strong emphasis on environmental determinants and quantification of risks. This led to the development of a long-term cross-sectoral programme on transport, health, and environment in the European region,[9] as well as the development of tools to quantify health impacts of transport, and model expected health risks, benefits, and related costs and savings from urban transport policies.[10] HIAs were also conducted to look into the impacts on health of adopting the EU Common Agriculture Policy by accession countries.[11]

The Rome centre also worked to integrate health into the new SEA[12] Protocol at the United Nations Economic Commission for Europe convention on EIAs. The WHO experience of environmental and social determinants of health, and of HIA for healthy public policies, informed the negotiations of the protocol text. The final text includes a broad health perspective and makes health a key part of the SEA, specifying ways to include health (e.g. consider health at different stages of the SEA process, consult health authorities, consider health goals, etc.).[13]

During the same period the WHO European Centre for Health Policy in Brussels developed a project to learn from HIA experience in developed countries and clarify the basic concepts, definitions, principles, approaches, and methods used in HIA in the context of the development of healthy public policies. A series of expert reviews and meetings were used to achieve this, and support for continuing learning was provided to a network of decision makers in Europe. This work led to the publication of the Gothenburg consensus[14] and other papers. Later the office focused on assessing the effectiveness of HIA and the role of HIA for HiAP.[15]

An HIA website at WHO HQ[16] was established in 2003 and a special theme issue of the *WHO Bulletin* (*International Journal of Public Health*) was dedicated to HIA experience at that time.[17] Recent developments in the use of HIA by the WHO have focused on applications at the strategic level, including in the extractive industry, as well as on the Rio+20 sustainable development and climate change debates.

Climate change

WHO have used HIA to assess the co-benefits and risks of policies proposed to mitigate climate change in the last report of the International Panel on Climate Change (IPCC). The panel reviewed mitigation policies for the housing, transport, agriculture, household energy, and healthcare sectors.[18] The impact assessment of these policies estimated some of them to have negative health impacts (for example using diesel fuels as a measure to reduce CO_2 in the transport sector is expected to increase PM_{10} air pollution and cause respiratory and heart disease) while other policies, such as the promotion of rapid bus transit systems coupled with infrastructure for safe cycling and walking, which were less prominent in the IPPC review, had large health co-benefits. In conclusion the WHO reports called for policymakers and stakeholders to use HIA to identify health co-benefits in sector and national policy making for climate change, not only because health is a societal goal in itself, but also because health and health equity gains tend to be local and to occur soon, benefiting those who contribute to the climate policies, while the gains from CO_2 reductions are diffuse and occur many years later.

Sustainable development

The WHO background documents for the Rio+20 Sustainable Development Summit (June 2012) identify that health should be an outcome of all policies. They state 'WHO has developed tools and indicators to assess the impact of policies in different sectors and their potential impact on peoples' health' and that 'health is both a contributor and beneficiary of sustainable development, health indicators will be a critical component to how we track the progress and impact of sustainable development after Rio+20'.[19] The paper on health in Rio+20 prepared by WHO for its Executive Board states that 'global governance for sustainable development can also be improved by enhancing awareness of, and accountability for, the health impacts of policy decisions. This can be promoted by the wider use of health impact assessment, and monitored by process indicators that measure inclusion of health into decision-making processes: for instance—proportion of sector policies and projects for which a Health Impact Assessment has been conducted'.[20]

In the Rio Political Declaration on Social Determinants of Health countries pledged to 'assess the impacts of policies on health and other societal goals, and take these into account in policy-making', as well as to 'work across and within all levels and sectors of government by promoting mechanisms for dialogue, problem-solving and health impact assessment with an equity focus to identify and promote policies, programs, practices and legislative measures that may be instrumental ... to adapt or reform those harmful to health and health equity'. The same declaration exhorts countries to 'promote awareness, consideration and increased accountability of policy-makers for impacts of all policies on health', and acknowledges the importance of '... reviewing and, where appropriate, strategically modifying policies and practices that have a negative impact on people's health and well-being'.[21]

In 2008 the Commission on Social Determinants of Health (CSDH) recommended that WHO supports 'health equity impact assessments' of major global, regional, and bilateral economic agreements, as well as of all government policies, including finance, as a way to address health inequalities and for member states to redesign their health sectors to integrate a focus on the social determinants of health across relevant sectors.[22] Recommendations included that countries should adopt and perform HIAs for policies and projects, focus further on health equity aspects (doing health equity assessments and developing disaggregated data systems, not assuming that public participation per se can ensure addressing of equity issues), build capacity, and exchange experience.

Extractive industries in developing countries

Natural resource extraction can be a key driver of development but many countries have been unable to harness this potential and have instead been plagued by the 'resource curse'—where oil or minerals neither benefit local populations nor lead to economic growth. Such large-scale development projects can trigger rapid population in-migration, with implications for competition for health and social services, increase in traffic injuries and can also affect communicable disease patterns (e.g. sexually transmitted diseases, HIV/AIDS) and increase social tensions, which can result in mental health problems, increased violence, alcohol consumption, and so on. These health impacts are also borne by those living in the proximity of extractive industry operations, including poor women and children. Industry often contributes to address certain health issues, such as vectors and HIV/AIDS, but does not engage with the breath of health issues, which end up posing a risk to the community and potentially to the project itself.

EIAs and SIAs tend to address a part of these issues, and are often done on a project-by-project basis, which limits the understanding of the overall impacts of the industry and decisions on how best to manage these. WHO headquarters is developing a strategic level HIA project to support government's capacity to foresee the health risks and benefits, and to plan and implement appropriate mechanisms to manage them, in connection with other relevant actors, such as government departments, industry, and the local health system. This is aimed at strengthening governance, oversight, and accountability for the health impacts of extractive industry operations at the national level. Results from field implementation are very encouraging.

A cooperation with multilateral development banks to support the inclusion of health goals as part of development lending for all sectors of the economy was begun by WHO headquarters in 2007.[23] Development banks expect their borrowers to integrate certain environmental and social aspects into the planning and implementation of the investment projects they support. A series of impact assessments are required by the banks to facilitate compliance, including on environment, safety of dams; pest management, indigenous peoples, involuntary resettlement, cultural property, and occupational health and safety.[24] Following the adoption of a new safeguard for community health and safety by the IFC in 2006, development banks have cooperated to mainstream a broad health perspective through HIA for development lending. This is continuing as part of the banks' work on safeguards and performance standards, and has the potential to influence large public and private sector investments in developing countries, including for example, natural resource extraction (oil, mining, forestry) infrastructure, and tourism. For further discussion of these issues see Chapter 29.

Healthy cities and Health in All Policies

The WHO European network of healthy cities developed an initiative to support implementation of HIA, engaging about 25 cities.[25] This involved development of an HIA toolkit for cities and implementation/capacity building of HIA in many of those cities.

Using HIA as a tool for HiAP was successfully implemented by WHO headquarters in a cooperation to examine the health impacts of policies on small-scale agriculture in Thailand, livestock raising among pastoralists in Uganda, and water management options in water-scarce areas in Jordan over the period 2003–2005.[26] The same project also generated extensive reviews of the health and environment impacts of policies in different sectors of the economy, and analysed the role of HIA, EIA. and economic analysis in bringing health and environment considerations into policy making.

HIA and the work of WHO

HIA has been a long-standing focus of WHO's work. The applications of HIA are reflected on the technical level in the practice and expertise existing in member states and expert groups. On the policy level, WHO has been able to respond to opportunities presented by international debates, such as the environmental health movement in Europe, the International Commission on Dams, issues raised by natural resource extraction in developing countries, and movements towards a green economy and sustainable development. WHO used an HIA framework to formulate the response to global issues so as to include health in these policy debates, with the overall goal of prevention of disease and health promotion through policy decisions and investments in those sectors. HIA has been a useful framework for achieving HiAP, as it includes focus on the evidence base (for health impacts of a policy decision), on facilitating participation in the policy debate (through access to tangible information on the project/policy expected impacts), and on encouraging baseline assessments, monitoring, and evaluation of policy and project performance.

The practice of HIA is closely linked to WHO's core functions: 'providing leadership on global health matters, shaping the health research agenda, setting norms and standards, articulating evidence-based policy options, providing technical support to countries and monitoring and assessing health trends'. As WHO's website states 'In the 21st century, health is a shared responsibility, involving equitable access to essential care and collective defense against threats.'[27]

Considering the broad range of social, environmental, and occupational determinants of health and the enormous potential for prevention through influencing policies in different sectors of the economy, one would expect that WHO and the health departments of member states would dedicate a large part of their efforts to HIA and HiAP, as is the case in places like Quebec and Thailand, but not yet the norm.

In WHO awareness of the importance of HiAP and HIA as tools is wide. Tools and field applications of HIA have been developed in WHO mostly by departments of environmental health and to some extent by healthy cities probably because environmental health issues are cross-sectoral issues. EIAs are widely used as a tool to mainstream environment into all policies, and have a policy and legislative framework. The contribution of WHO has been to bring a broader perspective of health determinants into those debates, as the environmentalists tended to focus only on environmental risks to health, such as pollution, and disease vectors. WHO's work has focused on broadening the understanding of all health determinants, social, environmental, and occupational, as an integral part of HIA. The extensive efforts to raise awareness and sensitize the parties negotiating the SEA protocol is one example where this succeeded. Environmental health departments in WHO have had a good focus on quantification of environmental risks to health and development of guidance (e.g. air pollution, noise, contaminated industrial sites, etc.) that relates the risks to their origins. This has helped to make the case for connecting sector policies with health.

The other area of work in WHO that has contributed to HIA implementation for HiAP is the healthy cities movement. This was conceived with cross-sectoral action for health as one of its basic objectives, and has a history of engagement and experimenting with different ways to promote health involving actors from different sectors at the local level. It is possible that this cross-sectoral work has more often happened at the local level due to closer contact of actors in different sectors with the population, greater personal accountability over policy decisions, and mayoral oversight and control of decisions in housing, transport, land-use planning, waste, water management, and other sectors.

Looking ahead

Looking ahead, the further development, integration, and wider application of HIA should be key to the strengthening of HiAP as a core function in health systems. Increasing knowledge about health impacts of policies and projects in specific sectors of the economy, along with implementation of HiAP in the same sectors, should provide a solid basis for development. Focusing HIA and HiAP work on priority development policy issues should be central to making it part of governance for sustainable development, which was the subject of global debate at Rio+20. The health sector and WHO as the global public health agency have a unique contribution to make through a robust capacity to anticipate and manage health risks and benefits from development initiatives. Human health impacts are easily understood by all, and access to reliable information from a trusted source on the health impacts of policies and investments should be central to the engagement and participation of different social groups in policy making.

HIA can be the key tool used by the health sector to contribute to the global governance of sustainable development for several reasons. First, because its wider adoption can influence different sectors of the economy to adopt strategies and implement projects that protect and promote health. Second, because the monitoring and reporting of health impacts of sector policies, based on an HIA framework, can bring transparency and accountability to those decisions, and enable feedback and revision of those decisions to produce better impacts on human health and well-being. Third, because the health sector has the knowledge, the evidence base, and the information systems that can be used to demonstrate the health impacts of policies, while WHO has the mechanisms to develop guidance on risks and benefits to health in the context of conflicting interests.

National health systems and WHO as part of the global health governance apparatus need to articulate a response commensurate to the opportunities opened by the global crises and emerging challenges in sustainable development. The jury is still out regarding whether or not the health sector will effectively create the space in international policy making to make its unique contribution to the global governance of sustainable development.

References

1. Birley MH. Guidelines for forecasting the Vector-Borne Disease Implications of Water Resource Development. World Health Organization, Panel of Experts on Environmental Management for Vector Control (PEEM) Guidelines number 2, WHO/ CSW/91.3, 2nd edn, Geneva, WHO, 1991.

2. Colson E. The social consequences of resettlement. Manchester: Manchester University Press, 1971.

3. World Health Organization. Sub-commission to the World Commission on Dams. Human health and dams. Geneva: WHO, 1999.

4. Inter-sectoral decision making skills in support of health impact assessment of development projects. Final report on the development of a course addressing health opportunities in water resources development 1988–1998. Geneva/Chalottelund: WHO, 2000.

5. Tiffen M. Guidelines for the incorporation of health safeguards into irrigation projects, through intersectoral cooperation, with special reference to vector-born diseasess. Geneva, WHO, 1989.

6. Hassan AA *et al.* Environmental health impact assessment of development projects: A practical guide for the WHO Eastern Mediterranean Region, Cairo, Eastern Mediterranean Regional Office WHO, 2005.

7. Weitzenfeld, H. Manual básico sobre evaluación del impacto en el ambiente y la salud de acciones proyectadas. Metepec: ECO, 1996, xiii, 244 p.

8. Intersectoral decision-making skills in support of health impact assessment of development projects: final report on the development of a course addressing health opportunities in water resources development. Geneva: WHO, 2000. WHO/SDE/WSH/00.9.

9. Dora C, Racciopi F. Including health in transport policy agendas: the role of health impact assessment analysis and procedures in the European experience. Bulletin of the World Health Organization 2003; 81: 399–403.

10. Health Economic Assessment Tool. Available at http://www.heatwalkingcycling.org/. Accessed 14 February 2012.

11. Lock K, Gabrijelcic M, Martuzzi M, *et al.* Health impact assessment of agriculture and food policies: lessons learned form the republic of Slovenia. Bulletin of the World Health Organization 2003; 81: 398–403.

12. Dora C. HIA in SEA and its application to policy in Europe, in Kemm J, Parry J, Palmer S (eds), Health Impact Assessment: Concepts, theory, technique and applications. Oxford: Oxford University Press, 2004.

13. United Nations Economic Commission for Europe Protocol on SEA. Available at http://www.unece.org/env/eia/sea_protocol.htm. Accessed 26 February 2012.

14. Diwan V, Douglas M, Karberg I *et al.* (eds). Health impact assessment from theory to practice. Report on the Leo Karpio workshop, Gothenburg, 28–30 October 1990, WHO and the Nordic School of Public Health. NHV-report 2000: 9, 2000. Gothenburg; WHO and Nordic School of Public Health.

15. Wismar M, Blau J, Ernst K, Figueras J. (eds). The effectiveness of health impact assessment: Scope and limitations of supporting decision making in Europe. Brussels: WHO European Observatory on Health Systems and Policies, 2007.

16. World Health Organization Health Impact Assessment. Available at http://www.who.int/hia/en/. Accessed 26 March 2012.

17. Dora C, Shademani R. Issue devoted to Health Impact Assessment. Bulletin of the World Health Organization 2003; 81: (6): 387–472.

18. World Health Organization. Health Impact Assessment—Health in the green economy. Available at http://www.who.int/hia/green_economy/en/index.html. Accessed 26 March 2012.

19. RIO+20 United Nations Conference on Sustainable Development. Available at http://www.uncsd2012.org/rio20/index.php?page=view&type=510&nr=287&menu=115. Accessed 26 March 2012.

20. World Health Organization. Executive Board United Conference on Sustainable Development RIO+20. Available at http://apps.who.int/gb/ebwha/pdf_files/EB130/B130_36-en.pdf. Accessed 26 March 2012.

21. World Health Organization. Rio political declaration on social determinants of health. Available at http://www.who.int/sdhconference/declaration/Rio_political_declaration.pdf. Accessed 26 March 2012.

22. Resolution passed by the WHO 124th Executive Board on 23 January 2009. 'Reducing health inequities through action on the social determinants of health' related to agenda item 4.6 for consideration by the World Health Assembly in May 2009. Available at http://apps.who.int/gb/ebwha/pdf_files/A62/A62_R14-en.pdf.

23. Pfeiffer M, Dora C. HIA and development lending; a guide for oversight. WHO, 2009 unpublished document.

24. World Bank Safeguard policies. Available at http://www.worldbank.org/safeguard. Accessed 26 March 2012.

25. World Health Organization. Urban Health—Health Impact Assessment. Available at http://www.euro.who.int/en/what-we-do/health-topics/environment-and-health/urban-health/activities/health-impact-assessment. Accessed 26 March 2012.

26. World Health Organization. The Health and Environment Linkage Initiative (HELI). Pilot projects: Action at country level. Available at http://www.who.int/heli/pilots/en/. Accessed 26 March 2012.

27. World Health Organization. About WHO. Available at http://www.who.int/about/en/. Accessed 26 March 2012.

Index